Studies of Brain Function, Vol. 5

Coordinating Editor
V. Braitenberg, Tübingen

Editors
H. B. Barlow, Cambridge
H. Bullock, La Jolla
E. Florey, Konstanz
O.-J. Grüsser, Berlin-West
H. van der Loos, Lausanne

Han Collewijn

The Oculomotor System of the Rabbit and Its Plasticity

With 128 Figures

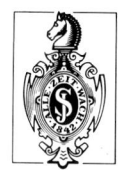

Springer-Verlag
Berlin Heidelberg New York 1981

Dr. H. COLLEWIJN
Department of Physiology I, Faculty of Medicine
Erasmus University Rotterdam, P.O. Box 1738,
3000 DR Rotterdam / The Netherlands

ISBN 3-540-10678-2 Springer-Verlag Berlin Heidelberg New York
ISBN 0-387-10678-2 Springer-Verlag New York Heidelberg Berlin

Library of Congress Cataloging in Publication Data
Collewijn, H. The oculomotor system of the rabbit and its plasticity.
(Studies of brain function ; v. 5) Bibliography: p. Includes index.
1. Eye--Movements. 2. Nystagmus. 3. Rabbits--Physiology. I. Title. II. Series.
[DNLM: 1. Eye movements. 2. Rabbits. W1 ST937KF v. 5 / QL 737.L32
C6980]   QP477.5.C64   599.01'823   81-2650

This work is subject to copyright. All rights are reserved, whether the whole
or part of the material is concerned, specifically those of translation,
reprinting, re-use of illustrations, broadcasting, reproduction by photocopying
machine or similar means, and storage in data banks. Under § 54 of the
German Copyright Law where copies are made for other than private use
a fee is payable to "Verwertungsgesellschaft Wort", Munich.

© by Springer-Verlag Berlin Heidelberg 1981.
Printed in Germany.

The use of registered names, trademarks, etc. in this publications does not
imply, even in the absence of a specific statement, that such names are
exempt from the relevant protective laws and regulations and therefore free
for general use.

Offsetprinting: Julius Beltz, Hemsbach/Bergstr.
Binding: Konrad Triltsch, Geographischer Betrieb, Würzburg
2131/3130-543210

Foreword

The invitation to contribute a volume to the series Studies in Brain Function offers me a welcome opportunity for a comprehensive presentation of my research on the eye movements of the rabbit, and for a review of the older results in the perspectives offered by the progress of my own work, but even more of the field in general. Characteristically this monograph emphasizes the views of the author, which may not always be generally accepted. Although connections with the work by other investigators are discussed as much as possible, I have not attempted to be complete in reviewing all publications related to oculomotor function in the rabbit.

While presenting an overview of current understanding of a system, it is always wise to trace the historical roots of our knowledge and concepts. On the one hand, we may find that many established concepts derive their strength more from convention and convenience than from rigorous evidence. Such traditional ideas should be challenged by critical experiments, using the best available techniques. On the other hand, some of the older publications remain a source of inspiration, because they contain valid ideas which generate fruitful experiments even today. A remarkable example of this category is Ter Braak's work on optokinetic nystagmus, published in 1936. It was a landmark in the development of oculomotor science and established many of the concepts that have become popular only in recent years, such as the distinction between optokinetic nystagmus and smooth pursuit, the interaction between visual and vestibular signals, the study of open-loop conditions and even modeling. Being written in German, this paper – although widely quoted – is not easily accessible to the majority of present-day oculomotor investigators. Its continuing value justifies a better availability and I am happy that the Editors of this series and Springer Verlag accepted my suggestion to include an English translation of this article as an appendix in the present book. Thanks are due to the copyright owners, the Hollandsche Maatschappij der Wetenschappen, Haarlem, The Netherlands, for their permission to reprint this paper in translation. No changes have been made in the original text, except completion of citations up to current standards, as far as possible.

I am most grateful to all my colleagues who collaborated with me in the research, and to the many others that provided discussion, inspiration, and much needed criticism. Finally, I should like to thank Miss S. Markestijn, Mrs. J. Dames, Prof. O.J. Grüsser and the staff of Springer Verlag for their assistance and support in the preparation of this book.

Rotterdam, Spring 1981 H. Collewijn

Contents

1	**Introduction**	1
1.1	Orientation of the Eyes	2
1.2	Retinal Organization	4
1.3	Visual Acuity	4
2	**Eye Movements in Spontaneous Behavior**	7
2.1	Techniques	7
2.2	Spontaneous Activity	8
2.3	Structure of Saccades	12
2.4	Intersaccadic Gaze Stability	20
2.5	Active Pursuit	22
2.6	Vergence	24
2.7	Conclusions	27
3	**Eye Movements During Passive Oscillation**	28
3.1	Rotation Around the Three Principal Axes	29
3.2	Properties of the Horizontal Canal-Ocular Reflex	32
3.3	Visual Suppression of the VOR	38
3.4	Maculo-Ocular Reflexes	41
3.5	Conclusions	48
4	**Optokinetic and Postrotatory Nystagmus**	49
4.1	The Nature of the Optokinetic Reflex	49
4.2	Optokinetic Responses to Sinusoidal Stimulation	51
4.3	Optokinetic Nystagmus	54
4.4	Open-Loop Optokinetic Nystagmus	60
4.5	Optokinetic Reactions in Different Directions	65
4.6	Vestibulo-Ocular and Optokinetic Responses During and After Rotations at a Constant Velocity	69
4.7	Conclusions	74

5	**Signal Processing**	75
5.1	Retinal Motion Detection	75
5.2	Relevance of Different Primary Optic Projections for OKN	77
5.2.1	The Geniculo-Cortical Projection	78
5.2.2	The Superior Colliculus	79
5.3	Direction-Selectivity in the Nucleus of the Optic Tract	83
5.4	Direction-Selectivity in the Posterior Accessory Optic System	90
5.5	Efferent Connections from the Nucleus of the Optic Tract	92
5.6	Effects of Bilateral Labyrinthectomy	98
5.7	The Effect of Cerebellectomy on OKN	100
5.8	Modeling of the Rabbit's Optokinetic System	106
6	**Adaptation and its Limits**	110
6.1	Unilateral Labyrinthectomy	111
6.2	Dark-Rearing	115
6.2.1	Responses to Sinusoidal Movement in Darkness (VOR)	116
6.2.2	Responses to Sinusoidal Movement with Eyes Open (VOR and OKN)	117
6.2.3	Optokinetic Nystagmus	120
6.3	Long-Term Adaptation of VOR and OKN	124
6.3.1	Adaptive Phenomena in the VOR	125
6.3.2	Conditions for Visual Adaptation of the VOR	129
6.3.3	Adaptation to Inverted Motion Vision, Restricted Visual Field	136
6.3.4	Adaptation to Inverted Motion Vision, Whole Visual Field	137
6.3.5	Adaptation by Visual Stimulation Only	138
6.3.6	Frequency Specificity of Adaptation	140
6.3.7	Adaptation in Synergic Operation of VOR and OKN	144
6.3.8	Conclusions on Adaptation	145
6.4	Optokinetic Anomalies in Albino Rabbits	147
6.4.1	Inverted OKN in Albino Rabbits	148
6.4.2	Anomalous Receptive Fields in the Nucleus of the Optic Tract in Albino Rabbits	154
6.4.3	Adaptation Experiments in Albino Rabbits	156
6.5	Conclusions	159
	References	161

Appendix

1	Introduction	181
2	**The Optokinetic Nystagmus in the Rabbit**	182
2.1	The Conditions for the Eliciting of OKN	184
2.1.1	Size of the Moving Field	184
2.1.2	Velocity of Moving Contrasts	186
2.1.3	Nature of the Stimulus	189
2.2	Slow and Fast Phase	195
2.3	Quantitative Relations Between Stimulus and Effect	197
2.3.1	Equilibrium Between Stimulus and Nystagmus, at Different Velocities of the Moving Contrasts	198
2.3.2	Behavior of Nystagmus at the Beginning and End of Stimulation	201
2.4	A Theoretical Model of the Central Mechanism of Stare Nystagmus	204
2.5	Optokinetic and Vestibular Nystagmus	206
3	**Stare Nystagmus in Other Species of Animals**	214
4	**The Localization of Stare Nystagmus in the Central Nervous System**	217
5	**Look Nystagmus**	225
6	**The Localization of Look Nystagmus in the Central Nervous System**	229
	References	236

1. Introduction

A unique feature of the oculomotor system is its commitment to a single constant load: the eye. In contrast to the motor apparatus of trunk and extremities, the eye muscles do not have to comply with a whole range of load variations imposed by joint angles, orientations with respect to gravity and external and internal forces. Eye movements are only made to serve vision, at least in the absence of any pathological condition.

This specialization may restrict the usefulness of the oculomotor apparatus as a general model for motor systems. For instance, the absence of a stretch reflex in the eye muscles may indicate that the oculomotor system lacks the machinery for peripheral load compensation found in spinal systems. On the other hand, many general motor functions such as postural reflexes and detailed movements are well developed in the oculomotor system and because of the relatively simple mechanical relations, they are more easily investigated in this than in other systems.

Eye movements controlled by the vestibular apparatus (vestibulo-ocular reflexes), proprioceptive input (cervico-ocular reflexes) or global motion of the visual surroundings (optokinetic reflexes) are essentially postural in character. They contribute to the stability of eye position in visual space and are found in some form in all animals with spatially organized visual perception.

On the other hand, in man and some other species the eye is capable of fine detailed movements related to the fine structure of visual patterns. These movements are to a large extent independent of general posture, head movements and even the visual background and are guided by specific, selected visual targets. Such movements might be compared to skilled, independent finger movements.

The present book is devoted essentially to the oculomotor system of the rabbit. The motor behavior of this animal is restricted largely to posture, locomotion and stereotyped movements. The eye movements are no exception and indeed it is commonly assumed that the rabbit rarely — if ever — makes any eye movements which could be called spontaneous, in the sense that they are not triggered by postural reflexes. This is generally true in experimental situations in which the animal is restrained and the head immobilized. Among the mammals usually studied in the laboratory, the capacity for independent control of eye movements is better developed in the cat and extremely well in primates. Interestingly, this trend is paralleled by the development of the capacity for skilled and independent movements of the extremities, which may indicate profound similarities in the control of ocular and other motor systems.

The clear limitations of the rabbit's oculomotor system do not make it uninteresting, but offer instead a very convenient model for the study of the *basic, mainly postural elements* of the system. In cats and primates these are more difficult to study because of the continuous interference by higher order control systems. Thus, in the rabbit it is possible to study the vestibulo-ocular and optokinetic reflexes in their pure form, uncontaminated by voluntary saccades or smooth pursuit.

The rabbit has been an important animal in the history of oculomotor research. As early as 1874, Hitzig discovered that stimulation of the cerebellum elicited eye movements in a rabbit. A major part of the investigations by Magnus (1924) and his coworkers on posture was concerned with the rabbit's oculomotor reflexes. Ironically, the existence of optokinetic eye movements in the rabbit was denied for a long time by such authorities as Bartels (1931), due to a misunderstanding of the nature of this reflex, and it remained for Ter Braak (1936) to correct this view with his classical investigations. The rabbit's brain stem circuits related to vestibulo-ocular reflexes were extensively investigated by Lorente de No (1931) and more recently by Ito and his colleagues. In a wider sense, the rabbit has been important in visual science in general. Brouwer's (1923) original discovery of retinotopic central visual projections was made in the rabbit, and more recently, fundamental discoveries such as direction-selectivity as a trigger feature of retinal ganglion cells (Barlow and Hill, 1963) were made in the same animal. In ophthalmological research the rabbit's eye is frequently used as a model, and the topographical anatomy and histology of the eye and orbit have been well described (see Prince, 1964).

The rabbit's eye and oculomotor apparatus are built in accordance with the general mammalian plan for these structures. However, for an appropriate interpretation of oculomotor performance, it is useful to summarize the features which are characteristic for this species.

1.1 Orientation of the Eyes

The rabbit has laterally implanted eyes. The topography of the optical axis and visual fields has been extensively described by Hughes (1971), whose summarizing diagram is reproduced in Fig. 1. His observations were

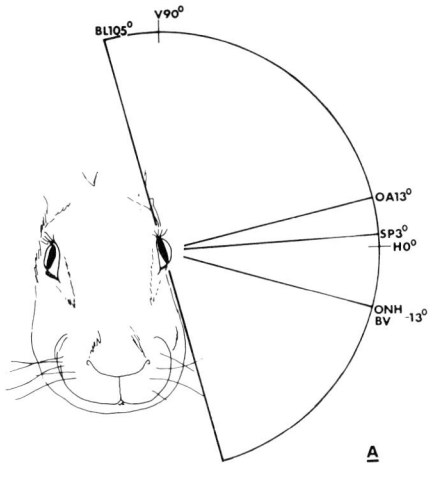

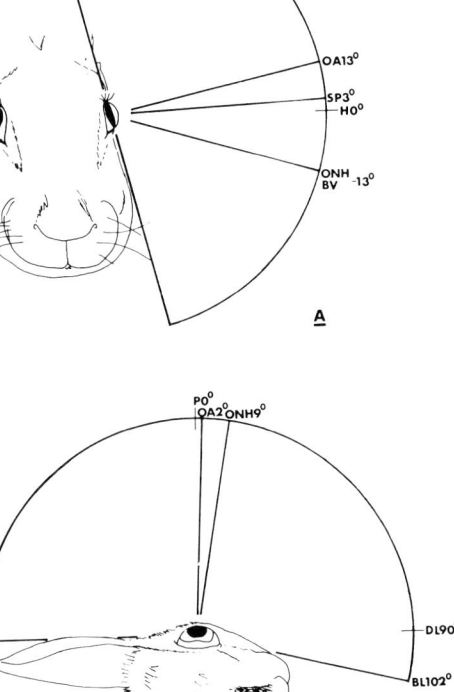

Fig. 1. Projection of retinal landmarks in the visual field of the rabbit in the freeze condition: **A** in the vertical plane, **B** in the horizontal plane. *BL* binocular limit; *V* vertical; *OA* optic axis; *SP* streak peak ganglion cell count; *H* horizontal parallel; *ONH* and *BV* optic nerve head and blood vessels; *DL* presumed projection of the decussation line; *P* perpendicular to long axis of head. (Hughes, 1971)

carried out in the "freezing state" in which rabbits crouch motionless with the nasal bone about 35° away from the vertical. In the "freezing" condition, the optical axis of each eye is directed about 2° anterior to the transverse plane. The monocular visual field extends 90° temporally and 102° nasally of the optical axis, thus the total extension is 192° in the horizontal direction. Vertically, the visual field extends about 105° superiorly and 75° inferiorly. Thus, the two eyes together cover practically the whole of the animal's surroundings, with only a negligible blind zone under and behind the head. Frontally the visual fields of the two eyes overlap in a potentially binocular zone with a width of about 24°.

1.2 Retinal Organization

The retina is afoveate, but certainly not homogeneous. Ganglion cells and other elements show a horizontal zone of elevated density, the visual streak, which was first described by Chievitz (1891). Recent quantitative descriptions of ganglion cell distribution have been given by Hughes (1971), Vaney and Hughes (1976) and Provis (1979). Hughes (1971) found a peak count of 7000 ganglion cells/mm^2 centered on the optic axis in the region under the optic nerve head. This peak diminished gradually in the inferior retina (which deals with the sky above the horizon), but more steeply in the superior retina, where the blind spot is formed by the optic nerve head with possibly a more elongated zone of inferior visual acuity due to the band of radiating myelinated fibers. Furthermore, Hughes (1971) described an upward bulge in the 1000-4000 ganglion cells/mm^2 isocount lines in the temporal retina, which he interpreted as a special zone serving the frontal binocular field. Provis (1979) does not confirm this upward bulge, but on the other hand describes a specific concentration of large ($> 20\mu$) ganglion cells in the temporal retina. This circumscript zone is centered around the decussation border. Provis (1979) offers several arguments for speculating that this temporal end rather than the center of the visual streak may represent the rabbit's analog of an area centralis. Some of Provis' (1979) diagrams are reproduced in Fig. 2 A-C. This retinal architecture seems readily interpretable in terms of the rabbit's natural behavior (see Lockley, 1975). As prey rather than hunter, this ground animal is surrounded by enemies. The visual streak will cover most of the perimeter of the horizon to detect potential dangers. On the other hand, the binocular zone may be specialized in different visual tasks, such as the ones related to food recognition and eating.

Visual streaks of some kind are found in many animals and may be related to a terrestrial (as opposed to arboreal) life style (Hughes, 1975a). Even in the retina of the cat the distribution of ganglion cells has features of visual streak organization, although a central area is also clearly developed (Stone, 1965, 1978; Hughes, 1975b; Wässle et al., 1975).

1.3 Visual Acuity

Visual discrimination tests using gratings with bars of various widths have demonstrated a resolution of 40 (occasionally 20) min arc cycle width in Dutch belted rabbits (Van Hof, 1967) and identical values for Wild European rabbits (Vaney, 1980). The validity of these psychophysically determined thresholds is supported by a study of visual evoked potentials by Kulikowski (1978) who calculated a resolution limit of 18 min arc for half-lop rabbits.

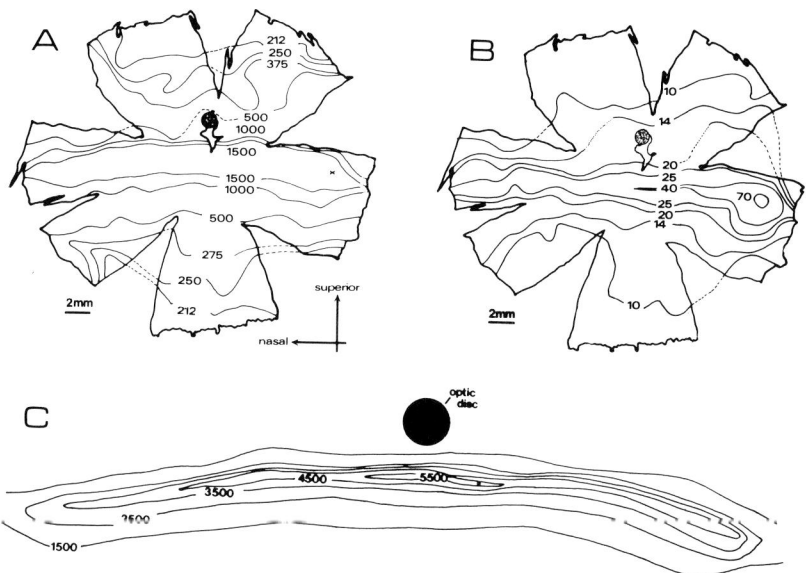

Fig. 2. Retinal ganglion cell density distribution maps of the left eye of a pigmented rabbit. Iso-density lines are *dashed* where counts of the ganglion cell layer were interrupted, either by cuts in the retina or by the myelinated fiber band. *Numbers* represent the density of ganglion cells/mm^2. The optic disc is *shaded*. **A** survey of the total population of ganglion cells. A *cross* in the temporal retina marks the position of the maximum density of large ganglion cells. **B** same retina, distribution of large ganglion cells (diameter > 20 μm) only. **C** part of the same retina but mapped using a higher sampling frequency to show the steep ganglion cell density gradients which occur in the visual streak. An *asterisk* in the temporal visual streak marks the peak ganglion cell density recorded in this retina (6500 ganglion cells/mm^2). (Provis, 1979)

There is general agreement on the absence of accommodation (Meyer et al., 1972; see also Prince, 1964), but some controversy exists about the refractive state. De Graauw and Van Hof (1978), using objective refractometry, found a systematic gradient in the refraction. In the optical axis a small hypermetropia was found (0.7 D), which gradually changed into a strong myopia (4.5 D) in the most anterior parts of the visual field. This would mean that without any accommodation the rabbit's refraction is adequate for distant objects in the lateral visual field and for nearby objects (e.g., food) in the anterior direction. Hughes and Vaney (1978), using similar methods, have been unable to confirm this myopia and found a small hypermetropia throughout the visual field.

Unless otherwise stated, the experiments descibed in this monograph were done with young adult, pigmented Dutch belted rabbits. This strain is medium-sized (adult weight about 2 kg), easily bred and kept and performs well in behavioral experiments, which indicates the general health of its neural systems.

Since this text is primarily a personal account of the investigations and views of the author, it will not present a comprehensive review of all aspects of oculomotor organization in the rabbit, although references to other workers will be made as much as possible. Firstly, I shall examine the spontaneous oculomotor behavior in freely moving animals, to give a global impression of the characteristics of the system (Chap. 2). Subsequently, I shall describe the vestibulo-ocular (Chap. 3) and optokinetic reflexes (Chap. 4). Some pathways will be examined in Chapter 5, and finally, some investigations on adaptivity of vestibulo-ocular and optokinetic reflexes to altered conditions will be described in Chapter 6.

2. Eye Movements in Spontaneous Behavior

Eye movements are usually equated with the rotations of the eye in the orbit, effected by the six extraocular muscles. However, with regard to vision it is more appropriate to define eye movements as the displacements of the eye with respect to the (largely stationary) world. Certainly, under the usual conditions in an oculomotor laboratory, where the head of the animal is mostly immobilized, this distinction is academic. In this situation, which is often imposed by technical limitations of the measuring equipment, eye position in the orbit is equivalent to eye position in space (– gaze). However, in a free situation, *gaze is the resultant of the positions of the eye in the orbit, the head on the body and the body in space.* As a result, practically every muscular action in the body tends to cause gaze changes, and the first problem seems to be how to avoid gaze movements rather than how to make them. An appropriate analogy (Whitteridge, 1960) would be a telescope aboard a rolling ship. Any precision under such conditions requires the development of stabilizing systems. Thus, the first task of the oculomotor apparatus is to stabilize the eye in space rather than to move it. Only when this has been achieved, can there be a meaningful addition of commands for intentional gaze changes. These too are often effected by combined eye and head movements.

Stabilizing eye movements consist essentially of rotations of the eye in the orbit, in the opposite direction to those of the head in space and about equal in magnitude. Since the eye can only rotate, linear displacements of the head cannot be really compensated in this way, or only for a specific distance. As a result, forward locomotion will be accompanied by backward flow of the visual surroundings, particularly in animals with laterally directed eyes, such as the rabbit. An interesting solution to this problem has been developed in some walking birds (e.g., chicken and pigeons) which show a visually induced linear head nystagmus during walking (Friedman, 1975; Frost, 1978).

2.1 Techniques

We recorded eye and head movements (relative to space) in unrestrained, freely behaving rabbits (Collewijn, 1977a) with a newly developed electromagnetic eye position measurement system.

The principle of this technique was conceived by Hartmann and Klinke (1976). Two horizontal a.c. magnetic fields of equal magnitude and frequency are arranged in spatial and phase quadrature to generate a magnetic vector of a constant magnitude which rotates 360° every period of the field frequency (600 Hz) at a uniform angular velocity. The phase of the potential induced in a sensor coil in the field will vary linearly with the horizontal angle of the coil in the field. Thus, by a simple procedure of phase detection the angular orientation of any object to which a coil can be attached can be measured.

To use this principle in freely moving animals, the magnetic fields have to be homogeneous in direction and magnitude throughout the space in which the animal can move. By a special configuration of the field coils (Rubens, 1945) homogeneity was achieved within a cube of 80 cm on a side. Scleral induction coils were permanently implanted on one or both eyes through procedures as described by Fuchs and Robinson (1966) and connected to a miniature socket on the skull. A coil for measuring head position was attached to the connector through which the animal was connected (by very flexible cables) to the measuring equipment. The rabbits could move freely on a square wooden platform (80 x 80 cm). A schematic diagram of the measuring principle and the experimental apparatus is shown in Fig. 3 A, B. Further technical details can be found in (Collewijn, 1977a) where some sources of artifacts are also discussed, as well as an extension of the measurement system to three dimensions. This extended system has been successfully implemented recently, along with a computer program for the correction of nonlinearities and interactions between the horizontal, vertical, and torsional components (Van der Steen, unpublished). The system is completely insensitive to linear displacements.

2.2 Spontaneous Activity

The typical pattern of eye and head movements of a rabbit exploring its new surroundings on the platform is shown at low sensitivity in Fig. 4. The essential feature of this movement pattern is that changes in gaze are effected by saccadic steps, between which the gaze angle is relatively stable. The

Fig. 3. A A rotating, homogeneous a.c. magnetic field is produced by two special arrays of coils in spatial and phase quadrature. The phase of the signal induced in a sensor coil in this field is a linear function of the horizontal angular position (360° around). The phase of these signals (e_2 in positions A, B) is detected with respect to a reference signal (e_1). Zero crossings of the signals trigger the setting and resetting of a square wave signal. The duration of the squares is proportional to the angular position of the coil.
B Schematic view of the rabbit on the platform and the two sets of five parallel coils. (Collewijn, 1977a)

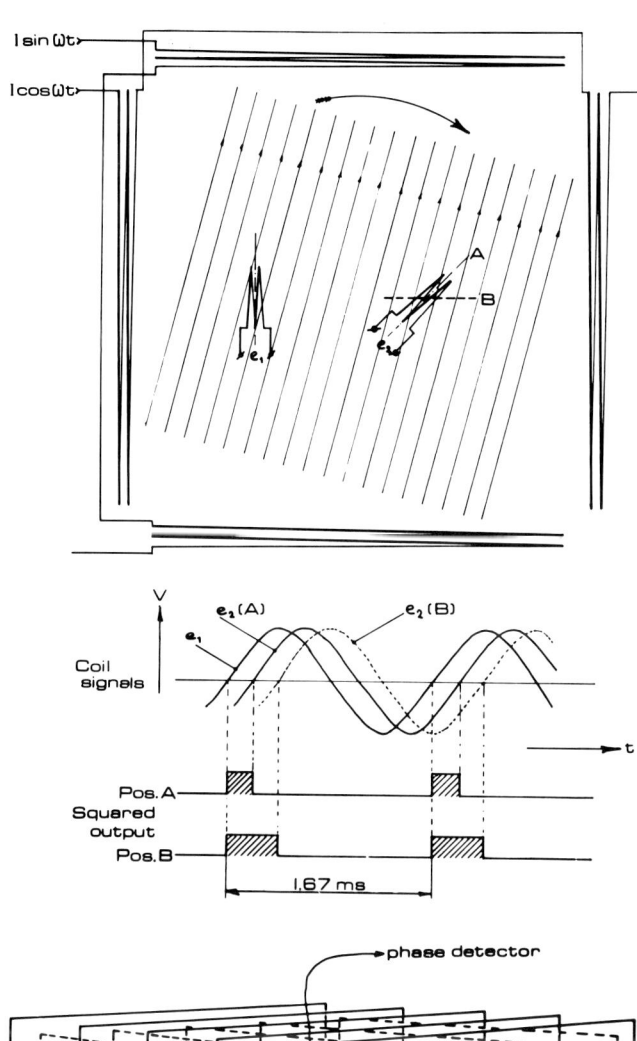
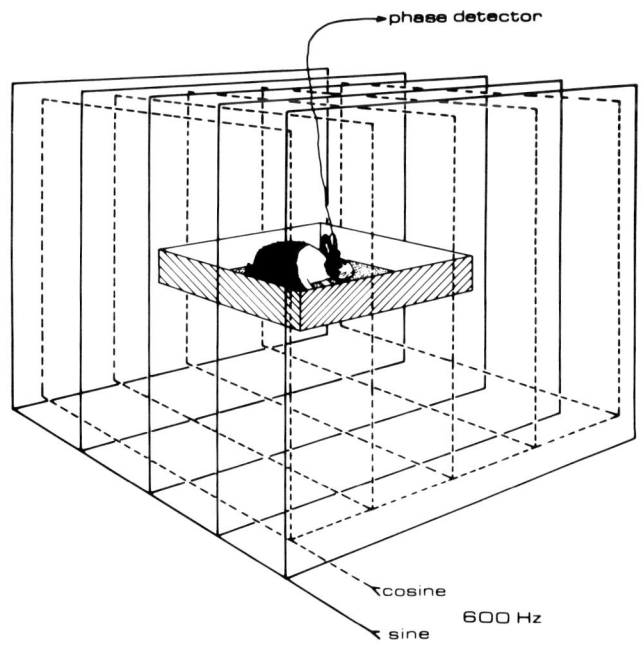

Fig. 3 A, B

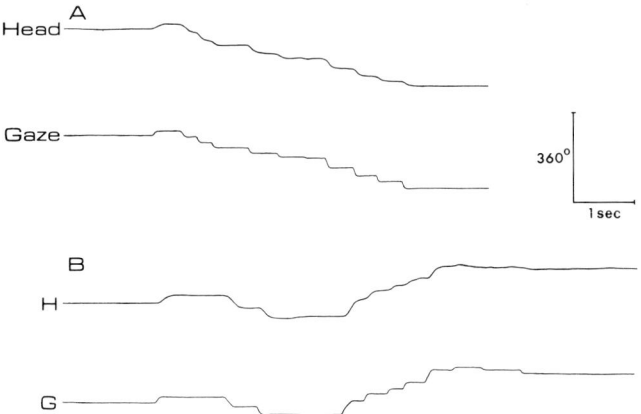

Fig. 4. Two examples of spontaneous, coordinated movements of head and gaze (= position of eye in space) in exploratory behavior, recorded at low sensitivity over the full 360° of rotation. Downward displacement represents rotation to the right (clockwise) in this and all other illustrations. (Collewijn, 1977a)

head follows a similar pattern and moves with the eye (but at a lower velocity) in combined eye and head saccades. The same type of movement is shown at higher sensitivity in Fig. 5 A. In this figure, position and velocity (obtained by suitable differentiation) are shown for the head in space, the eye in the head and the eye in space (gaze). Perfectly coordinated eye and head saccades are seen, in which the head is typically displaced by an angle similar to that of the eye, only at a slower rate. As a consequence, the excursions of the eye in the head are mostly transient and never very far from the midposition. Obviously, a recording of eye position in the head alone, as could also be obtained by traditional electro-oculography, would reveal very little about the actual gaze shifts. The pattern of Fig. 4 and Fig. 5 A is typical for active exploratory behavior.

This precise coordination between eye and head movements is not preserved in all behavioral states. Figure 5 B shows an episode when the rabbit was sniffing around the platform. The head movements were irregular and not organized in steps. Head velocity fluctuated and was rarely zero. However, the eye movement in space remained saccadic and between saccades the eyes executed compensatory movements in the orbit to balance the head movements. In Fig. 5 C head movements were even more erratic, because the animal was gnawing at the edges of the wooden platform, yet ocular stability was maintained quite well, with only saccadic gaze shifts. Figure 5 D shows a transition from violent head movements with frequent saccades to a quieter state and finally a state of complete rest (freezing).

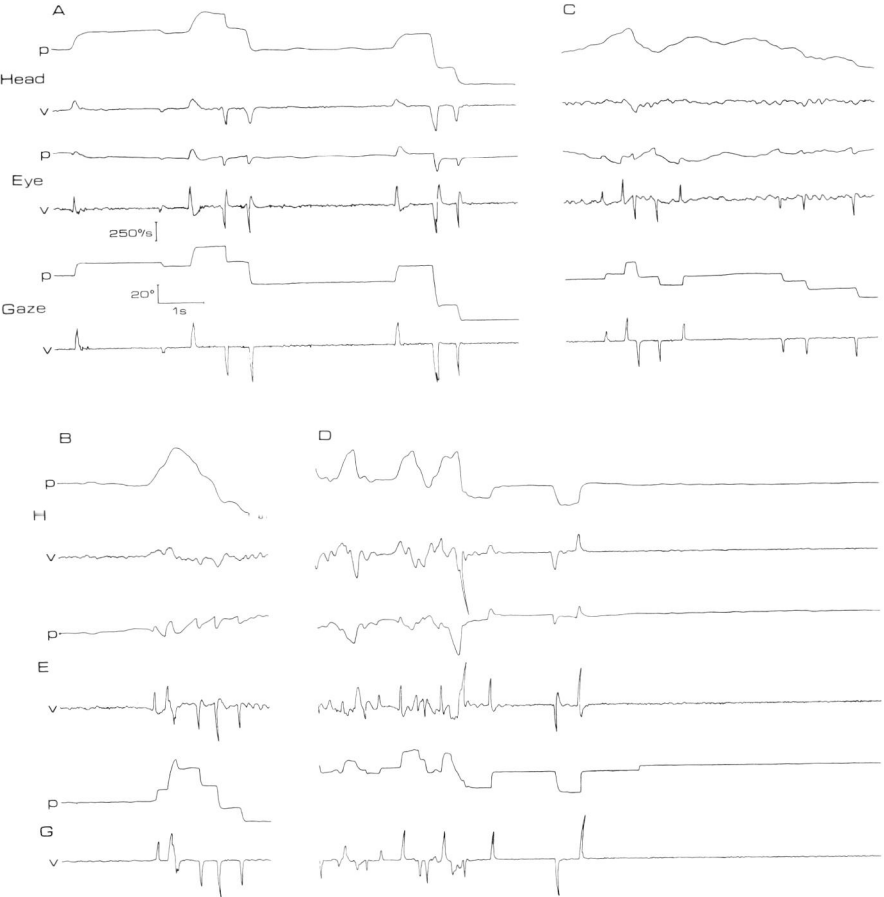

Fig. 5. Movements of the head, eye in the head (*Eye*) and eye in space (*Gaze*) in different behavioral states. Position (*p*) and velocity (*v*) are shown. **A** exploratory behavior with coordinated fast eye and head movements. **B** sniffing, with smooth head movements but saccadic gaze movements. **C** gnawing, with erratic head movements but saccadic gaze displacements. **D** transition from erratic head movements through coordinated eye- and head saccades to a quiet (freezing) state. (Collewijn, 1977a)

To convey a qualitative impression of the similarities and differences in the oculomotor behavior of the rabbit and other species recorded with the same apparatus, Fig. 6 shows exploratory behavior in a free rabbit (A), cat (B) and man (B). The species are similar in showing only saccadic gaze displacement and relatively stable inter-saccadic gaze intervals ("fixation periods"). The main differences are that from rabbit to man the saccadic gaze shifts become smaller, more frequent and more independent of the head

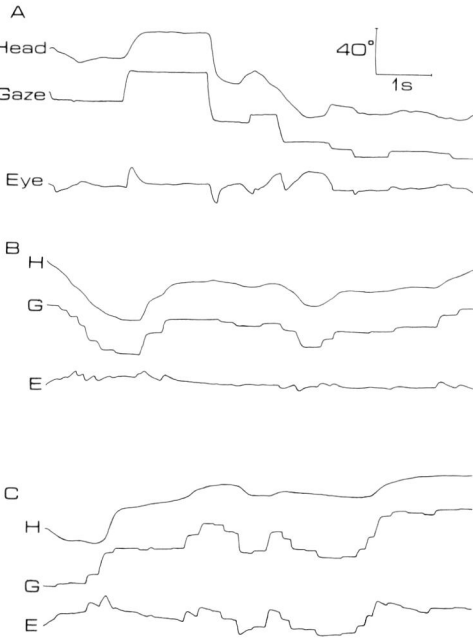

Fig. 6. Typical recordings of head, gaze and eye movements in freely moving subjects of different species. **A** rabbit; **B** cat; **C** man. (Collewijn, 1977b)

movements. The rabbit rarely makes a saccade without some accompanying head movements, whereas such events are rather common in the cat and very frequent in man.

2.3 Structure of Saccades

When an animal is passively rotated, e.g., to the right side, the eye will make compensatory (slow) eye movements to the left (with respect to the head) to stabilize gaze and fast (saccadic) movements to the right. Thus, saccadic gaze shifts are made in the direction of head rotation. These eye movements are largely caused by the vestibulo-ocular reflexes. Recordings of the type shown in Fig. 5 B can be interpreted in this way. In this case, the eye position deviates from the previous rest position in the orbit during the slow movements and is returned to it by the saccades. A similar relationship is seen during passive rotation. On the other hand, the coordinated eye and head saccades shown in Fig. 5 A are not clearly triggered by (and certainly not commensurate with) any preceding deviation of the eye in the head. Free rabbits very frequently make these large combined eye and head saccades, which are initiated independently of smooth head rotations and probably represent voluntary gaze shifts.

Figure 7 shows the structure of a typical combined eye and head saccade, with an amplitude of 20°, initiated while the head was stationary. Several

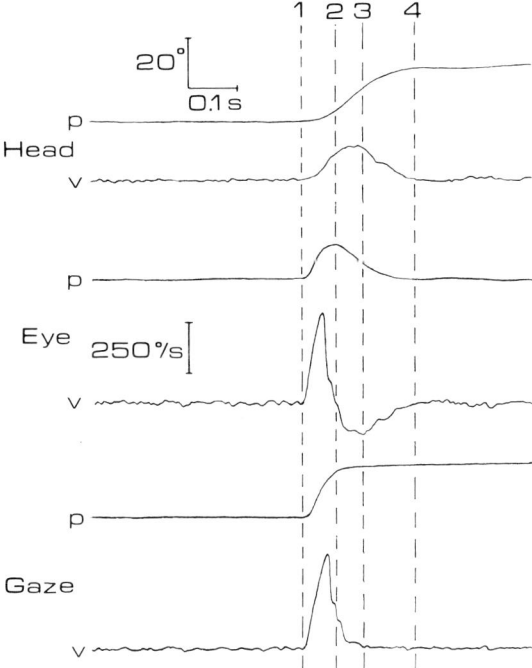

Fig. 7. Time course of a typical saccade, not preceded by a head movement. Position (p) and velocity (v) are shown. t_1 start of eye- and head movement; t_2 reversal of eye movement relative to the head; t_3 the eye reaches its final position in space; t_4 the head reaches its final position. (Collewijn, 1977a)

moments of interest (1-4) are marked by the vertical lines. At t = 1, the eye starts to move in the orbit and in space. This beginning is defined most clearly in the velocity traces. Head velocity starts to increase at the same moment, but at a much slower rate than eye velocity. The peak velocity of the eye in the head is reached rapidly (in this case 440°/s after about 27 ms). Peak velocity of the eye in space (gaze) is reached slightly later and is somewhat higher (in this case 460°/s after 40 ms), since head velocity is added to eye velocity. While head velocity continues to increase, eye velocity in the head declines sharply. At t = 2 (after 70 ms) the velocity of the eye in the head crosses the zero level and becomes opposite in direction to head velocity. From this point, head velocity is larger than gaze shift velocity. For human eye and head saccades as well it has been found (Bartz, 1966) that the compensatory backward movement of the eye in the head begins before gaze has reached its final position. At t = 3 (after 125 ms) gaze reaches its final position and remains steady thereafter. The head continues to rotate around the stationary eye for another 105 ms until 230 ms after the start of the saccade (t = 4). The amplitude of head and gaze rotation are approximately equal. The excursion of the eye in the head is only transient. The main characteristics of a typical eye and head saccade can thus be summarized as follows: (1) head and eye movement start simultaneously; (2) head movement is much slower and lasts much longer than gaze movement; (3) amplitudes of gaze and head position changes are similar; (4) the direction of the eye movement in the head inverts before gaze has reached its final angular position.

A collection of saccades of commonly found sizes and shapes is shown in Fig. 8. Saccades A through K were initiated while the head was stationary. A, B and C are *"single saccades"*, similar to those shown in Fig. 7. They may be called "single" because gaze velocity shows only one single peak. Other shapes were commonly seen among larger saccades. A similar shape with increasing amplitude would require a proportional increase in the maximal eye velocity, but apparently this cannot rise above a certain saturation level, and either a broadening (Fig. 8 D, J, K) or a splitting into two peaks (Fig. 8 G, H) occurs. The latter two are actually *double saccades*. These occurred frequently with intervals between the gaze velocity peaks as short as 40 ms. Such a double velocity peak was usually not seen in the head movement, but in a few cases splitting was also indicated (Fig. 8 G). Another common variant was a velocity peak followed by a lower "shoulder" (Fig. 13 E, F). Less common variants included bizarre forms with up to four velocity peaks.

Examples of saccades initiated when the head was moving are shown in Fig. 8 L, M and N. The eye movement in the head for these saccades consists of a slow (compensatory) and saccadic part, in opposite directions. Even in this situation the eye movements are not merely vestibulo-ocular reactions to the ongoing head movements, since the head movements are also accelerated during the saccades. The displacement of gaze (Fig. 8 L, M, N) is similar to that in saccades initiated with a stationary head (Fig. 8 A, B, C). Since gaze change is the only visually relevant parameter, a distinction between saccades with a stationary and moving head may not be very meaningful. A criterion for such a distinction might be arbitrary in any case, as head velocities occur in the whole range from zero to many degrees per second.

As shown in Fig. 9, the eye-head saccades are essentially similar in darkness, although the intersaccadic gaze stability is not as good as in the light. Apparently, visual information is not essential for the execution of coordinated eye and head saccades.

The link between eye and head saccades is not absolute, even in the rabbit, and Fig. 10, recorded at a higher sensitivity in a free rabbit, shows some

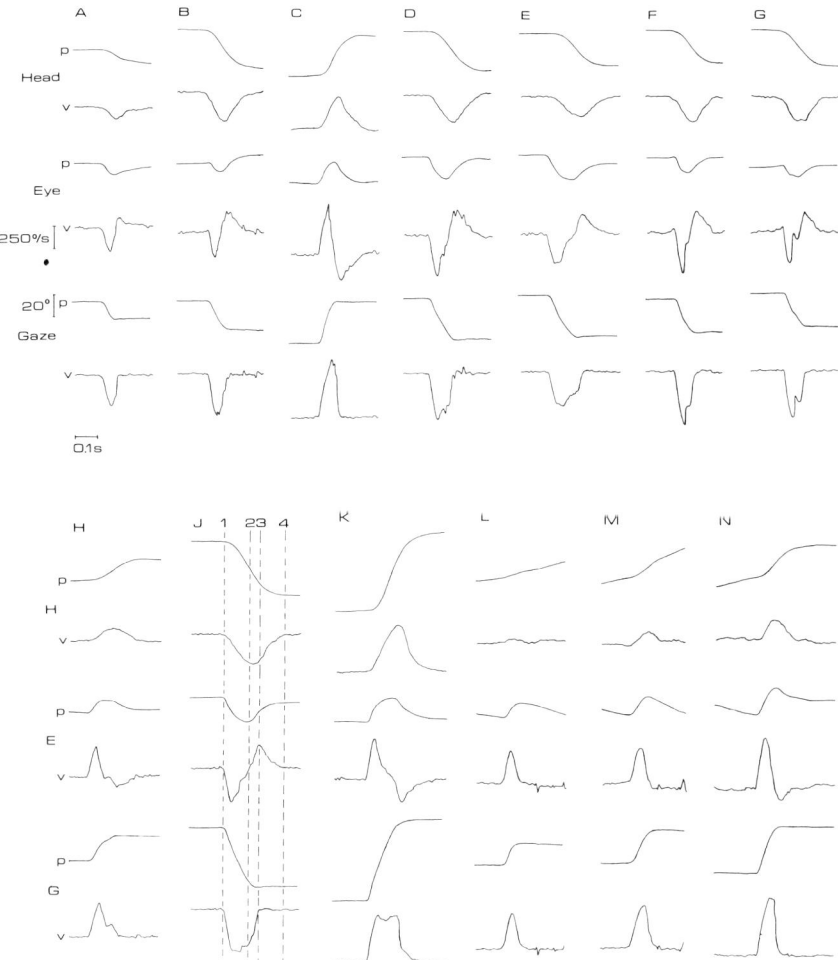

Fig. 8. Saccades of commonly occurring sizes and shapes, initiated with the head stationary (*A-K*) or moving (*L-N*). *A, B, C* straightforward saccades of increasing amplitude. *D, J, K* with increasing size duration may increase without a further rise in maximal velocity, and a plateau occurs in the eye velocity. Time marks (*1-4*) in *J* are equivalent to those in Fig. 7. In other cases large saccades show a velocity peak followed by a lower "shoulder" (*E, F*) or splitting with two velocity peaks (double saccades, *G, H*). *L, M, N* saccades preceded by a slow head movement. The gaze displacements are indistinguishable from those in *A-C*. (Collewijn, 1977a)

examples of spontaneous eye saccades initiated with the head at rest and accompanied by only minor (A) or no (B) head movements. Thus, independent eye movements can also be made by the rabbit, although they may be relatively rare.

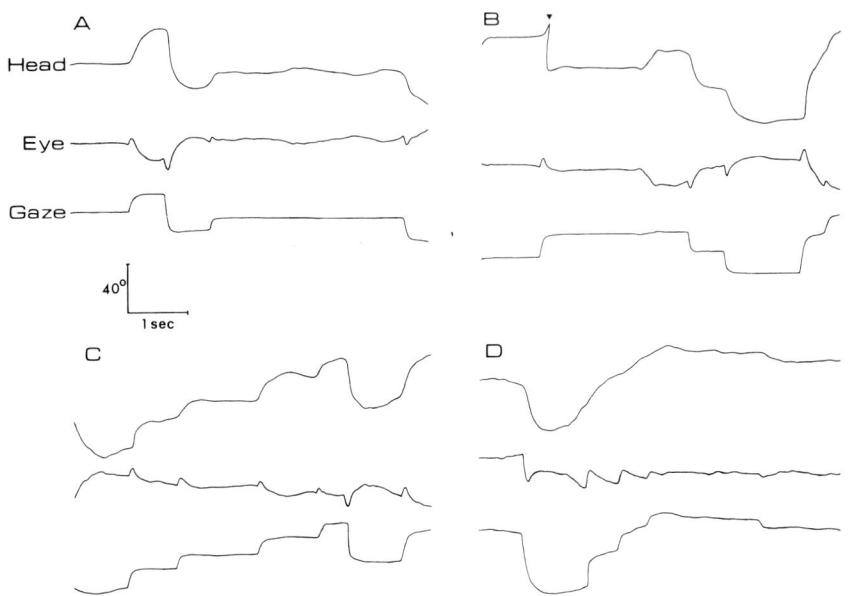

Fig. 9. Head, eye, and gaze movements in light (**A**, **B**) and darkness (**C**, **D**). The *triangle* in (**B**) indicates an automatic reset of the recorder to prevent overrange

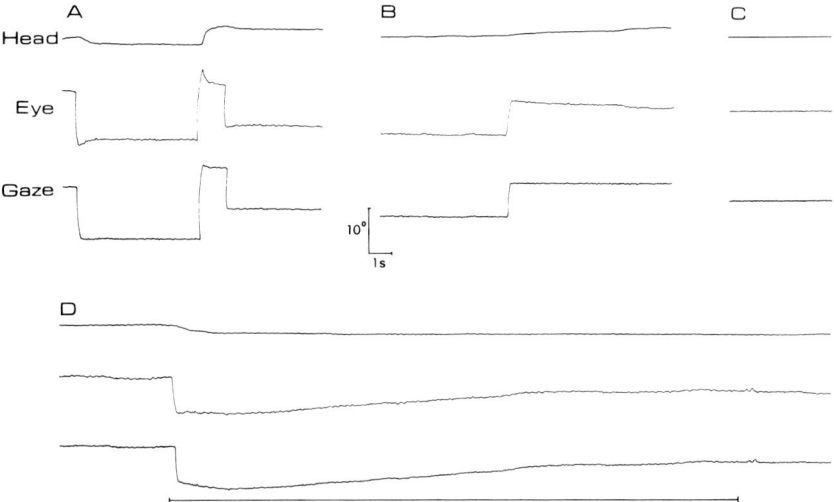

Fig. 10. Examples of gaze displacements made relatively independently of head movements. **A** eye saccades much larger than head movements. **B** eye saccades without similar head movement. Gaze stability was excellent and visual attention was probably maximal. In **B** the slow head drift was perfectly compensated and absent in the gaze. **C** noise level with a mechanically fixed sensor coil. **D** spontaneous drift of gaze in period of darkness (indicated by *bar*)

As stated, most of the saccades in the rabbit are fairly large. A distribution of the amplitudes of 5 x 125 consecutive saccades recorded in five active rabbits is shown in Fig. 11. All types of saccades were included. Double sac-

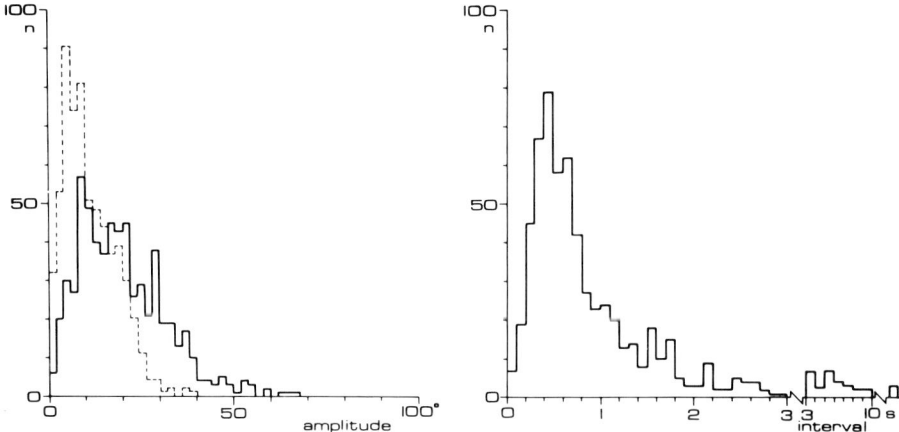

Fig. 11. Histograms of the distribution of saccadic amplitude (*left*) and intersaccadic interval (*right*) for 625 saccades (5 x 125 saccades from five rabbits). *Interrupted line* maximal deviation of eye in head; *continuous line* deviation of gaze. Periods of prolonged inactive (freezing) were not included in this sample. (Collewijn, 1977a)

cades with an interval shorter than 0.1 s were treated as single saccades. The solid line represents the amplitude of gaze shifts. The modal and median values were 10° and 19°, respectively. The dotted histogram shows the maximal displacements of the eye in the head for these same saccades. The modal and median values were 6° and 10°. Obviously, these movements (apart from their transient character) are smaller than the gaze shifts, due to the accompanying head movements. It is clear that small gaze shifts were rare. All saccades of up to 6° in amplitude amounted together to less than 10% of the sample. The smallest saccades observed measured about 1° and they were rare. The largest single saccade in this sample was 90°. The distribution of the duration of the intersaccadic intervals for the same sample (from which long periods of "freezing" were excluded) is also shown in Fig. 11. The modal and median values were 0.5 and 0.7 s, respectively, and the mean interval was 1.16 s.

It can be concluded that saccadic gaze shifts are frequent and relatively large in the active rabbit. Individual differences between the five investigated rabbits were very minor.

The diagrams of Fig. 12 show the maximal velocities and duration as a function of the gaze shift for a total of 199 saccades. In all cases a positive correlation between the parameters plotted on the abscissa and ordinate is

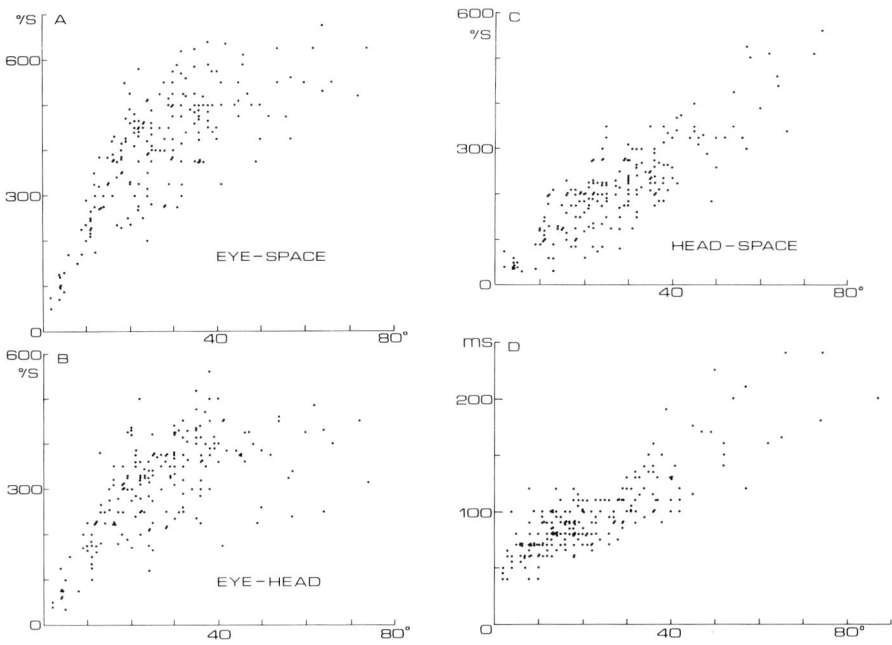

Fig. 12. Diagrams of maximal velocity of gaze (**A**), eye in head (**B**) and head (**C**) as a function of saccadic amplitude (gaze). The duration of saccades as a function of amplitude is shown in **D**. (Collewijn, 1977a)

clearly present, but the scatter is quite large. Linear and power functions have been fitted to these data (Collewijn, 1977a, b), but the correlation coefficients are rather low and it is probably more prudent to indicate only the general trends. Maximal gaze shift velocity (Fig. 12 A) is roughly proportional to the amplitude of the gaze shift for saccades up to about 30°, but in larger saccades a gradual saturation is seen for the velocity, which does not exceed about 625°/s. This effect was also discussed in relation to Fig. 8. As a consequence, the duration (Fig. 12 D), which has a minimal value of about 50 ms, seems to increase more steeply for saccades larger than about 30°. The maximum velocity of the eye in the head (Fig. 12 B) shows a similar distribution as Fig. 12 A, with a lower maximum. On the other hand the relation between maximal head velocity and amplitude of gaze shift (Fig. 12 C) seems to be essentially linear. No saturation effect is evident, and head velocities approached 600°/s for the largest saccades. The average duration of saccades in this sample was 89 ms. In combination with the mean interval of 1.16 s it may be estimated that in the active rabbit the intersaccadic intervals occupied about 93% of the total time.

The velocity amplitude relationship for saccadic gaze shifts in the rabbit does not differ greatly from that for human saccades measured with the head stationary (Baloh et al., 1975; Boghen et al., 1974), although velocities larger than 700°/s have been reported under certain conditions for man (Clark and Stark, 1974). In the monkey these higher velocities occur regularly (Fuchs, 1967). The minor differences in the dynamic properties of rabbit and human saccades are rather surprising in view of Barmack's (1976) finding that the stiffness of extraocular muscles in the rabbit is only about 0.11 g/deg, which is about one tenth of the values found for man.

It must be concluded that the free rabbit is able to make some independent eye saccades (in agreement with the observations of Hughes, 1971), but that most gaze changes are achieved by combined eye and head movements. In many of these, head and eye movements are both saccadic and initiated simultaneously. They are of the same type as described for the monkey (Bizzi et al., 1972), guinea pig (Gresty, 1975) and man (Bartz, 1966; Barnes, 1979).

For man, this gaze shift pattern was invariable whether it was elicited by visual targets or active or passive head movement in darkness, and an important role of the vestibulo-ocular reflex in the integration of eye and head movements seems likely (Barnes, 1979). For the monkey, a similar conclusion was reached by Morasso et al. (1973) and Dichgans et al. (1973a), who showed that gaze shifts elicited by visual targets were executed with equal precision whether the head was free, restrained, or unexpectedly arrested at the beginning of a saccade. This perfect coordination was severely disturbed after labyrinthectomy.

On the other hand, for the cat it has been found (Haddad and Robinson, 1977) that saccadic velocities increase when the cat is rotated, as if the head velocity were added to the eye velocity. Such evidence could be interpreted in favor of a suppression of the vestibulo-ocular reflex (VOR) during saccades. A rigorous test of this possibility in the rabbit has still to be made. The problems in doing this are that the rabbit makes few saccades without head movements, saccadic size increases with head velocities and gaze saccades are much faster than any normal nonsaccadic head movements. The time course of an eye and head saccade (Fig. 7) does not seem to argue for a suppression of the VOR at some time during the saccade. The gaze shift is effected largely between points 1 and 2, a period in which the head moves very little, so that any effect of the VOR would be relatively minor. In the period between points 2 and 3, the eye is moving opposite to the head, therefore the VOR must be working fairly well. In the final period, between points 3 and 4, gaze is stabilized while the head is moving, so the VOR must work perfectly. It seems that there remains little room or need for suppression of the VOR during saccades.

2.4 Intersaccadic Gaze Stability

Between saccades, gaze remains relatively stable and is not grossly affected by head movements (Figs. 5 and 9). A quantitative assessment of gaze stability in the rabbit has yet to be made, but the degree of stability probably varies a great deal with the behavioral conditions of the animal. Since the animal's own movements are the main sources of gaze instability one may expect a deterioration in stability due to increased motor activity. Darkness should have a similar effect by the interruption of the optokinetic loop. Furthermore, the level of functioning (gain) of the different stabilizing systems may vary with the animal's state of arousal and visual attention.

The lowest degree of stability is found in an active rabbit in darkness, as shown in Fig. 9 C, D in which retinal image slip of many degrees per second is seen. The best stability in the free condition is found when the rabbit is sitting quietly, but alert, with very little head movement. Such episodes are shown in Fig. 10 A, B at high sensitivity. A high level of visual attention is suggested by the occurrence of some independent eye saccades and in between them the drift of gaze was smaller than $0.1°/s$. The small fluctuations in head position (Fig. 10 B) were well compensated. Figure 10 D demonstrates the loss of this stability in the dark. Even though the head moved very little, gaze drifted in the dark with velocities up to about $1°/s$. In view of the noise level of the measuring system (Fig. 10 C) recordings at still higher sensitivity could not be made in the free rabbit.

Intermediate levels of stability are seen with nonsaccadic head movements in the light (Fig. 13). Grooming activity with rhythmic motion of the head is shown in Fig. 13 A. Most, but not all, of this movement was suppressed in the gaze. The same is true for Fig. 13 B, which shows a period in which the rabbit was sniffing the platform. During such activities as sniffing and grooming maximal visual stability may not be needed. In contrast, Fig. 13 C shows once more the coordinated eye and head saccades which seem to be characteristic of visual attention. Interspersed between the head saccades two periods of head shaking (possibly caused by awareness of the cables) occurred. In this case compensatory eye movements were good enough to practically eliminate these oscillations from gaze. Figure 13 D (recorded at higher sensitivity) shows small head vibrations (probably of circulatory

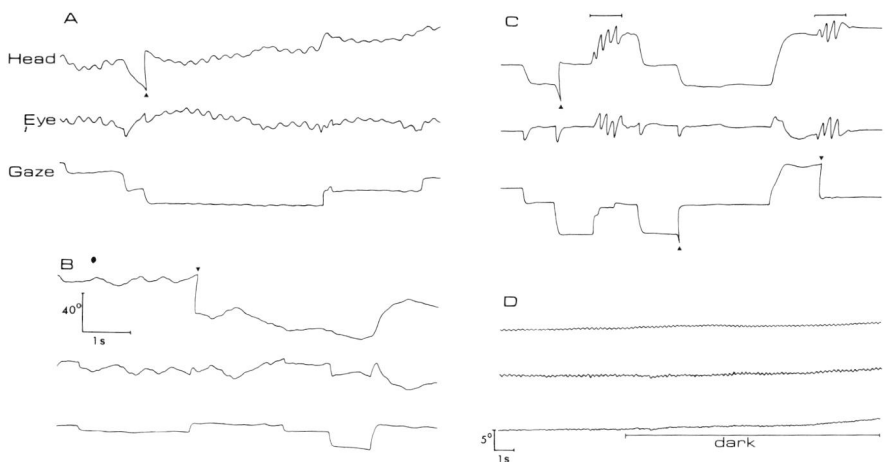

Fig. 13. Different levels of gaze stability. A grooming activity with rhythmic head oscillation which is largely, but not completely compensated. B sniffing activity with erratic head movements and relatively poor gaze stability. C violent head shaking with excellent compensation. D small head tremor with rather good compensation, also in darkness. (A-C from Collewijn, 1977a, calibration in B). *Triangles* resets of recorder to prevent overrange

and/or respiratory origin) in a quietly sitting rabbit. This small vibration (frequency about 4 Hz) was also largely compensated by the eye movements and was absent in gaze. Since this compensation persisted in darkness (Fig. 13 D, bar), is was probably effected by the vestibulo-ocular reflex. Notice that a slow drift (as in Fig. 10 D) did not occur in darkness.

When the head is immobilized, most sources of instability are eliminated and stability becomes maximal. This is shown in Fig. 14 for an alert rabbit, suspended in a hammock and with the head fixed by permanently implanted head screws. Figure 14 A and B shows that the eye remains immobile for extended periods in the light, although some infrequent saccades occur. In darkness stability is lost and drift with a typical velocity of 0.5°-1°/s, interspersed with saccades is seen. The stability of the rabbit's eye with the head fixed is recorded at high sensitivity in Fig. 14 C. The noise level (Fig. 14 D) is very low in these recordings due to the use of a different measuring system (Robinson, 1963). Thus, all the fluctuations in Fig. 14 C are real eye movements. A characteristic tremor with frequencies of about 3-7 Hz and an amplitude of about 0.1° (peak-to-peak) is seen. Drift (up to 1°/s) occurs again in darkness. To illustrate the contrasts with the fine grain of human eye movement Fig. 14 E shows a typical example of human fixations recorded with a scleral coil system (Collewijn et al., 1975) and the head restrained by chin and head supports. The main differences between man and

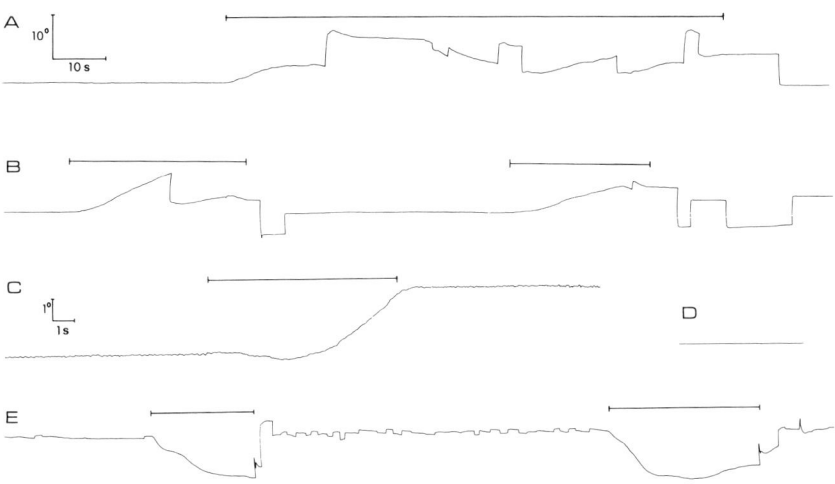

Fig. 14. Gaze stability with the head immobilized. The *bars* indicate periods of darkness in which stability is lost. **A, B** low sensitivity (calibration in **A**), spontaneous saccades in the light are rare but do occur. **C** higher sensitivity which shows spontaneous tremor and absence of microsaccades. **D** noise level shown by a mechanically immobilized sensor coil. **E** human fixation behavior (calibration as in **C**) which shows no tremor but frequent microsaccades and similar loss of gaze stability in darkness

rabbit "fixation" are the following. The human eye does not show the coarse tremor seen in the rabbit, but tends to make frequent small saccades (microsaccades). However, these microsaccades can be suppressed (Fig. 14 E, left part) as was described by Fiorentini and Ercoles (1966) and Steinman et al. (1967). In darkness, the human subject is as incapable as the rabbit of maintaining his eye position when he avoids making saccades. This phenomenon was first described by Skavenski and Steinman (1970). The overall stability of the eye is of the same quality in the rabbit as it is in man using slow control and better than in man using microsaccades. Recent data on human eye stability indicate that in the fixating human subject retinal slip increases to 20-40 min arc/s when the head is unsupported (Skavenski et al., 1979) and that it increases tenfold (to about 4°/s) during voluntary head oscillations (Steinman and Collewijn, 1980).

A final difference between rabbit and man is that reillumination after a period of darkness in man results in a refixation of the original target, while the rabbit will stabilize in any position reached during the drifting.

2.5 Active Pursuit

The oculomotor response of the rabbit to moving targets on a stationary background is limited. When the head is fixed, even "interesting" targets such as food do not elicit any smooth or saccadic eye movements. In the free animal definite reactions can be obtained. Figure 15 A shows the eye movements elicited by a mirror, which was rotated approximately sinusoidally in front of the rabbit. In the monkey and man such a stimulus produces

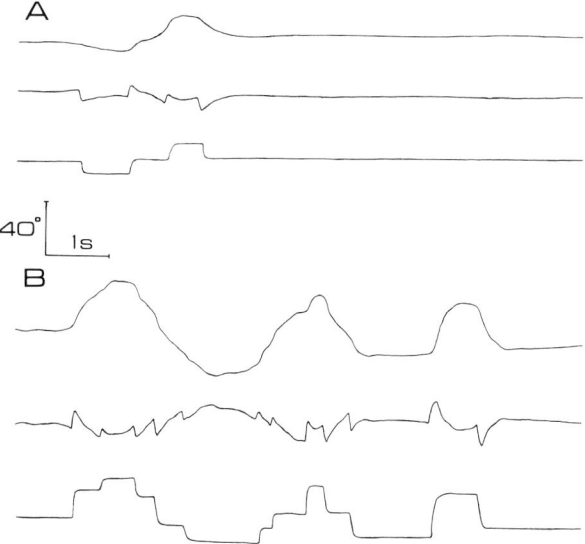

Fig. 15. Pursuit behavior in a free rabbit. **A** a mirror was oscillated in front of the animal. It was followed for a brief period after which interest was lost. **B** pursuit of a hand moved in front of the animal. In all cases the head movements are smooth, but gaze displacement occurs only with large saccades. *Upper trace* head, *Middle trace* eye in head, *lower trace* gaze

with great reliability smooth pursuit eye movements. The rabbit responded, but only briefly, by saccadic gaze displacements. Pursuit was elicited more reliably by moving a hand slowly to the right and left in front of the animal (Fig. 15 B). The animal clearly followed these movements with great interest. In this case as well, gaze was only shifted with large, saccadic steps and no smooth movements. However, a smooth component in both Fig. 15 A and B is found in the head movements, and it seems possible that the primary response consists of pursuit with the head and not with the eye. This would activate the vestibulo-ocular reflex with the generation of fast components as a secondary reaction. A somewhat similar hypothesis has been proposed by Barnes (1979) for human gaze shift to targets in the far periphery of the visual field. This might also explain the absence of any pursuit when the rabbit's head is fixed. On the other hand, the saccades in Fig. 15 B cannot be completely secondary to the head movements, since they are not only executed by the eye in the head but also in part by the head itself, so that the saccadic gaze shifts are larger than the saccades of the eye in the head.

2.6 Vergence

The recording system for freely moving animals also offered an opportunity to investigate the existence of vergence eye movements in relation to a visual task. For this purpose induction coils were permanently implanted on both eyes and the rabbits, reinforced by a food reward, were trained in a simple two-door discrimination box (Van Hof, 1966) to make the correct choice between vertical and horizontal striations. The forward locomotion of the rabbit during the approach to the doors was also recorded by connecting the head to a potentiometer with a fine steel cable. Some potential artifacts were avoided by restricting head rotations to the horizontal plane with levers attached to the head.

Unimpressed by all this instrumentation, the rabbits continued to perform reliably in their discrimination task and, to our surprise, convergence of the eyes was consistently recorded during the approach to the pattern and the collection of food (Zuidam and Collewijn, 1979).

Recordings of the relevant events in one approach are shown in Fig. 16 A. At point v, the patterns became visible. Approach and convergence started

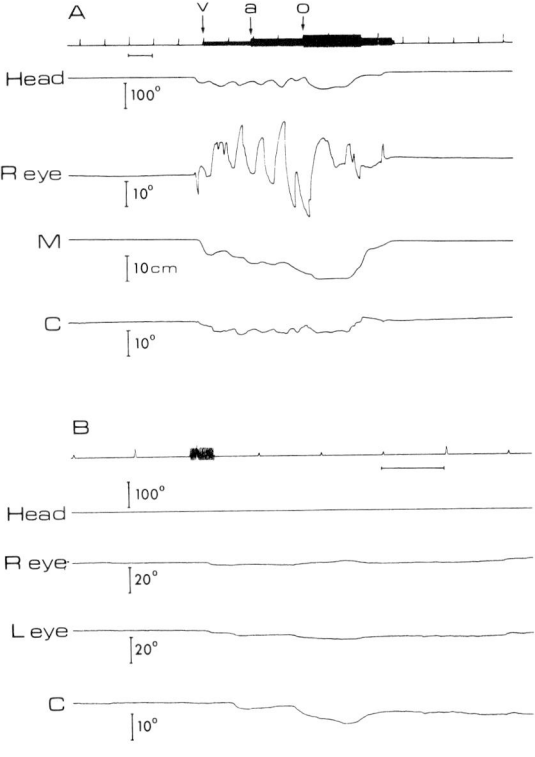

Fig. 16 a, b. Vergence in the rabbit. **a** Convergence during a visual discrimination task. *Upper graph* time scale (s) and event marks. *v* patterns visible; *a* doors accessible; *o* one door opened by rabbit. *M* forward motion of the rabbit (downward); *C* convergence (downward). **b** Convergence in a rabbit with the head immobilized, to which a food pellet was shown (*mark*) and fed

immediately and the correct door, which was accessible from point a, was opened at point o, after which a food pellet was consumed. This whole procedure took about 6 s, and the eyes diverged to the original position immediately afterwards. Not all responses were as neat as the one shown and sometimes vergence movements were absent or irregular. Therefore, averaging techniques were used to extract the mean vergence and locomotor response to 50 exposures of the patterns.

In all of the many sessions and for all of the 12 rabbits investigated, convergence was consistently recorded in this way. Figure 17 shows typical av-

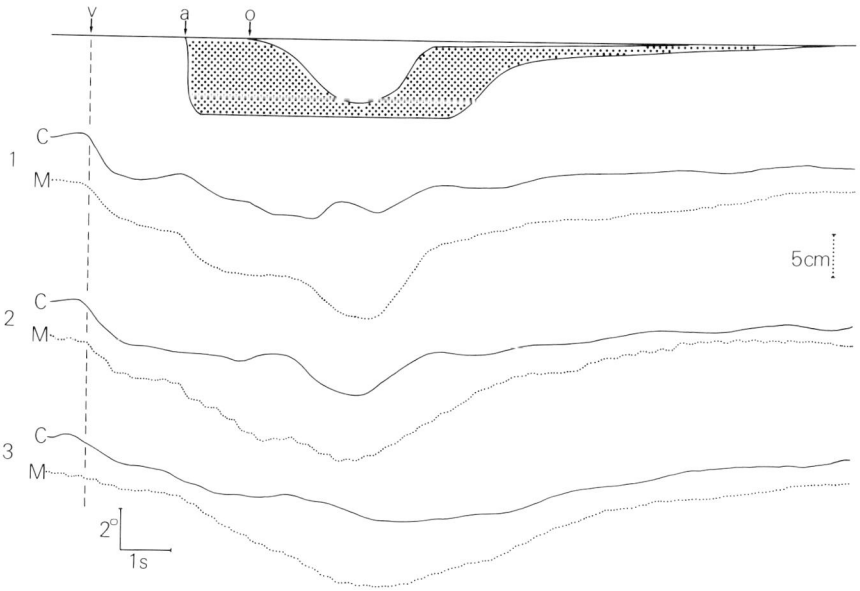

Fig. 17. Averages (50 trials) of convergence (*C*) and forward movement (*M*) in three rabbits. Averaged time windows in which doors were accessible (*a*) or open (*o*) are shown for rabbit *1*. Averaging is synchronized with the exposure of the patterns (*v*)

eraged responses for three rabbits. Convergence and approach to the patterns were strongly correlated. Typically, two stages could be distinguished. A first convergence movement was made as soon as the patterns became visible. A second, larger convergence usually followed when the animal proceeded through the door and took his pellet. When the approach to the patterns was blocked for some time after the exposure of the patterns, the second stage of convergence was delayed until the animal was released and moved forward. The convergence was not affected by the nature of the patterns and not abolished by the masking of one eye. Thus, disparity is not a necessary cue and a synergy with accommodation is also excluded since the latter is not found in the rabbit. The change in the size of the target during the active approach may be an important stimulus. In general, objects that were moved toward the resting rabbit did not elicit convergence, but a remarkable exception is shown in Fig. 16 B. A well-trained, hungry rabbit was restrained in a wooden box with the head immobilized by the implanted screws. A food pellet was shown at a distance of 30 cm and then put into the rabbit's mouth, where it was promptly eaten. This procedure elicited a marked convergence for a few times, after which the response habituated.

With the head rotations limited to the horizontal plane, the maximal convergence observed was 9°; with the head completely free the highest value was 18°. If it is assumed that at rest the rabbit's eyes are aligned for the projection of objects at an infinite distance on corresponding parts of both retinas, convergence would have to be 10.3° for a target at 25 cm distance and 25.3° for a target at 10 cm distance (interpupillary distance 45 mm). Our results show that convergence of this order of magnitude can be achieved, but that it is usually smaller. The value of these theoretical figures is limited. The distance for which the binocular parts of the retinas are aligned may be smaller than infinity, as De Graauw and Van Hof (1978) found that the rabbit is myopic in the binocular zone. The amount of tolerance in retinal correspondence for fused binocular vision (if present) in the rabbit is also unknown. Furthermore, the task required visual discrimination but not specifically binocular vision. This may explain the great variability between trials.

In cats, convergence cannot be demonstrated in all animals and, if present, it is only occasionally of the theoretically expected magnitude (Stryker and Blakemore, 1972; Hughes, 1972). Most responses were smaller and quick habituation was found.

A rigorous demonstration of vergence as an independent type of eye movement with a quantitative input-output study requires carefully controlled conditions and considerable understanding and cooperation on the part of the subjects. Such studies have only been done in man (Rashbass and Westheimer, 1961a, b; Alpern, 1962; Toates, 1974) and are hardly feasible in cats or rabbits. However, convergence clearly occurs in rabbits which have to look at nearby objects and this finding indicates that vergence is not limited to species with foveal, binocular vision and frontal eyes. This makes it more likely that cortical binocular units as described by Van Sluyters and Stewart (1974) can be stimulated by single objects in the visual world; this would actually require a convergence of 10°-20°.

2.7 Conclusions

The nearly panoramic visual field and lack of a fovea make it difficult to define the direction of gaze in a rabbit. Fixation in man implies the stabilization of the fovea on a selected target. The stabilization aspect is clearly present in the rabbit; selective aiming of a part of the visual field is a priori more questionable, since the animal sees most of its surroundings anyway. If the location of images on the retina were truly inconsequential, a rabbit would only need stabilizing oculomotor reflexes consisting of smooth compensatory eye movements and fast resets (saccades) to keep the eye within the mechanical limits of its rotation in the orbit. The prevalence of large saccades (Fig. 11) and their generally tight coupling with head movements points in this direction, as does the absence of a position correction after drift in darkness (Fig. 14 C). On the other hand, the structure of the retina is definitely inhomogeneous (Fig. 2). Van Hof and Lagers-Van Haselen (1973) and Vaney (1980) have observed that the posterior part of the retina, which has a relatively high density of large ganglion cells (Provis, 1979), is preferentially used in a food-rewarded visual discrimination task. With the frontal parts of the visual field masked, rabbits only learned such a task with great difficulty, although most of their visual streak was unobstructed.

It has been shown that rabbits can solve a discrimination problem for which the information from both eyes (separated by color filters) has to be used (Van Hof and Steele Russell, 1977). Zuidam and Collewijn (1979) recorded convergence in a similar discrimination task. Thus, the frontal (binocular) field may have a special function in discriminatory visual tasks such as food collection and inspection of objects (Fig. 15). An important function of saccadic gaze shifts (other than to recenter the eyes in the orbit) may be the redirection of the binocular zone toward targets of special interest. As the zone is much wider (about 30°) than a typical fovea (a few degrees), it is understandable that small saccades are relatively rare. Correct correspondence between the two retinal projections by appropriate vergence may be essential for a correct functioning of binocular vision.

3. Eye Movements During Passive Oscillation

In the preceding chapter, I have reviewed the spontaneous oculomotor behavior under unrestrained conditions as well as with the head immobilized. It was shown that between saccades gaze is stabilized to somewhat variable degrees of perfection. The rest of this text will be devoted mainly to the systems involved in this stabilization.

One important subsystem is the vestibulo-ocular reflex (VOR). This can be divided into the canal-ocular reflex which originates from the semicircular canals and the maculo-ocular reflex derived from the otolith organs, the utriculus and sacculus. The canals are activated by rotatory accelerations and thus changes in rotatory velocity. They do not respond to constant rotatory velocities or linear accelerations. The utriculus and sacculus respond to linear accelerations, among which gravity is probably the most significant because of its constant presence, considerable magnitude, and continuous pressure against which equilibrium and posture have to be maintained. A general review of mammalian vestibular physiology has recently been published (Wilson and Melvill Jones, 1979), while many details of vestibular neurophysiology have been described in a monograph in this series by Precht (1978). Neurophysiology of posture in general was recently reviewed by Roberts (1978).

A second subsystem is the optokinetic system (OKN) which is activated by a global drift of the retinal image.

In this chapter I shall describe the compensatory eye movements elicited by passive sinusoidal motion of the rabbit in the light (VOR and OKN) and in darkness (VOR only).

A third subsystem, the cervico-ocular reflex, is controlled by proprioceptive signals from the muscles and joints of the neck. As relative motion between head and body was excluded in our experiments with restrained animals, we have not obtained pertinent data on this system but some findings by other workers will be discussed.

The term *gain* will be used for the ratio between the velocities of the compensatory eye movements and the stimulus or the ratio between the amplitudes of the eye movement and stimulus movement. In the latter case, fast (saccadic) components are eliminated and the cumulative slow phase is reconstructed by joining the consecutive slow phases end-to-end (Meiry, 1971).

For stimuli which vary sinusoidally as a function of time, the *phase* of the adequate response with respect to the stimulus will be expressed in degrees (°); 360° stands for the length of a period.

Perfect compensation corresponds to a gain of 1.0 and a phase of 0°. As an introduction, I shall describe the compensatory eye movements of the rabbit elicited by rotation in three dimensions. This description will give an impression of the general level of the stability achieved in the three axes of motion and of the relative importance of canal-ocular, maculo-ocular and optokinetic reflexes.

3.1 Rotation Around the Three Principal Axes

Using the extended magnetic induction system (Collewijn, 1977a) compensatory eye movements around the vertical, sagittal, and transverse axis have been recorded recently in our laboratory by Van der Steen in alert rabbits. Vertical and horizontal scleral induction coils and skull screws were permanently implanted. The rabbit was suspended in a hammock and mounted in a normal position on a platform to which the head was rigidly connected with head screws. The platform was sinusoidally oscillated around the three principal axes with a range of frequencies, at an amplitude of 10°, except at the highest frequency for which the amplitude was 5°.

Figure 18A shows the results for oscillation in the horizontal plane (yaw), the direction in which oculomotor reflexes have been most often studied be-

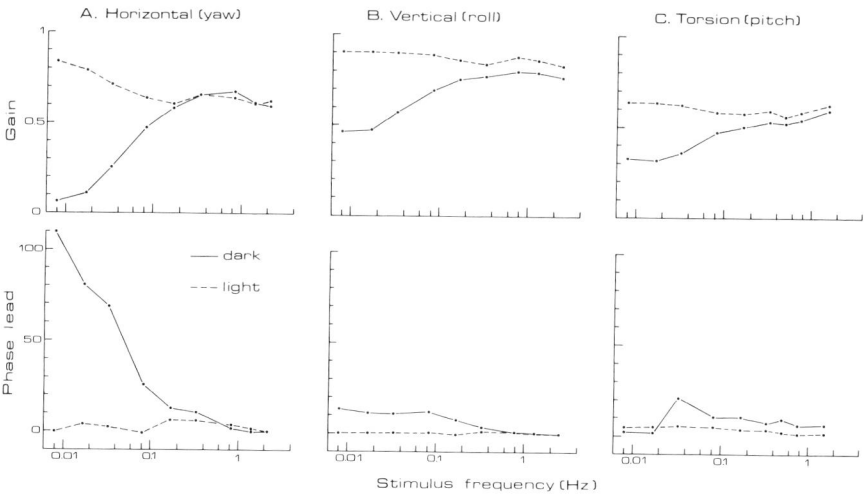

Fig. 18. Gain and phase of compensatory eye movements in three axes of motion (yaw, roll, and pitch) as a function of frequency, measured in the light (*interrupted lines*) and in darkness (*continuous lines*). Average values of three rabbits. (Van der Steen, unpublished)

cause of the relative ease with which horizontal eye movements can be recorded. These data agree largely with recent reports on the rabbit by Baarsma and Collewijn (1974) and Batini et al. (1979).

With normal illumination (interrupted lines), the gain is about 0.65 for frequencies of the order of 0.1-1 Hz and rises to about 0.8 for frequencies around 0.01 Hz. The phase is close to zero throughout the frequency range, which means that the eyes move in counterphase with the head. In darkness, responses are almost identical for frequencies above 0.2 Hz but decrease strongly and progressively with the lowering of the frequency. Gain is smaller than 0.1 for frequencies below 0.01 Hz and phase shows an increasing lead, which reaches a mean value of 110° at 0.008 Hz. The sense organs involved in these horizontal reflexes are the semicircular canals (mainly the horizontal ones) and the retina. In darkness, only the canal-ocular reflex is activated, which functions poorly at low frequencies. In the light, compensatory eye movements are induced by the optokinetic reflex (OKN) in addition to the canal-ocular reflex. The synergy between these reflexes extends the useful frequency range down to DC. For the higher frequencies, the contribution by the OKN is small.

Figure 18 B shows the results for the same rabbits oscillated around the sagittal axis (roll). Since the rabbit has lateral eyes, the adequate compensatory eye movements are vertical, so that when the head is tilted to the right side, the right eye moves upward and the left eye downward. With the lights on, gain is constant at 0.85 to 0.90 throughout the whole frequency range, with a phase angle not significantly different from zero. This performance in the vertical plane is remarkably good and superior to that in the horizontal plane (Fig. 18 A) at every frequency. This is also true in darkness. At the higher frequencies (> 0.2 Hz) the gain of the vertical vestibulo-ocular reflex is about 0.8 (horizontal only about 0.65), and for the lower frequencies it decreases to about 0.5 around 0.01 Hz (horizontal gain < 0.1). The phase error in darkness remains small (around 10°) as well. One important cause of these differences is undoubtedly the contribution of the maculo-ocular reflexes (originating from the utriculus and sacculus) to the compensatory eye movements. Particularly for the lower frequency range this macular input (which is sensitive to static tilt with respect to gravity) must be important.

Barmack (in press) has obtained very similar results for the horizontal and vertical VOR in the rabbit. Moreover, he has found that the low frequency (presumable otolithic) component of the vertical VOR could be abolished by positioning the rabbits with the nose pointing upward. In this orientation gravity does not interact with head rotation around the sagittal axis.

Finally, Fig. 18 C shows the performance of compensatory eye move movements when the same rabbits were oscillated around the transverse axis (pitch). The adequate eye movement in this case is torsion (counterroll) around the optical axis. In the light, gain is remarkably constant but at a level of only about 0.6, which is two thirds of the vertical gain. Phase errors are again very small (a lead up to 5°). In darkness, when only the canal-ocular and maculo-ocular reflexes were activated, gain of the torsional eye movements decreased in a similar way (but to a lower level) as for the vertical eye movements. A comparable increase in phase error (around 10° lead) also occurred.

Some general comments on these results have to be made. The gain is mostly considerably below unity so that retinal image stability is never achieved. One reason for this may be the behavioral status of the restrained animal. As has been discussed in Chapter 2.4, stability also fluctuates in the free animal and it may be maximal only in a state of high visual alertness. Barr et al. (1976) have described extreme variations in the gain of human VOR, which could be effectively controlled by various instructions to the subject. We have observed considerable differences between rabbits, and the responses from individual rabbits show also some fluctuation within or between sessions.

Flandrin et al. (1979) have described profound changes in the VOR related to the level of alertness in cats. During slow-wave sleep the VOR gain decreased to 40% or less and phase advances up to 90° were observed. In paradoxical sleep, the VOR disappeared entirely.

A second reason for a less than maximal gain in our experiments may be the absence of a stimulus for the cervico-ocular reflexes. These have been reinvestigated in the rabbit by Gresty (1976) and more recently by Barmack et al. (in press). Relative motion between trunk and head induces slow eye movements which are compensatory in direction and synergic with the VOR. In addition, fast (saccadic) eye movements are elicited in the same, compensatory direction. It is clear that only the smooth component can contribute to intersaccadic stability by decreasing retinal slip. However, Barmack et al. (in press) found that the smooth component of the cervico-ocular reflex has a significant gain only in the low frequency range. In the horizontal plane, the mean gain rose from 0.21 at 0.005 Hz to 0.27 at 0.02 Hz and declined to < 0.1 above 0.1 Hz. For the vertical cervico-ocular reflex (induced by rotation of the body relative to the head around the longitudinal axis) gains were even smaller by a factor of 2-3. A linear addition of these cervico-ocular responses with the VOR was also shown by Barmack et al. (in press), who suggest further that the relatively high gain in the horizontal plane may compensate for the absence of otolithic information in this plane.

Whatever the merits of the cervico-ocular reflexes, it is clear that they do not contribute significantly in the frequency range above 0.1 Hz, a range in which the majority of spontaneous head movements is made.

A third, more intriguing possible reason for the imperfect compensation in our measurements with sinusoidal stimulation is that these movements are rather artificial and unusual for a rabbit, but that after sufficiently long experience with this stimulus the responses improve. This adaptive process will be discussed further in Chapter 6.3.7.

3.2 Properties of the Horizontal Canal-Ocular Reflex

The pure canal-ocular reflex can be isolated by oscillating the animal in darkness in the horizontal plane. Some examples at three frequencies are shown in Fig. 19. The eye movement in the head (eye) as well as in space (gaze) are shown to illustrate the measure of stability achieved. For 0.05 Hz the gain of the VOR is still quite reasonable, yet gaze stability is extremely poor due to the appreciable phase lead of the VOR. This illustrates the overwhelming importance of correct phase relations in addition to sufficient gain

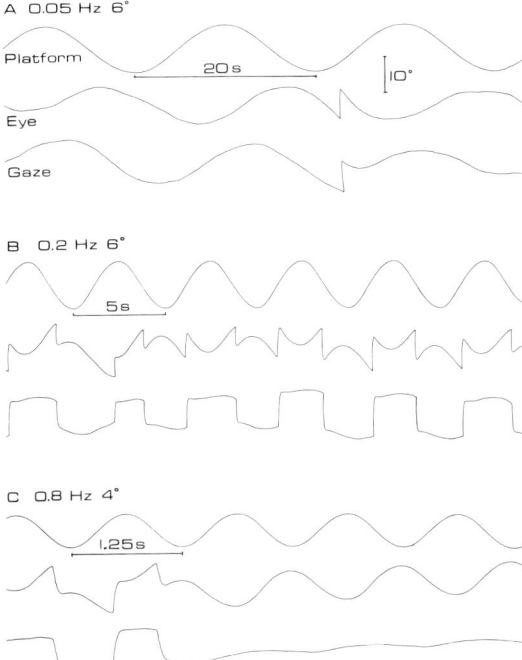

Fig. 19. Typical recordings of the horizontal canal-ocular reflex elicited by passive oscillation in darkness at 0.05, 0.2, and 0.8 Hz. At 0.05 Hz the effect of the VOR on gaze stability is almost nil, due to the large phase error

mains possible, of course, that the rabbit suppresses the VOR under other, as yet unidentified behavioral conditions.

3.4 Maculo-Ocular Reflexes

In addition to the canal-ocular reflexes elicited by rotatory accelerations, the rabbit possesses well-developed maculo-ocular reflexes, originating from the stimulation of the otolith organs by linear accelerations such as gravity. The utriculus and sacculus are multidimensional linear accelerometers. The neurophysiology and response dynamics of their afferent fibers have been recently investigated in great detail in mammals, particularly in the monkey (Fernandez et al., 1972; Fernandez and Goldberg, 1976a, b, c) and in the cat (Loe et al., 1973). The distinct feature of these fibers is that — in contrast to canal afferents — they show a tonic response to static tilt and are coded for linear accelerations in specific directions. These static properties are in agreement with the general structure of the otolith organs and the three-dimensional arrangement of the hair-cells in the utricular and saccular maculae (Lindeman, 1969). The dynamic properties of the otolith organs have been controversial (see Wilson and Melvill Jones, 1979), but the recent measurements by Fernandez and Goldberg (1976c) of primary macular afferent fiber responses to sinusoidally modulated linear accelerations have provided direct data on the frequency response of these units, two types of which are now distinguished. In *regular* units, gain was practically constant over a range from DC to 2 Hz, with no more than 10° phase change either side of zero. Thus, these regular units faithfully encode the imposed linear accelerations. *Irregular* units on the other hand increased their gain by about a factor of 20 when frequency was increased from DC to 2 Hz, with a somewhat variable phase lead of 20°-30°. These characteristics obviously would favor the transmission of higher frequencies and thus the changes in the linear acceleration vector. For otolith-dependent units in the vestibular nuclei, a somewhat similar differentiation into static and dynamic units has been made by Schor (1974) on the basis of gain as a function of frequency. However, in contrast to the peripheral units (Fernandez and Goldberg, 1976c), central otolith-dependent units have been reported to develop a strong phase lag with increasing stimulus frequency (Melvill Jones and Milsum, 1969). Phase was about zero at 0.1 Hz but lagged about 180° at 1-2 Hz.

To investigate maculo-ocular responses, stimulation of the neck proprioceptors or canals has to be avoided. This can be easily achieved in static conditions by tilting the animal (head and body) and measuring the steady-state responses. This was done a long time ago by Van der Hoeve and De Kleijn

(1917) and Fleisch (1922a). Lateral tilt (roll) produced compensatory vertical eye movements and nose down or up (pitch) resulted in torsional counterroll. The gain of these static responses was about 0.6. The function of these reflexes in maintaining the retina in a stable orientation during head tilt is clear. However, the macula is sensitive not only to gravity (g), but also to the linear accelerations associated with locomotion. For example, a forward acceleration of the head will affect the otoliths in the same way as an upward pitch of the head: the otoliths will be displaced backward. Among other postural adjustments which may be fully adequate this would also elicit a torsional counterroll of the eye with the upper pole moving forward. Acceleration to the side would induce a downward movement of the ipsilateral eye. A moving animal will experience a multitude of erratic linear acceleration in various directions; the "compensatory" eye movements elicited by these accelerations are obviously not adequate for vision and therefore investigation of the dynamic response characteristics of the maculo-ocular reflexes is highly relevant.

These dynamic characteristics have been investigated with sinusoidal linear accelerations produced by a horizontal parallel swing (Fig. 28 A) in the frequency range between 0.068 and 1.22 Hz and with acceleration steps (0.02-0.11 g) generated by a cart, running on a rail track (length 30 m) and pulled forward by the steady force of a falling weight (Fig. 28 B). The horizontal acceleration a was directly measured with a linear accelerometer on the cart and calculated for the parallel swing.

The otoliths will be affected by the vectorial sum of a and g which will deviate from the true vertical by an angle Θ:

$\Theta = \arctan a/g$

Values of Θ in the range of about 1°-44° were realized.

This change in apparent direction of gravity is considered as the stimulus for the compensatory eye movements. If these reach the amplitude Φ, the gain G will be defined as

$G = \Phi/\Theta$

For the sinusoidal movements on the parallel swing the phase angle between Φ and Θ is also calculated; phase is defined as zero when the compensatory eye movement (e.g., downward movement of the right eye for an acceleration to the right) is maximal when the acceleration is maximal (i.e., when the swing is deviated maximally to the left). These relations are rather complex and have been neglected sometimes in the literature. The mechanics of the parallel swing are further complicated by the presence of a vertical component (with the double frequency) in the swing motion, which has to be accounted for in a correct calculation of the total linear vector. This has

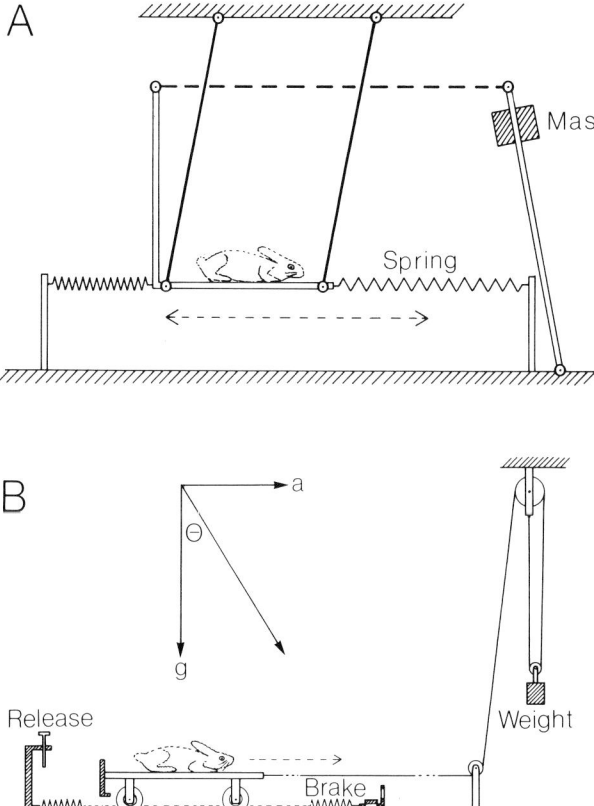

Fig. 28. Construction of **A** the parallel swing with variable frequency and **B** the linear acceleration track. The *inset* shows the linear vector which is the sum of the gravity vector (g) and the horizontal acceleration (a) and is rotated over an angle Θ with respect to the objective vertical. (Baarsma and Collewijn, 1975a)

been done for the data presented here. A derivation of the relevant equations and further technical details have been given in Baarsma and Collewijn (1975a) and will not be repeated here. A final complication is the change in *magnitude* of the total linear acceleration compared to g. It has been reported that an increased g-value causes augmented oculomotor and perceptual responses to tilt (Colenbrander, 1964; Schöne, 1964). For most of our stimuli this change in magnitude was small and it was neglected in the analysis of the results.

Since a meaningful interaction of maculo-ocular reflexes with visual stimuli could not be expected in our experiments, all measurements were done with the eyes covered. The eye movements (vertical and torsional) were measured with scleral coils as described by Robinson (1963).

In all rabbits, approximately sinusoidal eye movements were recorded on the parallel swing in the expected directions, i.e., torsional for swinging in the antero-posterior direction and vertical for swinging in the transverse direction. Gain and phase were calculated from the computer-averaged response to five periods of swinging. The most striking result was the generally low gain, i.e., the amplitude of the eye movements (Φ) was much smaller than the rotation of the linear vector (Θ). In general Φ was of the order of 1°. A systematic variation of the swing amplitude (10-30 cm) revealed no nonlinearities and therefore the results of all amplitudes and rabbits (n = 14) have been pooled in the Bode plots of Fig. 29 (vertical maculo-ocular responses to transverse swinging) and Fig. 30 (torsion, sagittal swinging). For both directions similar results were obtained. Gain was only about 0.25 for the lowest stimulus frequency used (0.068 Hz) and decreased rapidly as frequency was increased, to reach values of about 0.01 for frequencies around 1 Hz. The phase lag was about 10° at 0.068 Hz, but increased to about 180° at the highest frequency (1.22 Hz). These results indicate that the maculo-ocular reflex performs very poorly with a dynamic stimulus, except for very low frequencies (< 0.1 Hz).

The responses obtained with acceleration steps are shown in Fig. 31. All traces are the averages of ten runs on the linear track. The accelerations are shown in Fig. 31 A. The cart was released at t = 0. Frequencies above 3 Hz have been filtered out from the accelerometer signal, yet the record is very noisy due to the imperfections of the simple mechanical device used. The steady components of the accelerations (determined by the pulling force) were about 0.02, 0.04, 0.07, 0.09, and 0.11 g (durations 11, 8, 6, 5 and 4.5 s, respectively). These admittedly rather crude stimuli elicited reproducible eye deviations in the theoretically expected directions (Fig. 31 B, C). The eye movements were extremely slow (recordings with obvious disturbances such as saccades were discarded). The eyes started to move immediately when the rabbit was accelerated and reached a final position in several rabbits after 3-5 s. In the examples of Fig. 31 the movements were apparently not completed even after 5 s. Due to the limited length of the track the final eye positions could often not be determined. When the acceleration was terminated and the cart rolled on with a steady velocity, the eye started a return movement with an equally slow time course. When the cart was braked to a halt, the deceleration induced a strong oculomotor response opposite to the first one. The magnitude of the responses was about proportional to that of the acceleration, while the time course remained similar. This is more clearly shown when gain (Φ/Θ) is plotted as a function of time (Fig. 32). With the possible exception of the lowest acceleration (0.02 g) which was relatively more disturbed by noise than the higher ones, the time course of gain was similar for all accelerations. It reached a level between 0.5 and 0.6

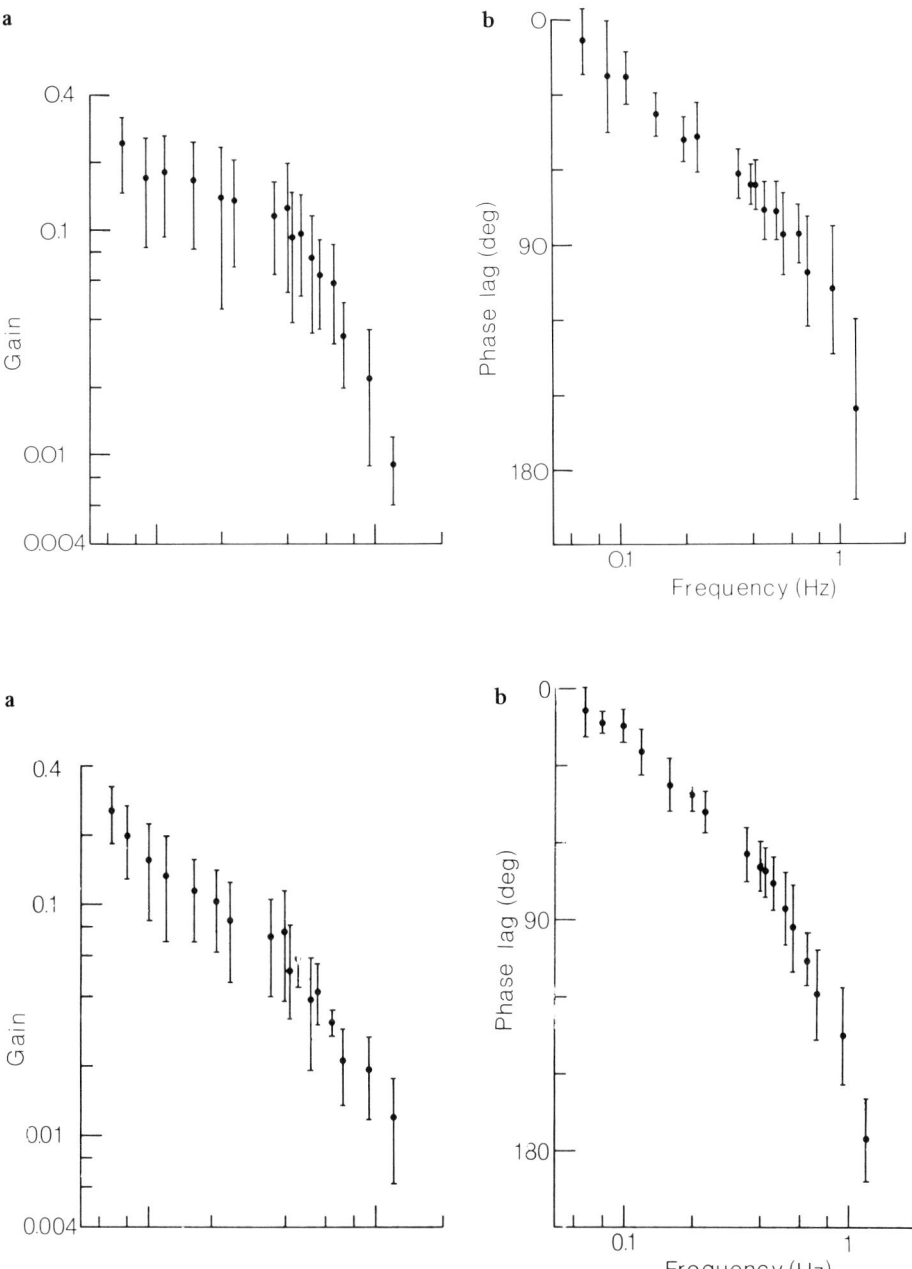

Fig. 29 a, b. Gain and phase of vertical eye movements elicited by transverse linear oscillation in darkness. Average values (± 1 S.D.) of 14 rabbits. (Baarsma and Collewijn, 1975a)

Fig. 30 a, b. Gain and phase of torsional eye movements elicited by antero-posterior linear oscillation in darkness. Average values (± 1 S.D.) of 14 rabbits. (Baarsma and Collewijn, 1975a)

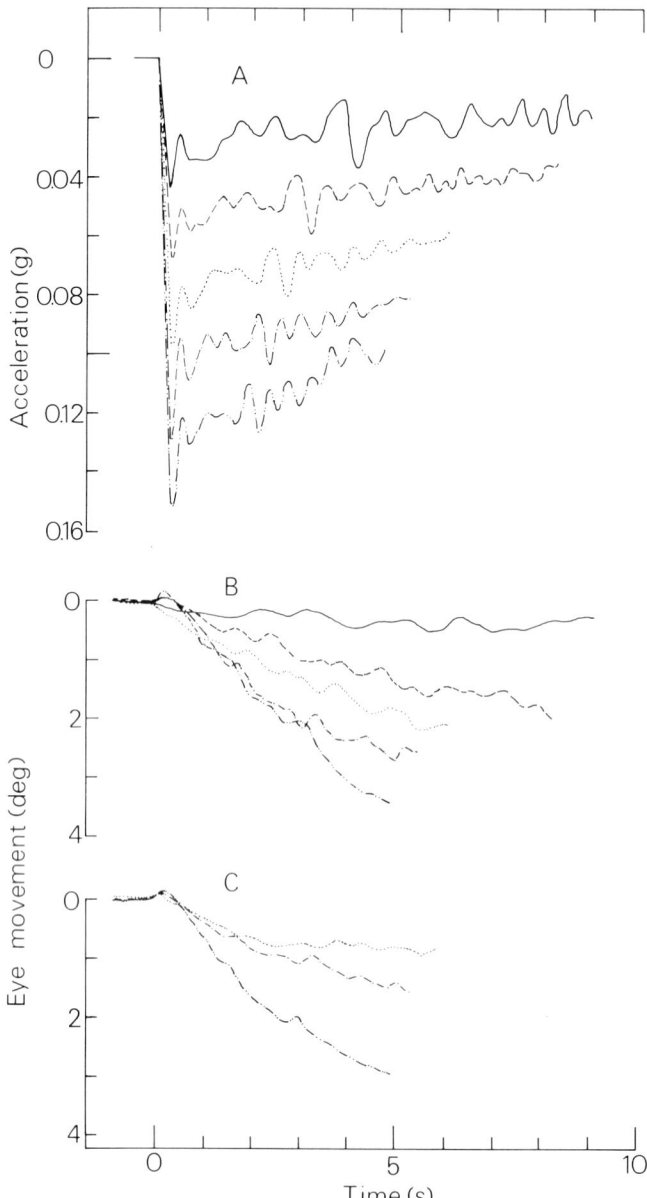

Fig. 31. A linear acceleration of the platform on the track as a function of time with different pulling weights (10, 20, 30, 40, and 50 kg). Frequencies above 3 Hz have been filtered out. **B** downward movements of the right eye due to application of these accelerations along the transverse axis (rabbit moving to the right). **C** nasal torsional eye movements due to acceleration of the same rabbit in the forward direction. All traces are averages of ten recordings in one rabbit. (Baarsma and Collewijn, 1975a)

after about 5 s. These values are substantially higher than those measured on the parallel swing.

The results of both sinusoidal and step linear acceleration stimuli show that maculo-ocular reactions are extremely slow. This confirms some old observations. Fleisch (1922b) accelerated rabbits on a short linear track (length 1.5 m) and found that the eye movements were small and could only be recorded by a sensitive optical lever technique; furthermore they were slow ("had a long latency"). Lack of a sensitive recording technique may account for De Kleijn and Magnus' (1921) failure to record similar responses. Lorente de Nó (1931) in his classical study elicited tonic vestibulo-ocular reflexes in rabbits after plugging the semicircular canals and emphasized the slow nature of these reactions.

It is now clear that this sluggishness is not due to the properties of the otolith organs or its afferent fibers (Fernandez and Goldberg, 1976c) which transmit the higher frequencies faithfully or even preferentially. In all probability, the otolith signals are subject to considerable modification before they are relayed to the oculomotor neurons. An indication of this is formed by the phase relations observed for otolith-dependent units by Melvill Jones and Milsum (1969), which are strikingly similar to the phase relations we found for the maculo-ocular reflex (Figs. 29 and 30).

Functionally these findings are satisfactory and readily interpretable. The fast otolithic responses are undoubtedly valuable in the rapid adjustments of posture but, as stated before, the compensating eye movements such as would be elicited by the erratic linear accelerations associated with locomotion are not adequate but on the contrary very harmful to visual stability. Most of these accelerations will be in the higher frequency range (see Wilson and Melvill Jones, 1979, Fig. 8.20) and fortunately these are hardly transmitted by the maculo-ocular reflex. As will be discussed in Chapter 6.3.1 these high frequency responses may even be actively eliminated by adaptive processes. If on the other hand the head is tilted slowly, the maculo-ocular reflex will become effective exactly in the low frequency range where the canal-ocular reflex fails (Fig. 18). The same is true for a fast tilt after which the head is kept in a tilted orientation. The canal-ocular reflex will take care of the initial correction, and while its response wears off the maculo-ocular response will build up to maintain the compensatory deviation of the eye.

Van der Hoeve and De Kleijn (1917) and Fleisch (1922a) measured maculo-ocular reactions in rabbits in a static condition and found a gain of about 0.6. Our data from the linear track experiments (Fig. 32) show that such a gain is indeed reached if the acceleration (equivalent to tilt) is maintained for about 5 s.

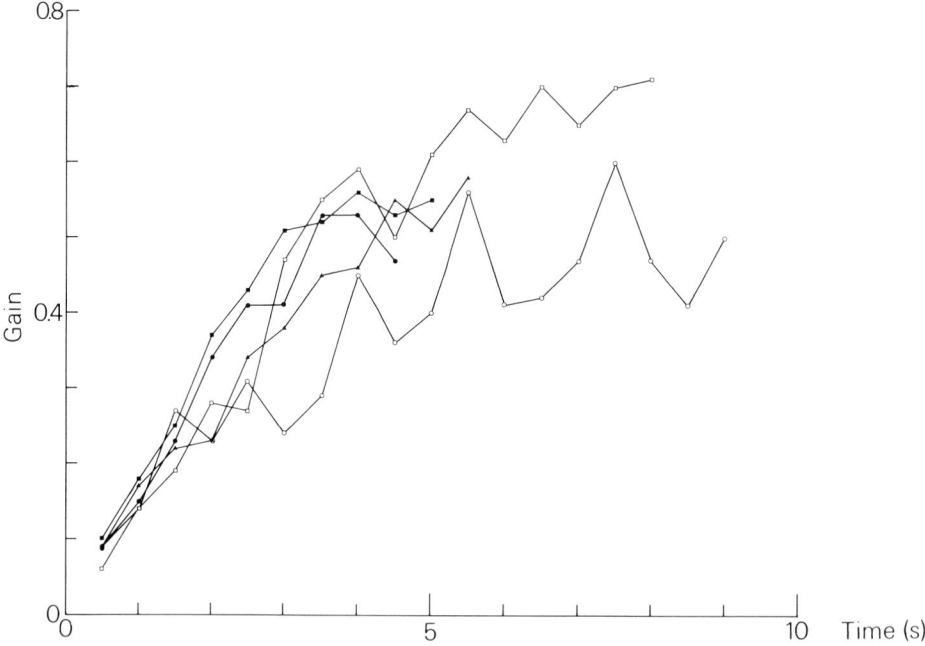

Fig. 32. Increase of gain with time during constant acceleration. Averages of seven rabbits for vertical eye movements. Approximate magnitudes of acceleration: 0.02 g (*open circles*), 0.04 g (*open squares*), 0.07 g (*triangles*), 0.09 g (*filled squares*), 0.11 g (*filled circles*). (Baarsma and Collewijn, 1975a)

3.5 Conclusions

In this chapter I have examined the compensatory eye movements elicited during passive (oscillatory) motion of a rabbit. Under suitable stimulus conditions, the properties of the canal-ocular and maculo-ocular reflexes have been identified and the significant contribution by vision has been shown. It was also demonstrated that the different systems complement each other in a meaningful synergy to achieve a rather constant gain and negligible phase errors throughout a wide frequency range.

One surprising result is that the total gain of all these systems usually remains below unity. In part this may be due to the experimental conditions, in which the movements were stereotyped, animals were restrained, and maximal visual performance was not behaviorally required or reinforced.

4. Optokinetic and Postrotatory Nystagmus

In this chapter I shall discuss some stimuli which are less natural than the ones discussed in Chapter 3 to elicit compensatory eye movements. The most important of these is the isolated optokinetic reflex (OKN), produced by rotation of the visual surroundings around the stationary animal. The responses to sinusoidal as well as constant velocity rotation will be examined. The responses of the animal to passive rotation at constant velocities and to velocity steps will also be investigated. Common to all of these stimuli is the fact that they never occur under natural behavioral conditions.

4.1 The Nature of the Optokinetic Reflex

The optokinetic system has been — and still is — surrounded by considerable confusion, because the term "optokinetic" has been loosely used for all pursuit eye movements elicited by moving objects, and often no distinction is made between selective foveal pursuit of targets on a stationary background on the one hand and stabilization of the eye on the global visual surroundings on the other. Nowadays, the first kind of tracking is called *smooth pursuit*. Obviously, its development is secondary to the presence of a fovea or central area. The second kind of response is the true optokinetic nystagmus, which is found in any animal with spatial vision. Even when the eyes cannot be moved in the head, as in insets (but also in the owl), optokinetic (or "optomotor") responses of the head or whole body can be elicited by suitable stimuli. Since both types of reactions are present in man, for whom such responses were first described, the understanding of the fundamental difference has developed very slowly.

The discovery of optokinetic nystagmus (OKN) is often attributed (Collins et al., 1970) to Purkinje who first observed it in a crowd watching a cavalry parade, while Helmholtz mentioned in 1866 that such eye movements were most readily observable in railway passengers looking at the moving landscape. Bárány (1908) introduced optically elicited nystagmus as a diagnostic tool in the clinic and used a small hand-held striped drum as a convenient stimulus in a bedside test. The first optical recordings of pursuit of a series of moving objects were made — again in the human — by Dodge in 1903. Most of these historical observations would now be classified as smooth pursuit, since in nearly all cases a relatively small target was seen on a stationary background. This type of stimulus does not elicit any reliable responses in rabbits, and the existence of OKN in the rabbit was firmly denied by Bartels (1931) in a review of the comparative physiology of these responses as understood at that time.

Ter Braak (1936) was the first to recognize that: (1) the adequate stimulus for OKN is movement of the surroundings *as a whole* with respect to the eye; (2) such movements are normally caused by rotation of the head and not by movement in the surroundings; (3) such visual stimuli will function in synergy with the signals from the semicircular canals. Ter Braak (1936) enclosed the rabbit in a striped drum and was successful in eliciting OKN by rotating the drum at moderate angular velocities.

The essence of OKN is not to aim the eye at any specific object, but to reduce the velocity of gaze displacement (drift) between saccades to an acceptable level. Traditionally, OKN is elicited by continuous rotation of a drum at a constant velocity. The eye will track such a movement with a smooth movement which is interrupted regularly by saccades (fast phases) in the opposite direction. This regular sequence of smooth and saccadic movements is the classical optokinetic nystagmus. The direction of the OKN is often (especially in the clinic) defined as that of the fast phase, which is more easily observable than the smooth component (slow phase). The smooth phase is seen in isolation when the stimulus amplitude is limited, as in oscillation of the drum instead of undirectional rotation. Foveal smooth pursuit may also take the form of a nystagmus, especially when the stimulus contains multiple target points or is repetitive in nature (such as the Bárány drum). Ter Braak (1936) called this "look"nystagmus ("Schaunystagmus") in contrast to the "stare"nystagmus ("Stiernystagmus") elicited by full field or peripheral field stimulation and later the terms "active" and "passive" nystagmus were used for the same distinction (Scala and Spiegel, 1941). The modern term *"smooth pursuit"* is adequate to describe the voluntary, selective pursuit of relatively small targets and the term *optokinetic nystagmus* should be reserved for responses to stimuli occupying the whole visual field.

Afoveate animals possess only the OKN system. Isolated moving targets are not smoothly pursued, except in the absence of any structured background. A single moving light-spot in darkness will elicit nystagmus even in a rabbit (Ter Braak, 1936) but this is OKN and not smooth pursuit, since no selection is involved and the nystagmus does not stabilize the target on any particular part of the retina.

Foveate species posses both systems. Smooth pursuit is easily isolated by presenting moving targets on a stationary background. However, OKN is usually mixed with smooth pursuit as the subject is inclined to pursue certain details (e.g., one stripe) in the pattern. Instructions to just look at the pattern and not voluntarily follow any detail may alleviate this admixture, but effective control of the type of response is difficult to obtain. A solution could possibly be found in the use of patterns without clearly identifiable details, such as certain types of visual noise.

4.2 Optokinetic Responses to Sinusoidal Stimulation

As OKN is the response controlled by a subsystem of the compensatory reactions associated with head movements, we shall first discuss the responses to sinusoidal movement of the visual surroundings, as a complement to the sinusoidal rotation of the animal studied in Chapter 3. Figure 33 illustrates some responses to sinusoidal oscillation of a drum (diameter 140 cm, height 125 cm) rotated around a vertical axis centered on the midpoint between the eyes of a rabbit. A scleral coil and head screws had been permanently implanted so that the rabbit could be immobilized comfortably with normal binocular vision. All equipment (including the magnetic field coils) was located outside the drum, so that vision was unobstructed and limited to the drum. The drum was lined with a random dot pattern (elements about 1°; Julesz, 1964). The animal and the frequencies illustrated are the same as shown in Figs. 19, 20, and 26. These figures indicated that the visual stimulus was especially effective in the low frequency range. This is fully confirmed by Fig. 33. At 0.05 Hz, a stimulus with an amplitude of 4° induced an almost perfect sinusoidal optokinetic response with few saccades; gaze is stabilized on the drum. An increase in the amplitude to 8° resulted in equally good slow pursuit, but due to the increased amplitude of the eye movements more saccades were introduced. An increase in the frequency to 0.2 Hz (Fig. 33 C, D) revealed another effect. For an amplitude of 4° the response was still rather good, although smaller than at 0.05 Hz. However, an increase in the stimulus amplitude to 8° did not cause an enlarged stimulus response at this frequency. This proves that the optokinetic system is nonlinear. Finally, at 0.8 Hz and 4° amplitude the responses are diminished considerably more (Fig. 33 E).

A survey of gain as a function of stimulus frequency at different stimulus amplitudes is given in Fig. 34 A. It shows a family of curves, each for a different amplitude. These (and other) results suggest that gain may be deter-

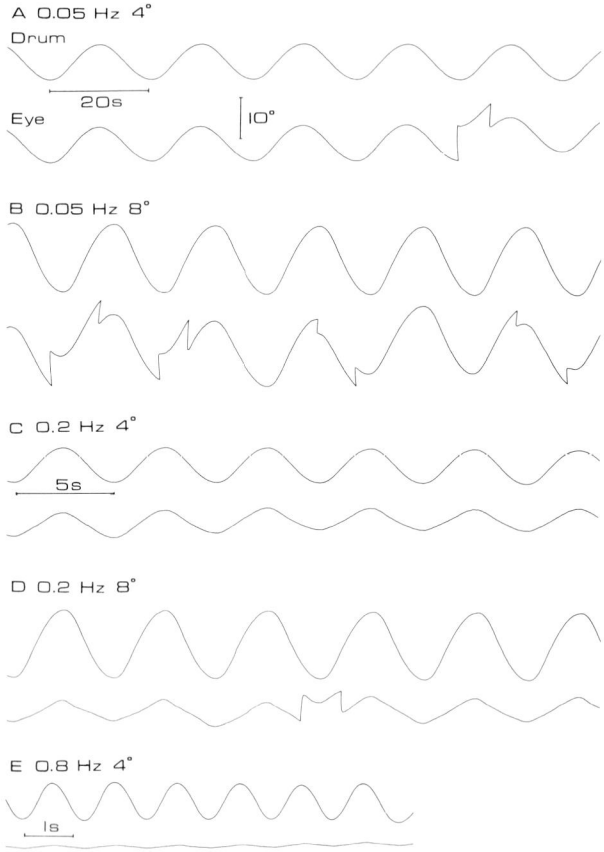

Fig. 33. Typical examples of horizontal optokinetic pursuit in a rabbit, elicited by sinusoidal rotation of a whole field drum (lined with a random-dot pattern) around the animal

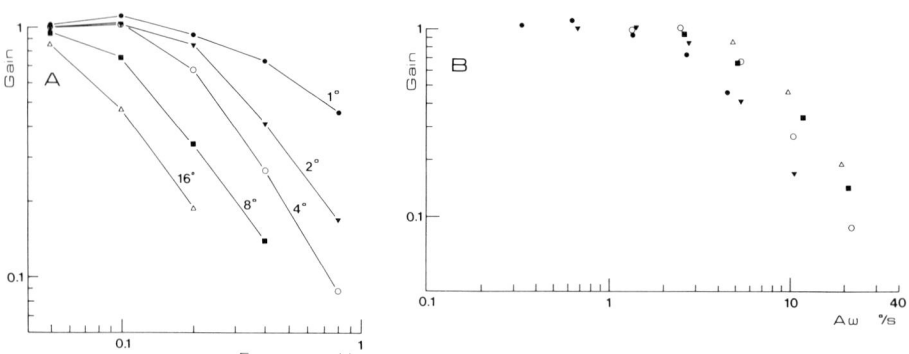

Fig. 34. Optokinetic gain for sinusoidal stimulation. **A** gain as a function of stimulus frequency for various stimulus amplitudes. Gain decreases strongly with the increase of amplitude. **B** gain as a function of the maximal velocity of the sinusoidal stimulus (A) for the different amplitudes (same symbols as in **A**)

mined by the velocity of the stimulus, which is proportional to both frequency ω and amplitude A:

$$p = A \sin \omega t \quad (\text{deg}) \qquad (1)$$
$$v = A\omega \cos \omega t \quad (\text{deg/s}) \qquad (2)$$

in which p = drum position, v = drum velocity, A = amplitude of drum motion, t = time, $\omega = 2\pi f$, f = frequency in cycles/s (Hz). The maximal drum velocity v_{max} is reached when $\cos \omega t = 1$, thus:

$$v_{max} = A\omega \qquad (3)$$

The data of Fig. 34 A have been replotted in Fig. 34 B with gain as a function of the maximal stimulus velocity $A\omega$. The family of curves of Fig. 34 A shows confluence into a single function. Gain is about 1 for velocities up to 2°/s and then falls with a slope of about 45°. This means that for stimuli faster than 2°/s gain decreases proportionately with the stimulus velocity, or in other words, the response will saturate at about 2°/s for sinusoidal stimuli. The agreement between the recent data of Fig. 34 B and an earlier published graph for the same relation (Collewijn, 1969, Fig. 6 A) fortunately shows a good consistency throughout the years of our experiments, notwithstanding the introduction of several improvements in the experimental techniques. The decrease in gain for higher frequencies and velocities is not accompanied by any significant shift in the phase of the responses (Fig. 33). Under all stimulus conditions, the OKN responses have a very small phase lag (Collewijn, 1969) which can be explained largely by a dead time of the system of about 75 ms (see Chap. 4.3 and Fig. 39).

The nonlinear relations shown in Fig. 34 are characteristic of the optokinetic system of the rabbit, which is essentially a low velocity system. In a way it is complementary to the canal-ocular system, which performs poorly in the low frequency range (Fig. 18 A). For physiological movements (which have limited amplitudes) low frequencies will correspond to low velocities and the two systems working in synergy will produce adequate compensatory eye movements in a wide (presumably the whole physiological) frequency range. The properties of OKN also account for the nonlinear characteristics of visual suppression of the VOR by rotation of the visual surroundings together with the head (Fig. 27). OKN can suppress the VOR only in the range where the eye velocities produced by the VOR are very low (Baarsma and Collewijn, 1974). Although these interactions between VOR and OKN are qualitatively clear, the precise mode of interaction is uncertain. The simplest, linear interaction would be the following. When an animal is subjected to a certain oscillation in darkness, the VOR will partly compensate this but some motion of gaze will be left; if the same stimulus is administered in the light, the VOR will give the same response as in the dark and the remaining gaze motion will be the stimulus for the optokinetic system, which will correct part of it. Assuming that the optokinetic gain (G_o) and vestibular gain (G_v) will vectorially sum in a linear way to the synergic gain (G_{syn}), we may write:

$$G_{syn} = G_v + G_o (1 - G_v) \qquad (4)$$

Similarly, for the suppression case the gain (G_{suppr}) can be expressed as the vector sum

$$G_{suppr} = G_v - G_o G_v \qquad (5)$$

These relations, deduced by Baarsma and Collewijn (1974), were recently found to satisfy measurements in albino rabbits by Batini et al. (1979) when the phase relations were duly taken into account (i.e., vectorial addition was correctly executed). Although definite departures from linearity in the interaction between VOR and OKN have not been clearly identified so far, future more elaborate measurements will have to show whether the relations (4) and (5) are really correct over a wide range of stimulus frequencies and amplitudes.

4.3 Optokinetic Nystagmus

The classical way to elicit optokinetic responses is to place the animal in the center of a striped drum rotating at a constant velocity (Ter Braak, 1936). When the drum starts to rotate, the rabbit's eyes will deviate with a smooth movement in the direction of the drum rotation, and after some time the eyes will quickly return toward the midposition by a saccade, after which the slow deviation is resumed. With continued rotation a regular nystagmus will develop in which the eyes are deviated in the direction of the slow phase (Collewijn, 1970a). The nature of the response is strongly influenced by the velocity of the stimulus. For low drum velocities (up to about 2°/s) the slow phase immediately reaches a steady velocity, which approaches the drum velocity and is maintained as long as the drum moves. For higher drum velocities (up to 30°-60°/s) the slow phase is initially not higher than 1°-2°/s, and only when rotation is continued does it gradually increase to a maximum. These differences are illustrated in Fig. 35 A, B and 36 A, B. The gain of OKN (slow phase velocity/stimulus velocity) is evidently time-dependent for velocities in excess of a few degrees per second. Therefore, an "initial" gain (arbitrarily defined as the gain reached after 3 s of stimulation) has been distinguished from a "maximal" gain (Collewijn, 1969). The gain values as a function of stimulus velocity are shown in Fig. 37 A. For

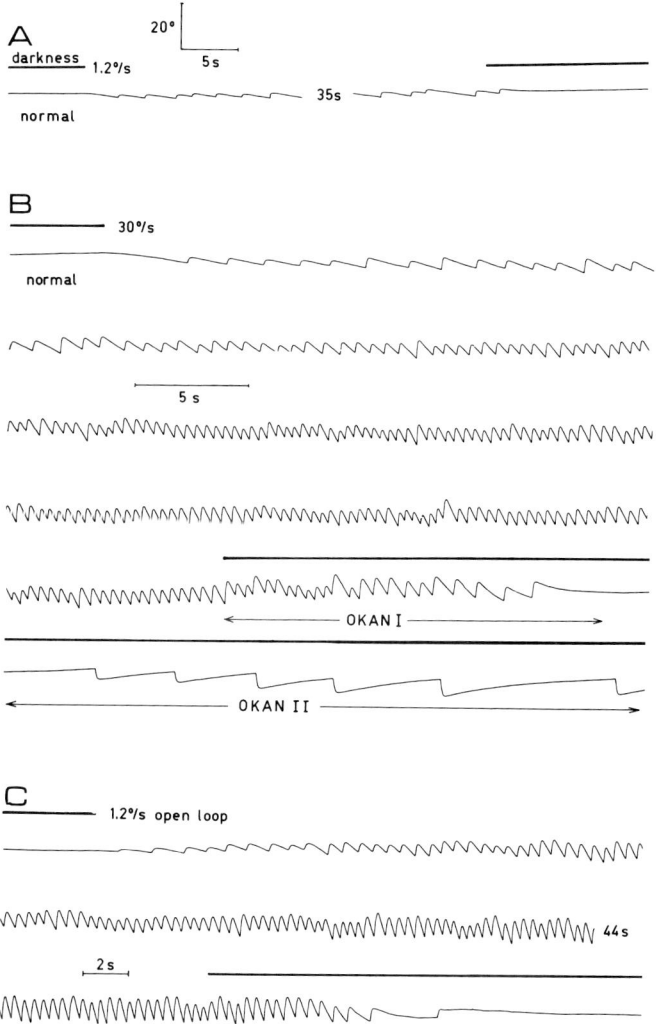

Fig. 35. Typical examples of OKN and OKAN in the rabbit. The *horizontal bars* mark periods of darkness. A stimulus velocity 1.2°/s. Immediate and sustained reaction, no afternystagmus. B stimulus velocity 30°/s. Gradual build-up of slow phase velocity; *OKAN I* and *II* in darkness. Continuous recording. C open-loop conditions: seeing eye immobilized, moving eye covered. Stimulus velocity 1.2°/s in anterior direction. Gradual build-up of slow phase velocity far in excess of stimulus velocity; afternystagmus in darkness

stimulus velocities up to about 2°/s, initial and maximal gain are identical and vary between 0.7 and 0.9. For higher stimulus velocities, initial gain decreases in proportion to the increase in the stimulus velocity, which means that the response saturates at about 2°/s. This result is consistent with that

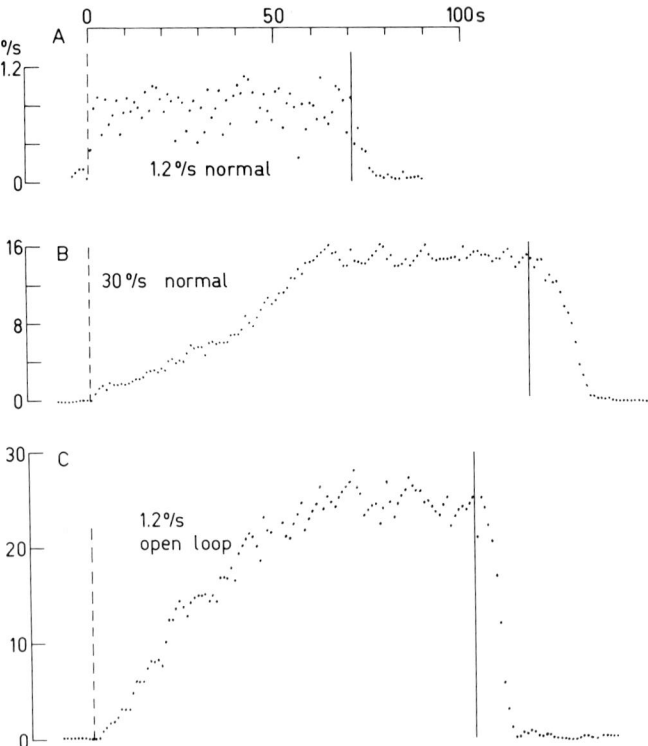

Fig. 36. Time course of slow phase velocity of the same three recordings shown in Fig. 35. Beginning and end of stimulation are marked by the *interrupted* and *solid lines*, respectively

obtained for sinusoidal stimulation (Fig. 34 B), in which the stimulus motion of course is most often not continued for very long in the same direction. When rotation is continued long enough, a steady state with the maximal gain is reached, which is considerably higher than the initial gain, but still lower than the gain at low velocities (Fig. 37). The increase to this maximum may take a period of the order of a minute for stimulus velocities of 30°-60°/s. For many rabbits 30°/s is about the maximum stimulus velocity for which an adequate velocity build-up is seen, but some rabbits will respond well even to 60°/s. For stimulus velocities from 60°-100°/s rabbits only show a very weak and irregular response (slow phase velocity about 1°/s) without any tendency to develop a faster response. (The velocity range to which the rabbit responds can be extended somewhat by accelerating the drum rotation gradually, which diminishes retinal slip velocities as the eye has more time to catch up with the drum).

Some recent results on maximal (steady state) gain of OKN in rabbits are shown in Fig. 38 A. The adequate range (after velocity build-up) extends to about 20°/s with gain values between 0.6 and 0.8. For 60° and 100°/s, even the maximal gain is too low for the responses to be of any practical significance.

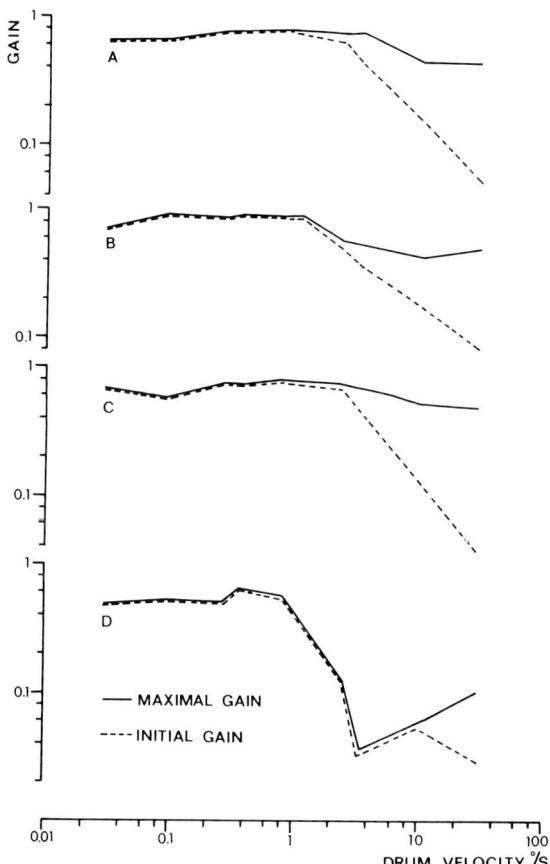

Fig. 37. Optokinetic gain for a constant velocity stimulus, as a function of stimulus velocity. Initial gain: measured after 3 s, maximal gain: measured when a steady state was reached. Averaged results of nine rabbits. **A** both eyes open, drum rotates to the right. **B** both eyes open, drum rotates to the left. **C** vision with left eye only, drum rotates to the right. **D** vision with left eye only, drum rotates to the left. (Collewijn, 1969)

For comparison, some gain-stimulus velocity relations for other species are also shown. Figure 38 B shows our (unpublished) data on cats with permanently implanted head coils, recorded with precise calibration in the rotating magnetic field (Collewijn, 1977a). Also shown are the data from Evinger and Fuchs (1978), recorded in a full-field drum when the cats could also see food, a condition resulting in optimal responses (calibration is approximate). Obviously, the cat's OKN velocity range is highly similar to that of the rabbit. It should be noted that the cat has an only moderately developed central area (see Chap. 1.2) and poor smooth pursuit (Evinger and Fuchs, 1978).

The performance of primates in the high velocity range is considerably better. Figure 38 C shows our own data on man (unpublished, precise calibration, instruction not to pursue any details), those of Zee et al. (1976b) obtained with DC electro-oculography and old data extracted from Grüttner (1939), who was one of the first to give a complete and profound descrip-

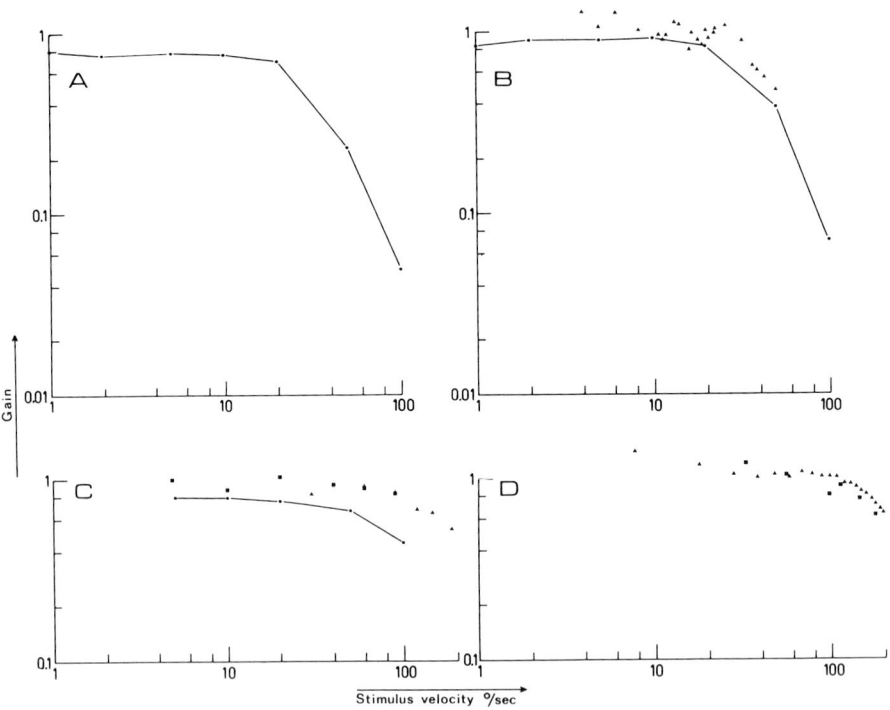

Fig. 38. Slow phase velocity gain of OKN as a function of stimulus velocity for different species. **A** rabbit. **B** cat. *Continuous line* Collewijn, unpublished data; *triangles* after Evinger and Fuchs (1978). **C** man. *Continuous line* Collewijn, unpublished data; *squares* after Zee et al. (1976b); *triangles* after Grüttner (1939). **D** monkey. *Triangles* after Igarashi et al. (1977); *squares* after Komatsuzaki et al. (1969)

tion of human OKN. In man the gain for high stimulus velocities is much better than in rabbit or cat and moreover maximal values are reached almost immediately after the onset of the stimulus. A quite similar picture is obtained in the monkey (Fig. 38 D) for which data are shown derived from Komatsuzaki et al. (1969) who used electro-oculography with approximate calibration and Igarashi et al. (1977) who also used electro-oculography with an unspecified calibration procedure. Precise calibration is lacking in practically all monkey experiments, and often it is just assumed that the monkey's OKN gain equals 1 with a stimulus velocity of 60°/s (Cohen et al., 1977). This may well lead to an overestimation of the gain. Nevertheless, the general shape of Fig. 38 C and D is similar and probably characteristic of primates with excellent foveal vision and smooth pursuit. It is tempting to speculate that the better performance at high velocities is due to the contribution of the smooth pursuit system.

The response of the rabbit to position- and velocity steps of the drum are shown in Fig. 39. Fast displacements of the drum to a new position do not elicit any response, even when the steps are small (0.5°-4°) in comparison to the wavelength of the visual pattern (grating of 10° black and 10° white bars). Such steps are much too fast to stimulate the OKN system (Fig. 38 A), but it is important to notice that the saccadic system as well is not activated by step displacements of the whole visual field (Collewijn, 1972a).

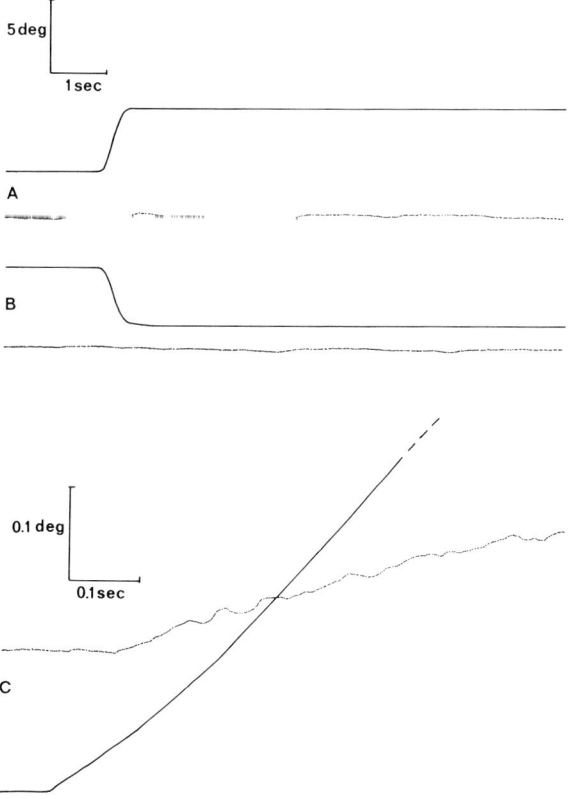

Fig. 39. Responses of the rabbit's eye (*dotted line*) to step-wise changes in position (**A**, **B**) and velocity (**C**) of a full-field stimulus consisting of black and white bars, each 10° wide (*continuous line*). Each recording is the average of 25 responses. (Collewijn, 1972a)

Although single position steps do not elicit pursuit, the system must be sensitive to a suitable sequence of small position steps, as it is possible to elicit OKN in the rabbit in a stroboscopically illuminated drum (Busch et al., 1979). When the drum suddenly starts to move at a constant velocity (Fig. 39 C), optokinetic pursuit starts after a well-defined latency of about

75 ms. This latency increases at very low stimulus velocities (of the order of 0.1°/s), which may indicate that the latency is the sum of a minimal signal transport time (dead time) of the system and the time required for the stimulus to cover a minimal visual distance. Previous measurements (Collewijn, 1972a) indicated that such a minimal distance is not larger than 0.007° or 1.2 µm on the retina, which is close to the distance between the centers of adjacent photoreceptors (about 1.7 µm; Sjöstrand and Nilson, 1964). The ability of the rabbit to detect extremely small position changes is also demonstrated by the positive optokinetic responses to very low stimulus velocities. The lowest retinal stimulus velocity tested by Collewijn (1969) was 0.003°/s; this was still quite effective but apparently not the lower limit, as Ter Braak (1936) found a response to a drum velocity of 6.4 s arc/s (= 0.0018°/s). At this velocity it would take about 4 s for the stimulus to travel through the interreceptor distance. The absence of spontaneous oculomotor activity in the immobilized rabbit makes it possible to detect systematic pursuit of such incredibly slow movements. This ultra-slow optokinetic pursuit is not unique for the rabbit, as similar slow tracking has been found in certain crabs (Horridge and Sandeman, 1964).

As stated, the striped drum is the traditional stimulus for OKN. Little research has been done on the sensitivity of OKN to the structure of the pattern, such as the distribution and width of stripes. It seems likely that the amount of moving contrasts will affect the gain of OKN, and indeed, an increase in the wavelength of the stripe pattern has been shown (Collewijn, 1970a) to decrease optokinetic responses to higher velocities. This is shown in Fig. 40, which was actually compiled to show the absence of a fixed relation between the positions of the visual pattern and the eye. The moving stripes of different widths have been projected on the nystagmus recordings with the proper time and space coordinates. The amplitude of the nystagmus is unrelated to the size of the stripes, but it increases with the velocity of the slow phase. Ideally, the slow phases should have the same slopes as the stripes (gain = 1); this is approached best with the finest grating used (4° black − 4° white). We found later (Dubois and Collewijn, 1979a) that a random dot pattern (Julesz, 1964) with elements of 1° was about twice as effective as this grating. A systematic investigation of the effects of texture, contrast and luminance of the stimulus pattern has still to be undertaken.

4.4 Open-Loop Optokinetic Nystagmus

Motion of a pattern on the retina (slip) elicits an optokinetic eye movement in the same direction. This will decrease the slip-velocity and thus the

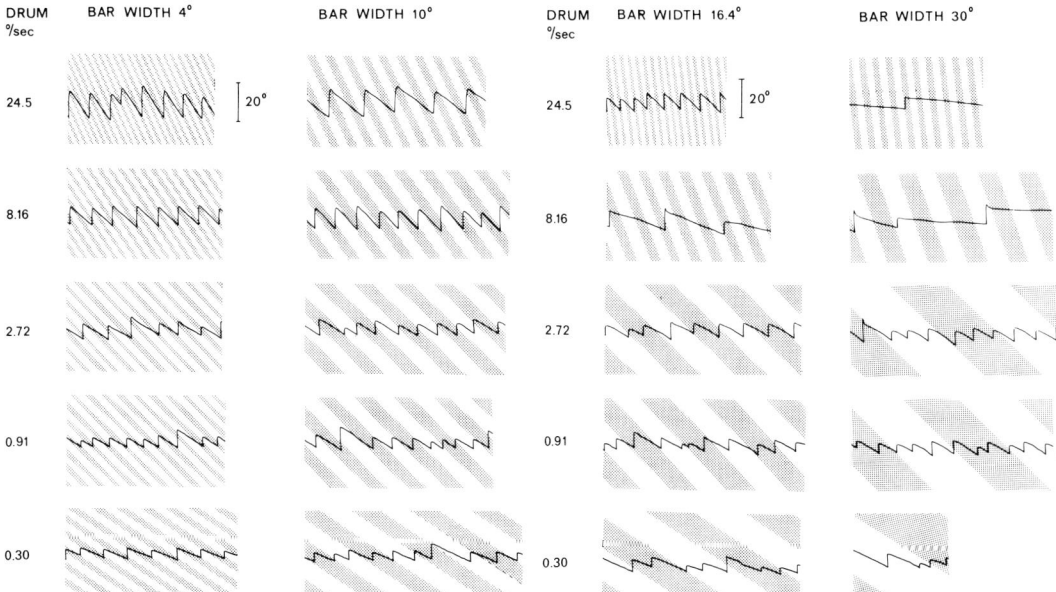

Fig. 40. Examples of OKN elicited by different stripe widths and stimulus velocities. The moving stripes have been projected with the appropriate width and slope (= stimulus velocity) on the nystagmus records. Calibration: 10°. (Collewijn, 1970a)

stimulus velocity. The response is fed back (with a negative sign) to the stimulus and therefore the OKN system is a negative (closed-loop) feedback system, in contrast to the VOR, as eye movements are not relayed back to the labyrinth (although head movements are), and the VOR is essentially a feedforward (open-loop) system.

The optokinetic feedback loop, combined with the nonlinear velocity sensitivity, makes the real stimulus-response relationship rather hard to understand. Therefore an attempt has been made to dissociate the response from the stimulus to study the OKN system under open-loop conditions. Classically, this situation has been studied in clinical cases with unilateral paralysis of the eye muscles and intact vision, as first described by Ohm (1926). When the paralyzed eye is stimulated with a moving pattern, optokinetic eye movements are elicited in the other eye, even when this is covered. This phenomenon has been confirmed in several patients (Körner and Dichgans, 1967; Hood and Leech, 1974), and it has been noticed that the slow phase eye velocity in this condition can exceed the stimulus velocity by a factor of 2 and more.

Experimentally, the same situation can be achieved by paralyzing or mechanically immobilizing one eye. This was done by Ter Braak (1936) and Collewijn (1969) in the rabbit, and by Koerner and Schiller (1972) in the monkey. An example of such a recording in a rabbit is shown in Fig. 35 C, and the time course of slow phase velocity in Fig. 36 C. With a constant slip velocity of 1.2°/s (about the optimal stimulus) the contralateral eye developed a nystagmus of increasing intensity with a maximal slow phase velocity of about 25°/s. The overall course was very similar to that of a normal OKN elicited by a relatively high stimulus velocity (Figs. 35 B, 36 B). Apparently a high OKN velocity can only be built up very gradually in the rabbit either in normal or open-loop conditions.

More recently, a similar dissociation was achieved with normally moving eyes in rabbit and man (Dubois and Collewijn, 1979a, b). A moving pattern was projected onto a screen in an otherwise dark room, with two perpendicular servo-controlled mirrors in the light pathway. The angle of these mirrors was controlled by the horizontal and vertical eye position signal. In this way the position of the moving pattern could be stabilized on the retina, independent of eye movements. The movements of the stimulated eye were measured, the other eye was covered. The method is nontraumatic; vision, movement and proprioception are normal and the switch between normal and open-loop conditions is easily made. The only limitation was the restricted size of the stimulus pattern (diameter 30°). The open-loop gain as a function of stimulus velocity measured with this technique is shown in Fig. 41 for rabbit and man, which show a remarkable similarity. The highest gain

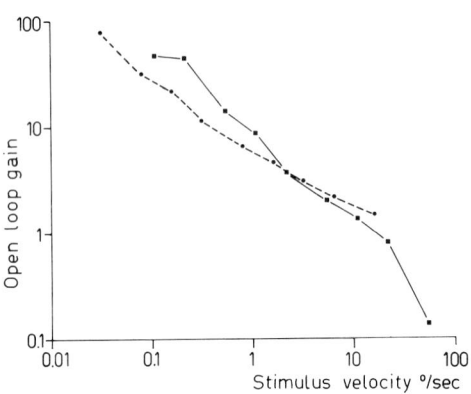

Fig. 41. Open-loop optokinetic gain as a function of stimulus velocity. The open-loop condition was achieved with servo-controlled mirrors controlled by the position of the seeing eye so that the stimulus outline was stabilized on the center of the retina. *Circles* man, *squares* rabbit. (Dubois and Collewijn, 1979a, b)

(about 100) is reached at stimulus velocities in the range of 0.01°-0.1°/s, with a decrease to about 1.0 at velocities around 10°/s and a further decrease at higher velocities. In monkeys with one paralyzed eye, a similar relationship was found by Koerner and Schiller (1972) and Körner (1975). In the open-loop situation with one eye immobilized, the gain-stimulus velocity relation was somewhat steeper than with the eyes unrestrained (Collewijn, 1969; Dubois and Collewijn, 1979a). This may indicate an influence of extraretinal (e.g., proprioceptive) signals.

One problem with these open-loop gains is that they are too high to be reconciled comfortably with the gain of normal OKN. In the latter, the difference *stimulus velocity – eye velocity = slip velocity* maintains the response, and the internal gain of the loop is equal to the quotient *eye velocity/slip velocity*. The latter is rarely larger than 5-10, while in the open-loop situation gains of 100 are not exceptional. This discrepancy has not been resolved and may indicate that the concept of OKN as a feedback system with only retinal slip velocity as input is too parsimonious.

The dissociation between vision and eye movements has also been used to demonstrate the efficacy of the optokinetic feedback loop in stabilizing the eye (Collewijn and Van der Mark, 1972). In the open-loop condition the moving covered eye shows the same instability as found in a normal rabbit in darkness (Fig. 42 A, E, see also Chap. 2.4), since these movements are not perceived by the immobilized (seeing) eye.

The animal was surrounded by a servocontrolled striped drum. The drum position was controlled by the position of the moving (covered) eye and the movements of the eye were reproduced with inverted direction by the drum and shown to the seeing (immobilized) eye. In this way the optokinetic feedback loop was externally closed and the result was an immediate stabilization of the moving eye (Fig. 42 B). When the sign of the feedback was incorrect, so that the drum moved in the same direction as the eye, a positive feedback loop was created which generated an intense spontaneous nystagmus (Fig. 42 C). It was also shown that the amount of reduction in drift obtained by the visual feedback can be approximately accounted for by the known open-loop gain/stimulus velocity relationship (Collewijn and Van der Mark, 1972).

Recently, the open-loop technique has been used to measure the efficacy of stimulating different parts of the rabbit's retina to elicit OKN (Dubois and Collewijn, 1979a). A moving pattern was stabilized on different parts of the retina and the open-loop gain was measured. The results are shown in Fig. 43. The optokinetic sensitivity is highest in an elongated zone just above and parallel to the visual horizon, with a maximum around the optical axis of the eye, i.e., lateral in the visual field. This distribution is markedly similar to that of the density of ganglion cells in the visual streak (Fig. 2). The total sensitive area extends 50° superior, 10° inferior, 75° posterior and 100° anterior in the visual field of each eye. Outside this area no OKN could be elicited even with very large stimuli. Especially remarkable

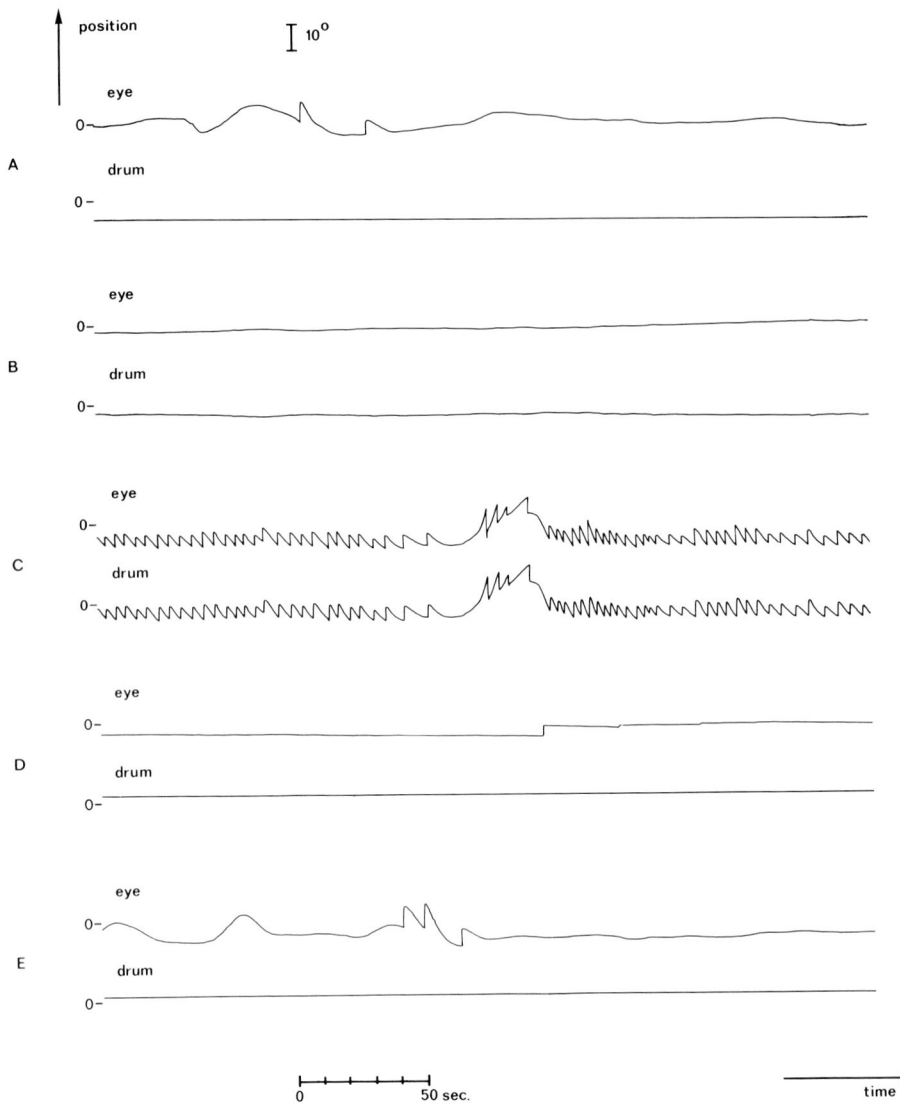

Fig. 42. Control of eye movements by an external optokinetic loop. The movements of the right (covered) eye were recorded (*upper traces*). The left (immobilized) eye looked at the drum, the position of which (*lower traces*) was controlled by the position of the right eye. **A** open-loop condition, drum stationary. **B** drum moving in opposite direction as right eye, negative optokinetic feedback loop. **C** drum moving in same direction as right eye, positive feedback loop. **D** both eyes freely moving, drum stationary (normal condition). **E** as **D** but in darkness. (Collewijn and Van der Mark, 1972)

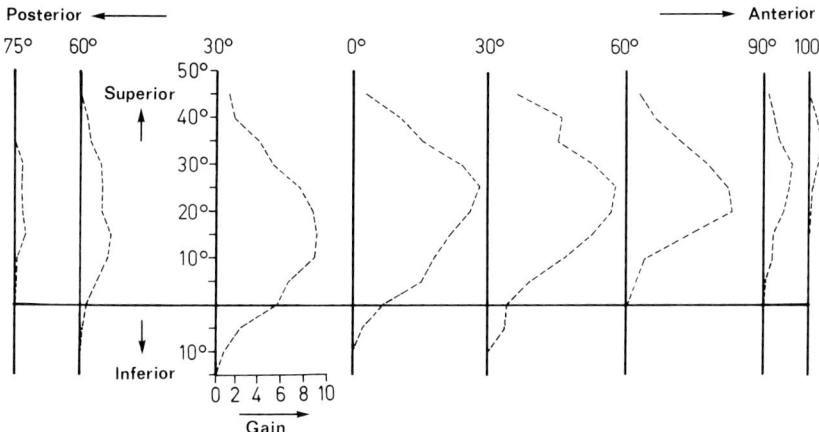

Fig. 43. Open-loop gain of slow phase of optokinetic nystagmus elicited by a random-dot pattern of 30° x 30° moving in the anterior direction at 0.55°/s. The retinal position of the stimulus outline was stabilized in different parts of the visual field of the left eye by servo-controlled mirrors. The movements of the same eye were recorded. The center of the stimulus was positioned in eight horizontal locations (*thick vertical bars*); the vertical position was varied in steps of 5°. Averaged results of six rabbits. (Dubois and Collewijn, 1979a)

is the total absence of optokinetic reactions in the inferior visual field and the poor sensitivity in the binocular zone. Experiments with corrective lenses have shown that this distribution is not an artifact of a faulty refractive state (Dubois and Collewijn, 1979a).

4.5 Optokinetic Reactions in Different Directions

So far, only horizontal OKN has been described and an important asymmetry in the horizontal optokinetic sensitivity has been neglected. This asymmetry is revealed as soon as one eye is covered and the monocular optokinetic responses to posterior and anterior motion are tested (Ter Braak, 1936; Collewijn, 1969). A strong preference is found for stimuli moving in the anterior direction (temporal to nasal). The optokinetic responses to posterior motion are very poor, particularly at stimulus velocities higher than 1°/s (Fig. 37 D), and not improved by continued stimulation. For anterior motion, the responses to monocular stimulation are equal to those for binocular stimulation (Fig. 37 C). The directional bias is also clearly demonstrated in open-loop experiments (Fig. 44). The rabbit shares this property with many other animals such as the pigeon (Mowrer, 1936a) and the guinea pig (Smith and Bridgeman, 1943). From observations on a great number of mammals, birds and reptiles, Tauber and Atkin (1968) concluded that in all cases this type of directional preference in monocular vision correlated with the absence of a fovea and bidirectional response with the presence of a fovea, irrespective of the proportion of optic nerve fibers crossing in the chiasm. The monocular preference was always for anterior movement. The cat's monocular OKN responses, which are normally bidirectional (in agreement with the presence of an area centralis) become asymmetric (preference for temporal to nasal motion) when the visual cortex is removed (Wood et al., 1973) and also when cats are reared from birth with monocular visual deprivation (Van Hof-Van Duin, 1976b). Atkinson (1979) has found that a similar asymmetric monocular OKN is present in infant monkeys and humans during the first few months after birth, after which OKN becomes symmetrical. This is possibly related to the maturation of foveal and/or binocular vision. Recently, Baloh et al. (1980) have reported monocular, temporal to nasal, directional preference of OKN in human rod monochromats, who are congenitally afoveate due to the maldevelopment of cone receptors. In addition to the asymmetry the OKN showed a slow build-up of slow phase velocity which made it quite similar to the OKN of the rabbit. We shall see that some cerebellar lesions can lead to a similar condition in human patients (Chap. 5.7). Schor and Levi (1980) have found asymmetrical monocularly elicited OKN in persons with strabismic or anisometropic amblyopia. Reduced velocity of the slow phase driven by nasal to temporal or upward motion was seen in the amblyopic as well as in the normal eye of some subjects. A sensory distrubance of the perception of motion could not be demonstrated. Van Hof-Van Duin (1976b) has suggested that the development of symmetrical OKN is closely associated with the development of normal binocular vision.

Vertical optokinetic responses have been recorded under normal (Collewijn and Noorduin, 1972a) and open-loop conditions (Dubois and Collewijn, 1979a). The gain under normal conditions was about equal to the initial gain for horizontal responses and is hardly improved by continued stimulation. There was no monocular preference for upward or downward motion. The open-loop gain in the vertical directions (Fig. 44) lies between the horizontal gain for anterior and posterior motion. Erickson and Barmack (1980) have compared horizontal and vertical OKN and found that gain for up-down stimulation was slightly greater than for down-up stimulation. Moreover, the vertical excursions were often very large (greater than 20°) before resetting occurred.

Torsional OKN (Collewijn and Noorduin, 1972a) has the same input-output relations as vertical OKN and is also symmetrical. The amplitude of the torsional nystagmus beats was often very large, with a total range up to 70° between the extreme deviations, whereas for horizontal OKN the total range rarely exceeds 30° (Collewijn, 1970a).

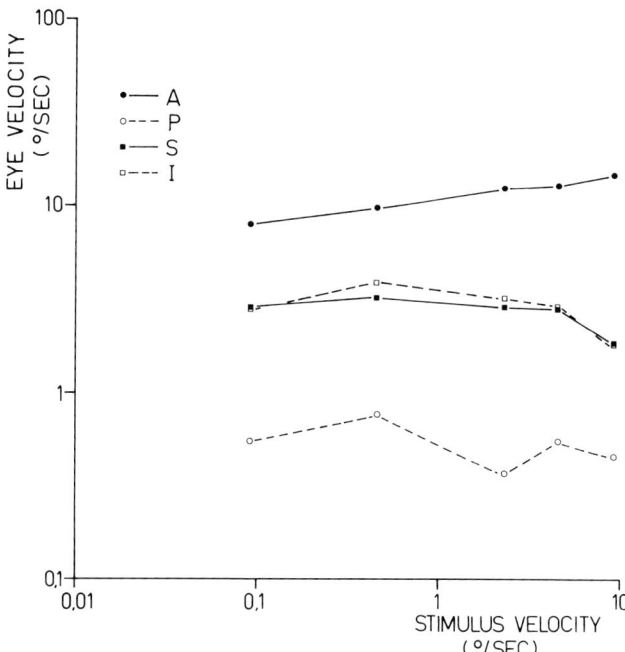

Fig. 44. Slow phase eye velocity as a function of stimulus velocity measured in open-loop conditions. Averaged results of five rabbits. Stimulation was given in four directions: anterior (A), posterior (P), superior (S) and inferior (I). (Dubois and Collewijn, 1979a)

All eye movements are largely conjugate but a systematic disjunctive component has been identified in the rabbit (Collewijn and Noorduin, 1972b). The rule is that the most adequately stimulated eye responds slightly better than the other eye. With both eyes open, horizontal stimuli faster than a few degrees per second only stimulate the eye for which the movement is in the anterior direction, and that eye will move faster than the other, indirectly driven eye (Fig. 45). In monocular vision, the seeing eye will respond better than the driven eye in all directions. As a result, a systematic disjunctive component is introduced to the OKN. Disjunctive OKN has also been deliberately induced (Collewijn and Noorduin, 1972b) in the convergent as well as in the divergent direction by presenting linear anterior or posterior motion ("tunnelmotion") to both eyes. Such a stimulus induces no conjugate eye movements. The difference between maximal convergence and divergence varied between 7° and 23° in eight rabbits, and the vergence movements were very slow. The vergence was mostly tonic in nature (Fig. 46 B-E) but a regular convergence nystagmus with even a number of saccades in opposite directions for the right and left eye has been recorded (Fig. 46 A).

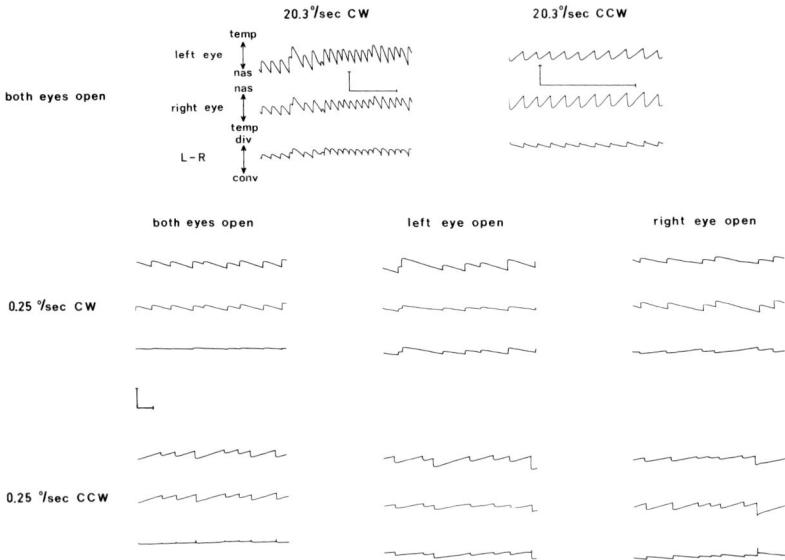

Fig. 45. Binocular recordings of OKN elicited by a drum rotating around the animal with both eyes seeing and either eye covered. The *lower traces* in each group show the difference between the movements of the left and right eye (vergence). Calibrations: 10° (vertical) and 10 s (horizontal). (Collewijn and Noorduin, 1972b)

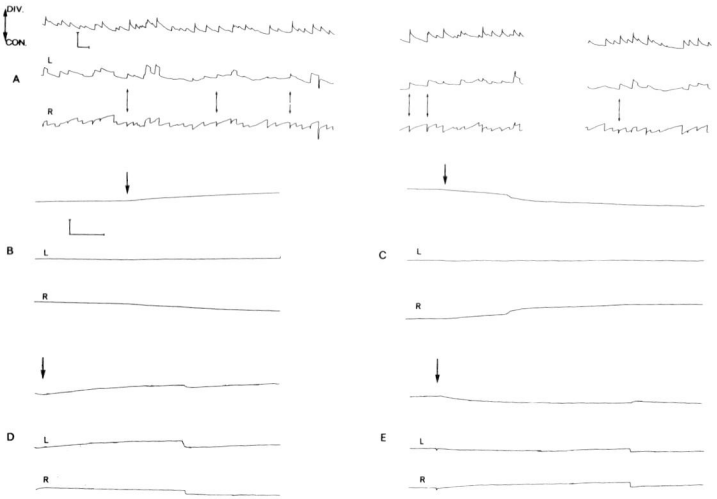

Fig. 46. Stimulation by equally directed translatory motion on both sides (tunnel-motion). **A** a rare case of regular vergence nystagmus with convergence during the slow phase and divergence during the rapid phase, elicited by forward motion of the patterns. Backward motion induced only divergence (as in **B** and **D**) but no regular nystagmus. The *double arrows* mark the occurrence of saccades which are oppositely directed in the two eyes. **B-E** usual reaction to backward (**B, D**) and forward (**C, E**) motion. *Arrows* mark the start of pattern motion. Calibrations: 10° (vertical), 10 s (horizontal). (Collewijn and Noorduin, 1972b)

4.6 Vestibulo-Ocular and Optokinetic Responses During and After Rotations at a Constant Velocity

In the rabbit, OKN with a slow phase velocity faster than a few degrees per second is built up slowly. A complementary phenomenon is found in optokinetic afternystagmus (OKAN), the persistence and gradual decrease of nystagmus when the stimulus is suddenly replaced by darkness. This primary afternystagmus (OKAN I) is identical in direction to the preexisting OKN; when it wears off it is sometimes followed by a secondary afternystagmus (OKAN II) in the opposite direction, and even further successive phases in alternating directions are sometimes observed in some species. The time course and several phases of OKAN have been extensively studied in the monkey (Cohen et al., 1977; Koerner and Schiller, 1972; Krieger and Bender, 1956; Büttner et al., 1976; Waespe et al., 1978) and in man (Mackensen and Wiegmann, 1959; Mackensen et al., 1961; Brandt et al., 1974) in which OKAN was first noticed by Ohm (1921). In the monkey, OKAN is generally better developed than in man. In the rabbit (Ter Braak, 1936; Collewijn, 1976; Neverov and Kissljakov, 1971) OKAN is a very marked phenomenon (Fig. 35 B, C; 36 B, C).

For the interpretation of this phenomenon we should return to the situation where the head is rotating in a stationary world. When an animal is rotating in darkness, the canal-ocular reflex will generate compensatory eye movements. If the stimulus is a velocity step (acceleration impulse) a force will only be exerted on the endolymph and cupula briefly. The cupula will be quickly deviated and then return exponentially to the neutral position with a time constant determined by the elasticity and viscosity of the cupula-endolymph system. Such a response for a rabbit is shown in Fig. 47 A.

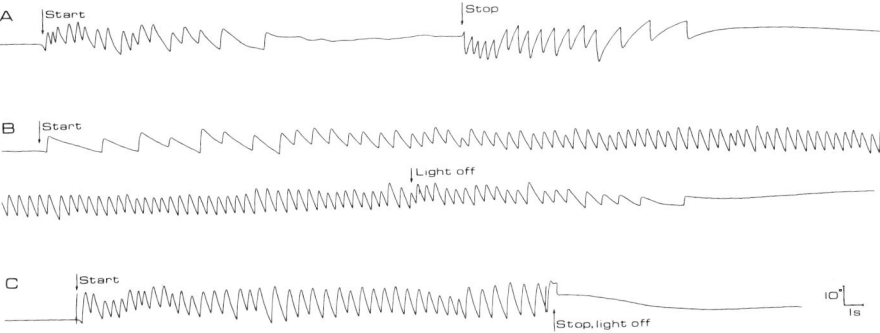

Fig. 47 a-c. Vestibular and optokinetic nystagmus and afternystagmus. **A** per-rotatory and post-rotatory vestibulo-ocular nystagmus elicited by passive rotation in darkness at 30°/s, followed by darkness. **B** OKN and OKAN elicited by rotation of drum, **C** passive rotation in the light at 30°/s to the right, followed by a sudden stop and darkness

The rabbit is first stationary in darkness and then suddenly rotated at 30°/s to the left. An intense nystagmus with the slow phase to the right is immediately generated (the per-rotatory nystagmus) and gradually dies out during continued rotation at a constant velocity. After this, a reverse velocity step is administered by suddenly arresting the rotation. The result is postrotatory nystagmus (PRN), which is the mirror image of the per-rotatory nystagmus and has been studied since the earliest times of vestibular physiology. Figure 47 B shows OKN and OKAN induced by rotation of a drum around the stationary animal at 30°/s to the right (corresponding to subjective rotation of the animal to the left). The time course of OKN is complementary to that of the VOR, as it starts slowly and builds up to a steady state which is reached at a time that the perrotatory nystagmus due to the VOR has died out. When the light is turned off, OKAN continues for some time in the same direction. The complementary action of VOR and OKN is confirmed by Fig. 47 C, where the rabbit is rotated in the light (to the left). Nystagmus is immediately fully developed and persists unchanged during the rotation. When the rotation is suddenly stopped and the light is simultaneously extinguished, the eye stops immediately due to perfect cancellation of the ORN by the OKAN. This interaction was recognized long ago (Ter Braak, 1936; Mowrer, 1937; Jung, 1948) and recently confirmed in a more quantitative manner for man (Koenig et al., 1978), rhesus monkey (Raphan et al., 1977, 1979) and squirrel monkey (Igarashi et al., 1978). It is equally valid for the rabbit, as long as velocities do not exceed the maximum for a sustained OKN (30°-60°/s).

Two problems arise in connection with postrotatory and optokinetic afternystagmus: their duration and their time course. If postrotatory nystagmus was dominated by the mechanics of the cupula, it should decrease exponentially with a time constant of a few seconds. We have seen (Sect. 3.2) that for sinusoidal oscillation the low frequency response of the rabbit (in contrast to several other species) is indeed dominated by a time constant of about 3 s. However, the duration of PRN in the rabbit is much longer than predicted by this time constant and moreover, the decay of the slow phase velocity is not exponential. For OKAN there is of course no clear a priori reason to expect an exponential decay. Typical examples of the slow phase velocity of OKAN and PRN as a function of time are shown in Fig. 48 (dots). The decay appears to follow a linear rather than an exponential course (Winterson et al., 1979b; Collewijn et al., 1980). The best-fitting exponential and linear functions for the data (calculated with a least-squares method) are also shown. In this and all other cases (n = 71) the exponential functions fit moderately at best: the predicted initial velocities are too high, the predicted decline is too fast in the beginning and too slow at the end, the predicted duration is too long. We have not observed a single case in

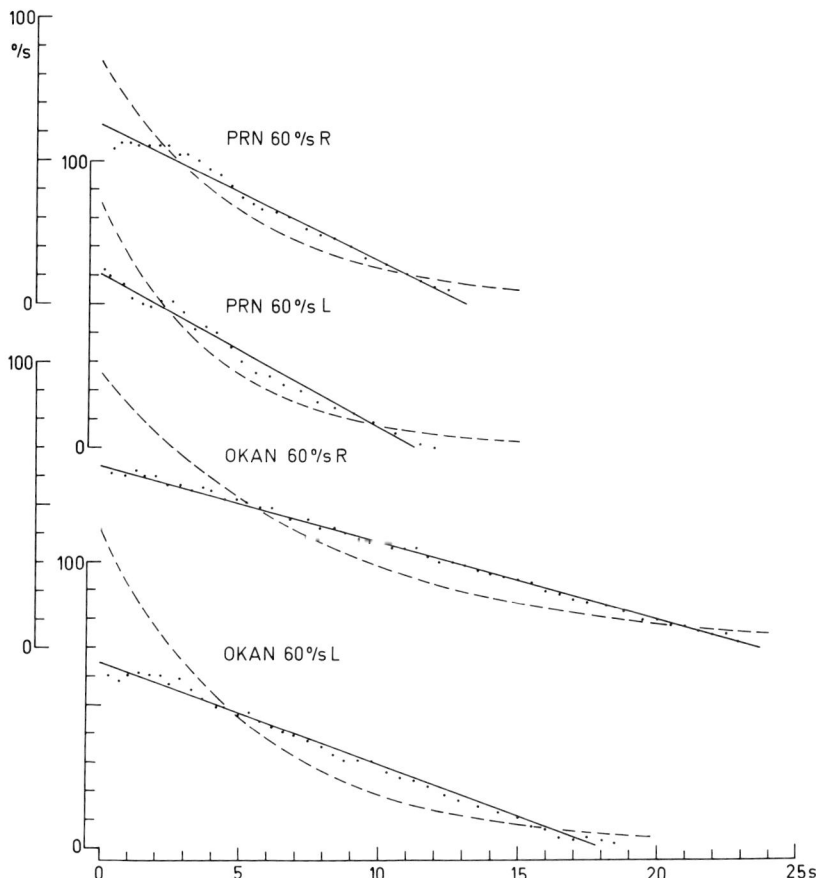

Fig. 48. Slow phase velocity of afternystagmus after stopping (*dots*) as a function of time with best-fitting linear (*continuous lines*) and exponential (*interrupted lines*) functions. Post-rotatory (PRN) and optokinetic afternystagmus (OKAN) were elicited by rotation at 60°/s

which the velocity decay was typically exponential. On the other hand in nearly all cases the data points could be fitted exceedingly well by a straight line. The most common variant of this monotonic linear decay, seen in about a quarter of the cases, was a plateau of constant velocity during the first seconds of afternystagmus, followed by linear decay. This is visible in Fig. 48, PRN 60°/s R and OKAN 60°/s L. This shape deviates even further from an exponential course than a straight line does. Another rather common feature was asymmetry between the responses in the left and right directions. The quality of the fittings was expressed in r^2, the coefficient of determination. It was usually between 0.94 and 0.97 for the linear and between 0.80 and 0.84 for the exponential functions. Paired t-statistics showed that the quality of the fitting was significantly better for linear functions ($p < 0.0005$).

The average calculated linear decay of OKN and PRN for stimulus velocities of 30°, 60° and 150°/s (only PRN) is shown in Fig. 49. These functions are of the form

$$V_t = a - bt \tag{6}$$

in which V_t = slow phase velocity at time t (°/s)
t = time (s) after velocity step or darkness
a = calculated velocity at $t = 0$
b = deceleration (°/s²)

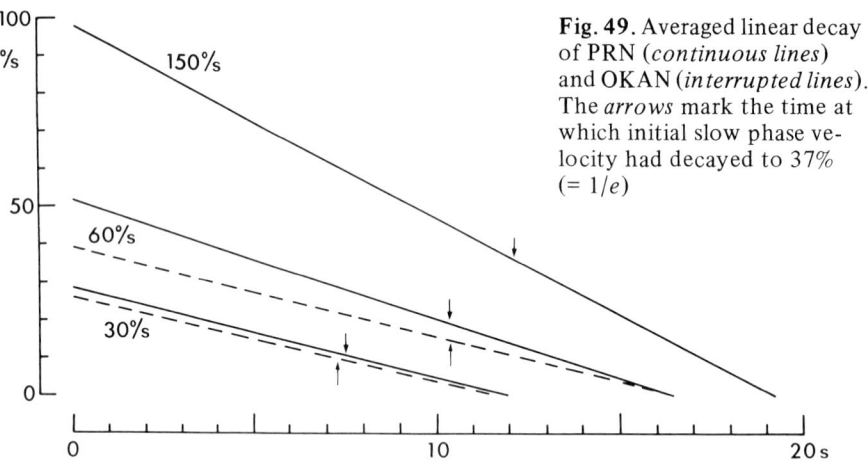

Fig. 49. Averaged linear decay of PRN (*continuous lines*) and OKAN (*interrupted lines*). The *arrows* mark the time at which initial slow phase velocity had decayed to 37% (= $1/e$)

The initial velocities are similar to the per-rotatory velocities of OKN and approach the size of the velocity step for PRN, except for a step of 150°/s after which postrotatory eye velocities are somewhat smaller. For the deceleration b average values varied between about 2° and 5°/s². The slope of decay is steeper for higher initial velocities, but similar for OKAN and PRN. Disregarding the linear shape of these functions, apparent time constants τ can be calculated after which the initial velocity has decayed to $1/e = 37\%$:

$$\tau = -0.63 \frac{a}{b} \tag{7}$$

The apparent time constants for the average functions (based on average a and b) are marked by arrows in Fig. 49. They vary between about 7 s for stimuli of 30°/s and about 12 s for steps of 15°/s. However, the scatter for individual values of b and τ was large. Certainly, the apparent time constants for the linear decay are not constant at all, but time-dependent, but the striking fact remains that they are longer by a factor of at least 3 than the time constants derived for the VOR during sinusoidal oscillation (Chap. 3.2). Even for sinusoidal oscillation, a nonlinearity was indicated by the increase in τ (decrease in phase lead) when the stimulus amplitude was enlarged (Chap. 3.2). These discrepancies and the nonexponential decay of afternystagmus are at variance with the description of the VOR as a linear system. For other species, these nonlinearities may be less prominent, although certain of our findings can be traced in the literature on cat and monkey.

For the cat, the cupular time constant is about 4 s (Blanks et al., 1975). Robinson (1976) found that the phase relations of the VOR in the low frequency range had to be described by two time constants, the shortest of which was at least 12 s, although Landers and Taylor (1975) calculated — with a similar system approach — a shorter time constant of 4.45 s. After a step in head velocity Robinson (1976) found a decay of slow-phase eye velocity to 37% in about 20 s. The shape of afternystagmus decay in the cat has not been described explicitly.

A much larger body of data is available for the monkey. The cupular time constant is about 5.7 s (Fernandez and Goldberg, 1971). For sinusoidal excitation of the VOR, considerably longer time constants have been reported. Skavenski and Robinson (1973) found it to be at least 43 s. Buettner et al. (1978) found somewhat lower values (11.9-29 s). Interestingly, anesthesia reduced these values to 4-7 s, the time constant of the cupula. Habituation, due to repeated stimulation, decreases the VOR time constant strongly as well. Blair and Gavin (1979) observed a decrease from about 40 to about 7 s in the course of repeated testing. Throughout the habituation process, they found that sinusoidal and velocity step tests of the VOR gave concordant estimates of the time constant and corner frequency.

In the alert monkey, slow phase eye velocity is closely paralleled by the discharge frequency of units of the vestibular nucleus during most manifestations of the VOR, OKN, PRN and OKAN (Waespe and Henn, 1977a, b, 1979; Buettner et al., 1978). These neurons may carry a common velocity signal for OKN, VOR and afternystagmus. The time constants of PRN, OKAN and neuronal activity always vary together.

Our results support the concept of a common velocity storage for optokinetic and vestibular eye movements, since the shape of OKAN and PRN for comparable velocities were indistinguishable and the phenomena interacted in a linear way in cancelling experiments (Fig. 47 C).

Although the shape of the velocity decay is not explicitly discussed by Waespe and Henn, some of their illustrations suggest a linear decrease (e.g. 1977b, Fig. 1 and 2; 1979, Fig. 4). In one of their figures (1977b, Fig. 3)

Waespe and Henn have even fitted the decay of OKAN and vestibular unit activity by *linear* regression functions.

Cohen et al. (1977) in their study of OKAN in the monkey treated slow phase velocity profiles as exponential, but exceptions to exponentiality were definitely observed. The authors stated that the decline of OKAN slow phase velocity appeared relatively linear at lower stimulus velocities (29° and 43°/s) and was close to exponential at higher velocities. Dominant time constants for OKAN varied with stimulus velocity and time (habituation) but were of the order of 5-20 s, which is not greatly different from our findings in the rabbit.

In a later study, Raphan et al. (1979) described the velocity decay in PRN in the monkey. Although they proposed a model which implies an exponential time course, several deviations from this assumption are obvious in their data. Many examples of linear decay can be seen in their illustrations. The occasional occurrence of a "plateau" of constant velocity in the first seconds of afternystagmus, similar to our data, is also shown. Clearly, linear decay as we find it in the rabbit is not uncommon even in the monkey, especially after initial velocities not higher than about 60°/s.

4.7 Conclusions

The optokinetic system of the rabbit is nonlinear. With short-term excitation it responds poorly to velocities above 2°/s, although with continued stimulation higher velocities can be built up in a period of seconds to a minute. When OKN with a high velocity has developed, optokinetic afternystagmus is observed when visual stimuli are suddenly eliminated. The optokinetic system is complementary to the vestibulo-ocular system in its response to low velocities, frequencies, and accelerations, its continued response to constant velocities, and the opposite afternystagmus after the arrest of head-rotation. The VOR and OKN, both of which show nonlinearities and ranges of poor response, produce adequate ocular stabilization throughout the physiological stimulus range when operating together in synergy.

5. Signal Processing

In the last decade, a wealth of data has been collected on the physiology and anatomy of oculomotor circuits and the control of gaze. To review this field comprehensively would go far beyond the scope of this monograph. For recent reviews I refer to (Robinson, 1975; Baker and Berthoz, 1977; Raphan and Cohen, 1978; Precht, 1978; Wilson and Melvill Jones, 1979; Granit and Pompeiano, 1979). In this chapter I shall deal mainly with topics which are related to my own research or in which the rabbit has been important for our understanding of the general physiology of oculomotor systems.

5.1 Retinal Motion Detection

A first step in the generation of optokinetic pursuit must consist in the detection of visual image motion on the retina. We have seen (Chap. 4) that the optokinetic system is sensitive to velocity, not position, of large visual patterns. A class of retinal ganglion cells suitable for this function was discovered by Barlow and Hill (1963). This type of unit is maximally excited by movement of a visual stimulus in a particular ("preferred") direction, but does not respond to or is even inhibited by movement in the opposite ("null") direction. These units have been called "direction-selective". Direction selectivity as a trigger feature for visual units has been subsequently identified in many species and at many levels in the visual system (Grüsser and Grüsser-Cornehls, 1973). At the retinal ganglion cell level, it has also been found in the cat (Stone and Hoffmann, 1972; Hoffmann, 1973; Stone and Fukuda, 1974; Cleland and Levick, 1974). In the rabbit, approximately one quarter of the retinal ganglion cells has direction-selective properties. The details of their receptive field properties have been investigated by Barlow et al. (1964), Barlow and Levick (1965) and Wyatt and Daw (1975). Subgroups of on-off and on-type direction-selective units were distinguished on the basis of their receptive field maps, but these types also differed in the velocity range to which they responded best. Oyster and Barlow (1967) first suggested that the output of the on-off units could be used as error signals for a visual servo-system which minimizes retinal image motion. The main argument for this hypothesis was that the preferred directions of on-off cells were concentrated in four principal directions (anterior, posterior, inferior, and superior) which roughly coincided with the lines of action of the four rectus muscles of the eye (Prince, 1964). On-type units on the other hand showed a three-lobed distribution of preferred directions: anterior, posterior-upward and posterior-downward. For both types, a relative abundance of units sensitive to movement in the anterior direction was found, which corresponds well with the preference of each eye for this direction as a stimulus for OKN. The distribution of these preferred directions and the velocity sensitivity ranges were described by Oyster (1968), and a collaborative effort followed (Oyster et al., 1972) to reconcile the findings on single units with the input-output properties of the OKN system (Collewijn, 1969). Large, moving stripe patterns similar to those of the optokinetic drum were used as a stimulus. On-off type units showed an initial response transient and later, a more or less steady firing level as the stimulus continued to move. The transient responses were more marked when the inhibitory surrounds of the receptive fields were masked. Below $1°/s$ the responses were quite small and increased only slightly as the stimulus velocity increased. Between $1°/s$ and $10°/s$ the responses increased dramatically and were roughly proportional to the stimulus velocity. Above $10°/s$ the responses saturated and did not increase up to $60°/s$, the highest velocity used. A fourth region of decreasing sensitivity for still higher velocities has been shown by Wyatt and Daw (1975). Thus, the on-off type cells do not respond at all well to velocities below $1°/s$, which is a retinal slip-velocity range optimal in eliciting OKN (Collewijn, 1969). The on-type units proved to be preferentially sensitive to this low velocity range. Maximal responses were obtained for velocities between $0.1°$ and $2°/s$. The lowest stimulus velocity used ($0.02°/s$) was still effective in exciting these units, but the responses fell to zero for velocities exceeding $3°-5°/s$. Thus, the two types of retinal direction-selective units are complementary in covering the whole range of velocities for which the rabbit's optokinetic system responds. Open-loop steady-state OKN velocities and unit discharge frequencies were plotted as a function of stimulus velocity, and the maxima were scaled to coincide (Fig. 50). With a stripe pattern as the stimulus, open-loop OKN responses show maxima for stimulus velocities of $0.4°$ and $30°/s$, and a minimum for about $3°/s$ (Collewijn, 1969). These maxima are replicated by the responses of the units and, particularly for the on-units, the correspondence with the eye movement data is close enough to suggest a prominent role for these units in the generation of OKN. Remarkably, the particular shape of the eye movement curve in Fig. 50 is changed into a flat relation (Fig. 44) when a random-dot pattern is used instead of a stripe pattern. The reality of this

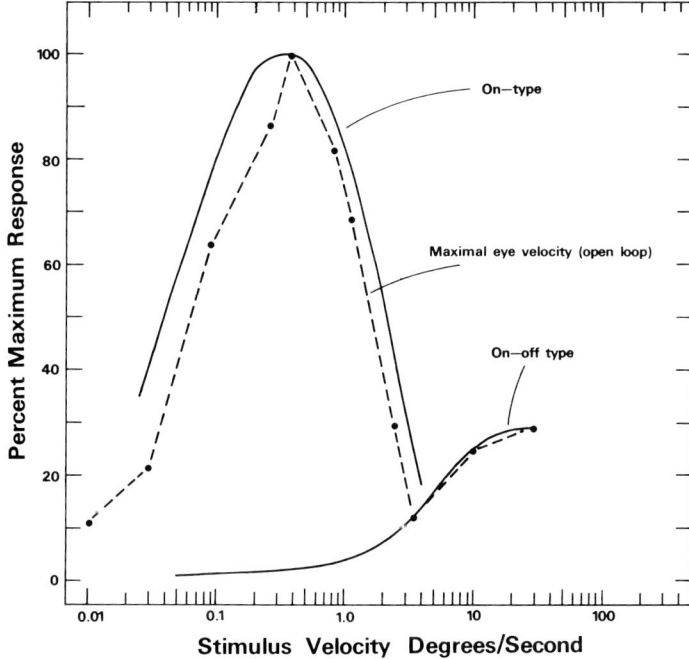

Fig. 50. Relationship of direction-selective ganglion cell responses to eye movement velocity. The *broken line* shows data replotted from Collewijn (1969). The *curve* shows how the velocity of the slow phase of optokinetic nystagmus (open-loop) varies as a function of stimulus velocity. The *ordinate* represents percent maximum eye movement velocity in °/s. The *continuous curves* show how the responses of direction-selective cells vary as a function of stimulus velocity. These curves have been rescaled (see text for details); they indicate a strong relationship between the firing rate of direction-selective ganglion cells and the velocity of the slow phase of optokinetic nystagmus. The on-type direction-selective cells are effective in the most important range of stimulus velocities, i.e., below 1°/s. (Oyster et al., 1972)

effect has been confirmed by testing both patterns to generate OKN in one and the same group of rabbits (Dubois, 1978). Possibly, the response characteristics of the direction-selective cells are also sensitive to the structure of the pattern, but this has not been tested directly.

5.2 Relevance of Different Primary Optic Projections for OKN

The retinal ganglion cells of the rabbit project to four major centers: (1) the lateral geniculate nucleus, (2) the colliculus superior, (3) the pretectum, (4) the posterior accessory tract and its nuclei. About 90% of the optic nerve fibers crosses in the chiasm and the projections are mostly contralateral. These connections have been investigated by degeneration techniques (Giolli and Guthrie, 1969; Scalia, 1972) and by autoradiography of ³H-leucine injected into one eye (Takahashi et al., 1977). Figure 51 shows some of the primary optic nerve projections at the meso-diencephalic junction as identified by the orthograde transport of horseradish peroxidase (Mesulam, 1978), injected into the left eye. These projections correspond very well to the description by Scalia (1972).

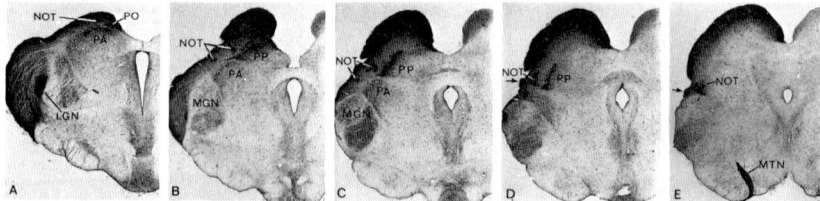

Fig. 51. Primary optic projections in the right meso-diencephalic junction as revealed by the anterograde transport of horseradish peroxidase, injected into the left eye and stained according to Mesulam (1978). The *dark stained zones* correspond to optic nerve terminations. A-E in rostro-caudal order. Specific endings are visible in the anterior pretectal nucleus (*PA*), the olivary pretectal nucleus (*PO*), the nucleus of the optic tract (*NOT*), the posterior pretectal nucleus (*PP*), the lateral geniculate nucleus (*LGN* only caudal part visible in **A**), the dorsal terminal nucleus (*arrow* in **D** and **E**), the medial terminal nucleus (*MTN*) and the colliculus superior. The projection to PA is weak and confined mostly to the anterior part. The projection to PP is much stronger and concentrated in the dorso-lateral part. The medial geniculate nucleus (*MGN*) is indicated but receives no optic projection. (Holstege and Collewijn, in press)

5.2.1 The Geniculo-Cortical Projection

An extensive projection is found in the dorsal lateral geniculate nucleus, mainly contralaterally, but with a distinct small ipsilateral projection. Levick et al. (1969) found direction-selective cells of the on-off type, but not of the on-type in the lateral geniculate. On the other hand Stewart et al. (1971) described both types of cells in the lateral geniculate. The dorsal lateral geniculate nucleus projects to the visual cortex (Giolli and Guthrie, 1971), in which direction-selective units have also been found (Chow et al., 1971; Murphy and Berman, 1979). Although nystagmus has been elicited by electrical stimulation of the lateral parts of the occipital cortex in the rabbit (Manni et al., 1964; Hobbelen, 1971), the cortex is certainly not essential for OKN, since OKN is present after complete decortication (Ter Braak, 1936), even immediately after the operation (Hobbelen and Collewijn, 1971). Spreading depression (Bureš et al., 1974) of the cortex has been found to increase the amplitude of OKN beats, without affecting the slow phase velocity (Hobbelen, 1971). This probably agrees with the findings of Neverov et al. (1976) who reported a decrease in fast phase frequency during spreading depression but did not record slow phase velocity. Although a modulating role of the cortex on OKN is not excluded, the main optokinetic pathway in the rabbit is evidently subcortical. In foveate animals, a much more explicit role of the cortex in OKN has been established. In the cat, monocularly elicited OKN is normally symmetric, but after removal of the cortex it becomes unidirectional with a preference for temporal to nasal motion, as in the rabbit (Wood et al., 1973). In the dog as well, OKN is still present after bilateral ablation of the hemispheres, but the maximal drum velocities (normally 400°/s) eliciting OKN are lowered to 40°/s (Ter Braak, 1936). The same result was found when only the visual cortex was removed. Smooth pursuit cannot be elicited after these operations, and one may hypothesize that the remaining OKN responses after visual decortication in the cat and dog represent the basic, rabbit-type OKN In the monkey as well, OKN can still be elicited by adequate full-field stimulation after bilateral visual decortication (Ter Braak, 1936; Ter Braak and Van Vliet, 1963), although Pasik et al. (1959) have been unable to confirm this finding. In human cases of occipital cortical damage which was extensive enough to cause permanent and complete blindness, positive OKN responses have only been reported in one case of long standing (Ter Braak et al., 1971) in which a rudimentary optokinetic response could be elicited about 4 months after the lesion, without any other recovery of visual function. Other adequately tested cases of cortical blindness (Velzeboer, 1952; Brindley et al., 1969; Brindley and Janota, 1975) revealed no evidence of a subcortical OKN in man. Thus, its existence remains doubtful. Of course, the degeneration of the massive descending projections from the cortex to the lower visual centers may profoundly disorganize the function of subcortical circuits that are normally operative. In general, the findings after decortication in animals support Ter Braak's (1936) hypothesis that smooth pursuit ("look-nystagmus") is cortically and OKN ("stare-nystagmus") subcortically mediated.

5.2.2 The Superior Colliculus

The superior colliculus in the rabbit receives a massive projection of optic nerve fibers, which is again largely contralateral with a minor ipsilateral component. Direction-selective receptive fields (both on and on-off types) have been described in the superior colliculus (Hill, 1966; Schaefer, 1966; Masland et al., 1971). The role of the colliculus in OKN and eye movements in general has been heavily debated, but may vary widely between species. In animals with foveal vision such as the monkey (Schiller and Stryker, 1972; Robinson, 1972) and the cat (Straschill and Rieger, 1973; Roucoux and Crommelinck, 1976), local electrical stimulation of the superior colliculus elicits conjugate, contralaterally directed saccades which tend to fixate the fovea on the part of the visual field represented at the stimulus site. Collicular lesions alone do not permanently interfere with the appropriate visual generation of saccades. Schiller et al. (1979) have shown that the collicular circuit in the monkey operates in parallel with the cortical circuit through the frontal eye field (area 8). Ablation of both structures permanently disorganized the saccadic fixation system. Smooth pursuit and OKN showed a narrowed range but were not absent. For a review of the visual-motor function of the primate superior colliculus, see Wurtz and Albano (1980).

In the rabbit, electrical stimulation of the superior colliculus of sufficient duration only elicits a horizontal nystagmus (slow phase ipsilateral) which is most intensive (Fig. 52) for rostral positions of the stimulus electrode (Blohmke, 1929; Arimoto, 1958; Collewijn, 1975a). A tonic vertical component is also present, with upward rotation of the contralateral eye on stimulation in the medial zones of the colliculus and downward rotation on more lateral stimulation. All these effects were best obtained in darkness, due to the stabilizing action of the OKN system in the light. The primary horizontal response was always smooth, not saccadic. Similar responses can be obtained by stimulation of the lateral pretectum, optic tract and lateral geniculate nucleus (Gutman et al., 1963), which casts doubt upon the specificity of these stimulus effects. Some of them could be caused by collateral activation of optic tract fibers branching and projecting to several terminal areas, as has been observed by Giolli and Guthrie (1969) and Hoffmann (1973). This effect was abolished by sectioning the right optic nerve, 8-30 days prior to stimulation (Collewijn, 1975a). In these animals, all primary optic tract fibers on the left side (except the few ipsilateral ones) had degenerated. Stimulation of the right superior colliculus gave the usual responses, but from the left colliculus no nystagmus could be elicited, except by stimulation near the rostrolateral edge, from where the responses were as vigorous as normally (Fig. 53). A systematic exploration of the left meso-diencephalic area in such hemideafferented rabbits showed that this trigger zone coincided with the nucleus of the optic tract (NOT), a pretectal nucleus which receives a dense terminal projection of optic tract fibers (Fig. 51). A second zone from which intensive nystagmus (slow phase velocity in steady state faster than 20°/s) was obtained was the lateral midbrain tegmentum (Fig. 54). No systematic oculomotor responses could be elicited in optically deafferented rabbits from the lateral and medial geniculate nuclei or the lateral posterior nucleus. Stimulation of the anterior and posterior pretectal

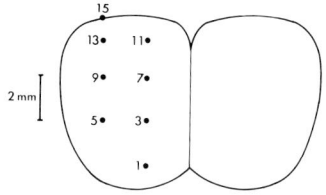

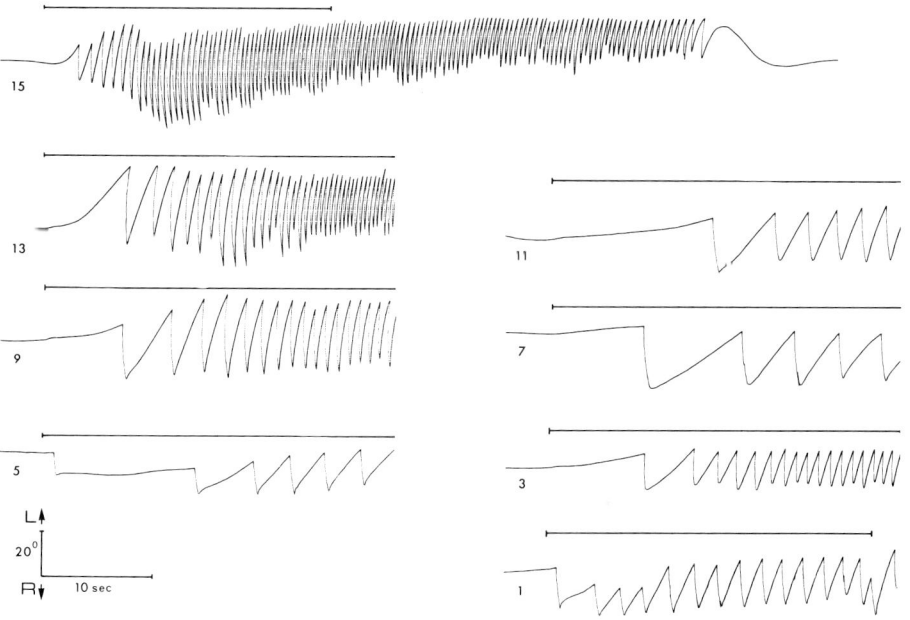

Fig. 52. Typical horizontal eye movements elicited by electrical stimulation of the left superior colliculus. The *inset* shows the stimulus positions in the colliculus, seen from above (rostral edge upward). Stimulus parameters: 20 pulses (2 ms duration) per second, intensity 0.1 mA, train duration marked by *horizontal bars*. Depth of stimulus electrode about 1 mm (Collewijn, 1975a)

nuclei also did not elicit eye movements. It is likely that the nystagmus elicited by stimulation of the normal rabbit colliculus is due to collateral excitation of the NOT, which may specifically mediate horizontal OKN. Responses drom the NOT area were equally positive after bilateral section of the optic nerves.

The probability of a role for the superior colliculus in OKN was further diminished by observations after careful ablation of this structure. Previously it has been stated (Hobbelen and Collewijn, 1971) that complete collicular ablation abolishes OKN. Also (spreading) depression of the colliculus (by application of concentrated KCl solution) strongly depressed OKN (Hobbelen, 1971; Neverov et al., 1976). All of these effects are presumably due to spreading of the lesion and the potassium depolarization to the nucleus of the optic tract, which is closely adjacent to the rostro-lateral edge of the colliculus. In two cases of complete collicular ablation with no pretectal damage OKN was still present (Collewijn, 1975a).

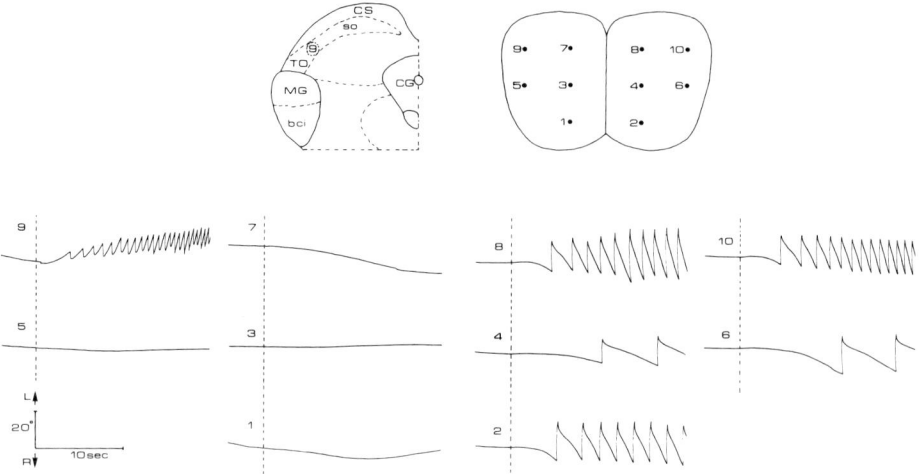

Fig. 53. Eye movements elicited from the left (deafferented) and right (normal) superior colliculus, 30 days after section of the right optic nerve. The *insets* show locations of the stimuli in the colliculus seen from above (*right*) and in a transversal section. Position 9 is shown to be inside the left optic tract. (Collewijn, 1975a)

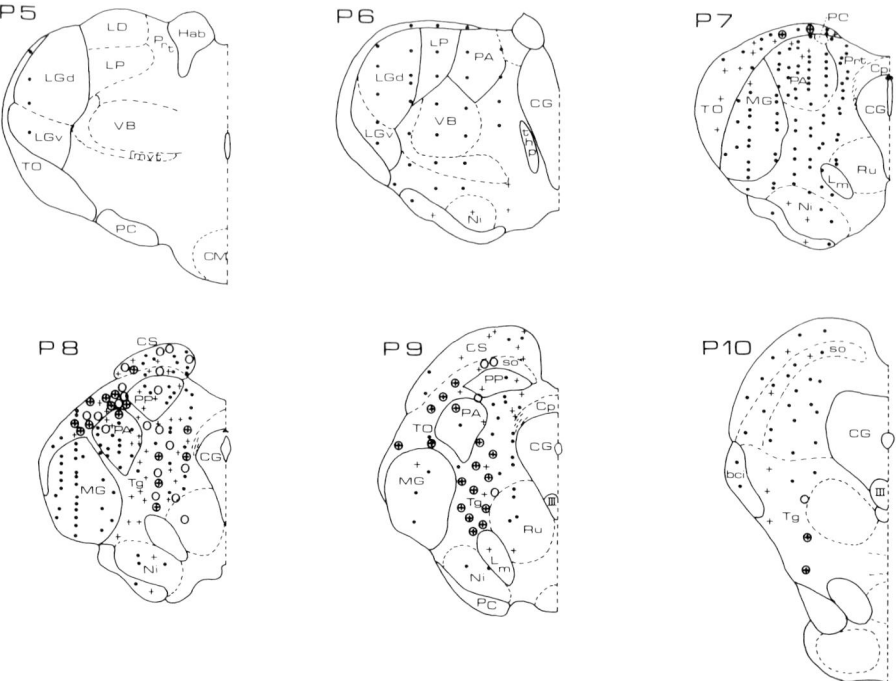

Fig. 54. Transversal sections through the left half of the brainstem, 5-10 mm behind the coronal suture. Pooled results of stimulation in nine rabbits, 8-30 days after transsection of the right optic nerve. Coding of the effects: *small dots* no effect; *plus signs* weak (up to 5°/s); *open circles* intermediate (5°-20°/s); *plus signs in circles* strong (> 20°/s). (Collewijn, 1975a)

As mentioned, no saccades were elicited primarily by stimulation of the colliculus, nor was this the case for any of the other structures mentioned so far. Saccades, however, could be easily and consistently elicited by stimulation in the mesencephalic central gray. As shown in Fig. 55, ipsilateral saccades were elicited by brief (e.g., 200 ms) stimulus trains. The latency was about 200 ms. A rebound saccade usually followed termination of the stimulus. Longer stimulus trains resulted in a sequence of saccades in the same direction with intervals of 0.5-1 s. These reactions could be obtained just as easily with the eyes open (Fig. 55 C, E, F) as with eyes closed (Fig. 55 A, B, D), in contrast to the slow responses from the colliculus, which were inhibited by the OKN system. A role for the central gray in eye movements has rarely been considered, but it may be important to investigate this structure more thoroughly.

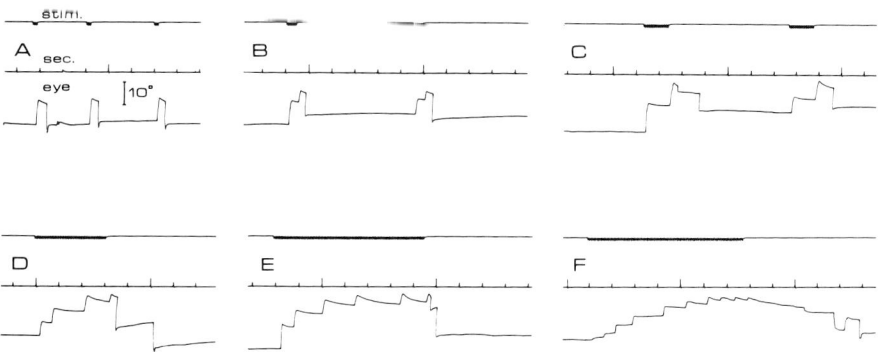

Fig. 55. Saccades elicited by stimulation of the midbrain close to the midline. Stimulus indicated by *horizontal bars:* **A, B, C** 40/s, 0.1 mA. **A, B, D** eyes closed; **C, E, F** eyes open. **A-E** were elicited from the same stimulus position, **F** from a different one. (Collewijn, 1975a)

5.3 Direction-Selectivity in the Nucleus of the Optic Tract

The hypothesis that the NOT is a link in the optokinetic pathway has been supported by the recording of the receptive field properties in this nucleus (Collewijn, 1975b). Units in the NOT showed a vigorous, rather regular spontaneous discharge of about 25-50 action potentials (AP) per second which was hardly affected by light or darkness or the presence of stationary patterns. They were strongly activated by slow motion in a preferred direction of relatively large patterns shown to the contralateral eye and inhibited by motion in the opposite direction (Fig. 56). The discharge was sustained

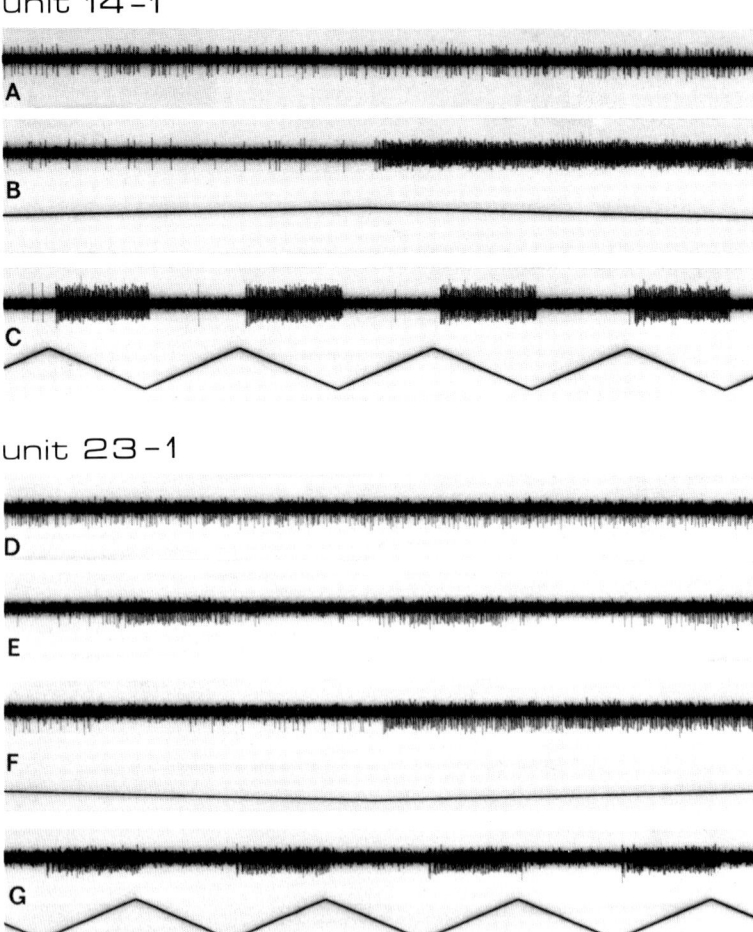

Fig. 56. Discharge pattern of two units (*14-1* and *23-1*) located in the nucleus of the optic tract. The *triangular waveforms* below the action potential traces indicate the position of a random checkerboard pattern, seen by the animal through a stationary aperture of 30° x 30°. The pattern was moved along the preferred-non-preferred axis. **A** and **D** resting discharge in darkness. **E** resting discharge with stationary pattern. A cyclic modulation (1/3 Hz) in synchrony with the respiration is seen. **B** and **F** pattern moving at 1°/s. **C** and **G** pattern moving at 20°/s. (Collewijn, 1975b)

for the duration of the movement. Transients at the onset or cessation of movement were absent or weak. Habituation was never observed, even when stimulation was continued for several hours. All units identified within the NOT were direction-selective and hardly showed any other trigger features.

Only some of them showed clear on or on-off reactions to flashed spots, and it was impossible to map the extent of the receptive field with such stimuli. Concentric or oriented receptive fields were never found. Some of the units could be driven above the resting discharge by diffuse strobe flashes at a frequency of 10-30/s, a finding which could possibly be related to nystagmus elicited by stroboscopic flicker (10-20 flashes/s) in the rabbit (Costin et al., 1965) and monkey (Pasik et al., 1970; Miller et al., 1979), but apparently not in man (Keane, 1972).

The only adequate stimulus was movement in the preferred direction. In the large majority of units, movement in the anterior direction was excitatory and motion in the posterior direction was inhibitory (Fig. 57). All units were excited by motion in four adjacent directions separated by angles of 45° and inhibited by motion in the four opposite directions. Thus, the excitatory response sector was about 180°, while the opposite 180° were inhibitory. The division between these sectors was often tilted up to 45° with respect to the vertical (Fig. 57). This inclination — which was not an artifact of variations in eye position — introduced a sensitivity to upward or downward motion. Only rarely was a unit encountered which was excited by posterior movement (1 unit in Fig. 57).

The direction preference was not affected by the nature of the pattern, but the response tended to decline when the number of contrast lines was

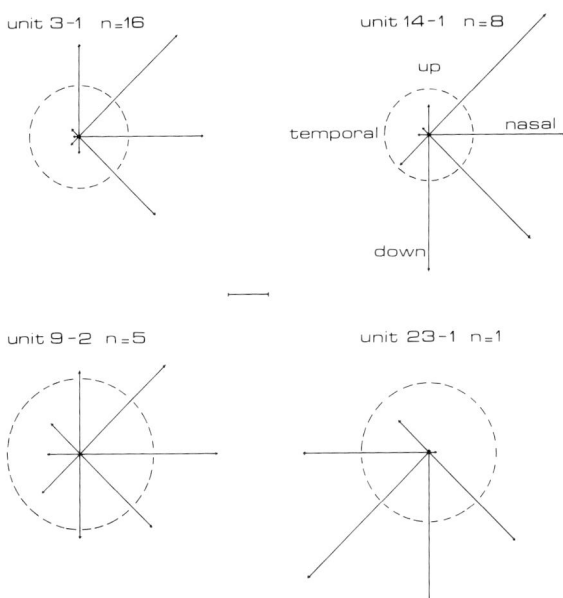

Fig. 57. Vector diagrams of direction selectivity. The *length of the arrows* represents the average discharge frequency during 40 s of stimulus movement in the *direction of arrow*. Random pattern, size 30 x 30°, velocity 1°/s. *Circle* maintained discharge in darkness. Calibration bar: 25 AP/s. All 30 units belonged to one of the four types illustrated; the frequencies (*n*) are indicated. (Collewijn, 1975b)

decreased. Figure 58 shows the response of 10 units to a random-dot pattern (elements 1°, Julesz, 1964), alternating black and white stripes each 4°, 2°, or 1° wide and a single white-black transition with the white or black edge leading (velocity in all cases 1°/s). In 8 of the 10 units, the random-dot pattern was the more effective stimulus and in only 2 units was a 4° white-4° black stripe pattern superior as a stimulus. This tendency agrees with the observations for OKN (Chap. 4.3). The effect of a single white or black leading edge was considerably lower (Fig. 58) but not different in nature, which shows that the direction selectivity was invariant for contrast direction. It was also not influenced by large variations in the brightness or contrast of the pattern.

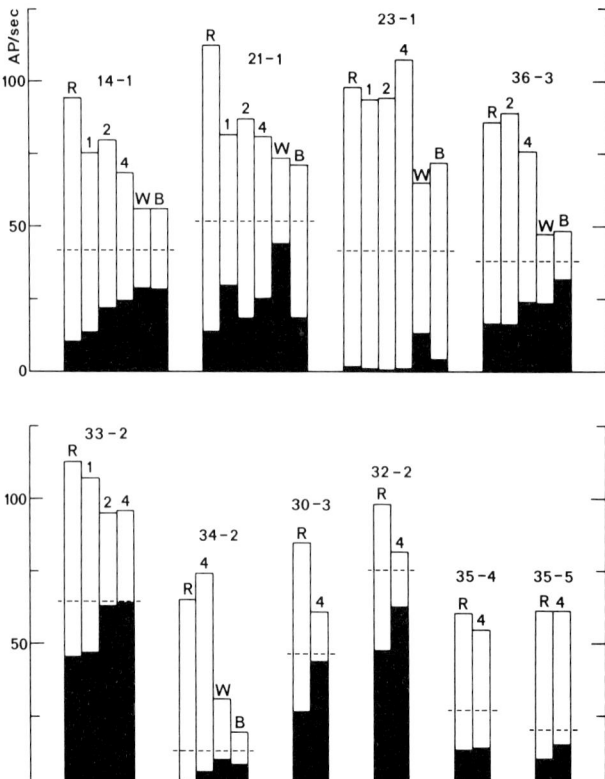

Fig. 58. Responses of 10 units to different patterns of 30° x 30°, moving at 1°/s. R = random pattern (elements 0.8°) *1, 2* and *4* grids of white and black bars, each 1°, 2° and 4° wide, respectively; *W* single white leading edge; *B* single black leading edge. *Open columns* discharge (averaged over 40 s) during motion in excitatory direction; *Black columns* discharge during inhibitory motion. *Interrupted horizontal lines* maintained discharge in darkness. (Collewijn, 1975b)

A further typical property of NOT units was the large size of the receptive fields. The strongest responses were usually elicited from a receptive field "center" which extended about 20° in the vertical and 30° in the horizontal direction. Peripheral to this zone the responses gradually decreased with increasing distance but without a change in the preferred direction. The horizontal dimension of the total receptive field was always larger than the vertical one. A size of about 90 x 40° was fairly typical, with extremes of 50 x 20 and 150 x 40°. All fields were located close to the visual horizon and slightly superior to it, as shown by the distribution of the receptive field centers and preferred directions (bisectrix of excitatory 180°) in Fig. 59. Also indicated are the extreme boundaries in the vertical and rostro-caudal direction in the visual field beyond which no direction selectivity was found in any NOT unit. Horizontally, the direction-selective zone extends throughout the visual field, including the binocular zone, with a relative paucity of elements more than 60° posterior. Vertically, the sensitive zone extends from about 15° inferior to 45° superior. These borders coincide remarkably well with the area in the visual field from which OKN can be elicited (Chap. 4.4; Dubois and Collewijn, 1979a) and with the projection of the visual streak (Fig. 2).

The influence of the size of the pattern was investigated by masks, centered on the most responsive part of the receptive field. Even with the smallest masks (2 x 2°) a clear response was obtained, although only a few elements of the random-dot pattern were visible. The responses increased steeply with the increase in stimulus area and were nearly saturated with a mask of 15 x 15°, both in the excitatory and inhibitory direction, although the total extent of the receptive fields was very much larger. No evidence for an inhibitory surround was found with larger stimuli.

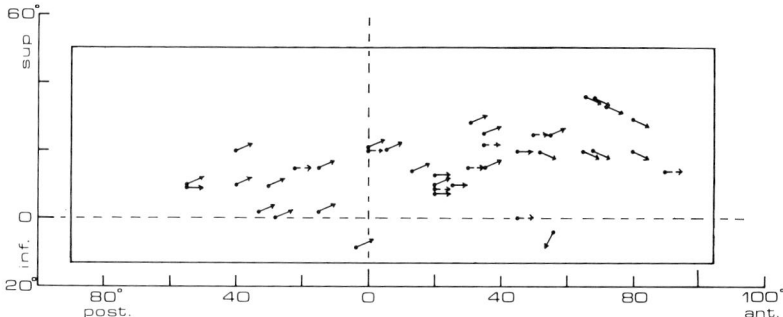

Fig. 59. Location of centers of receptive fields of 39 DS units, with the *arrows* pointing in the preferred direction, in Mercator's projection. The *interrupted arrows* were only determined by hand, the others by a complete vector diagram. The *rectangle* indicates the maximal extension of the combined receptive fields; it coincides fairly well with the visual streak. (Collewijn, 1975b)

The response of the units as a function of stimulus velocity (measured in 17 units) could be roughly divided into two types. In 11 units, a typical reaction as shown in Fig. 60 A was found. Responses increased with velocity up to about 10°/s and were slightly lower at 20°/s. Inhibition and excitation usually showed a similar velocity sensitivity. Up to 10°/s the responses above the resting discharge were approximately proportional to the logarithm of stimulus velocity. In 6 units, another function was found (Fig. 60 B). This type as well responded to all velocities tested, but the maximal excitation and inhibition were obtained at lower velocities (around 1°/s). Many transitions between the two types were encountered and Fig. 60 A and B probably represents the extremes of a continuum rather than a truly bimodal population. All responses mentioned have been obtained through the contralateral eye. The input from the ipsilateral eye has not been investigated in depth but appeared to be very limited in preliminary measurements.

All NOT units could be excited by electrical stimulation of the optic chiasm with single pulses (50 μs, 50-300 μA). The distribution of the latencies was narrow and unimodal, the average latency was 2.2 ± 0.3 (S.D.) ms. From the latency of the field potential presumably caused by the activation of presynaptic fibers, a conduction velocity of 13 m/s was estimated for the afferent fibers to the NOT. Recently, Semm (1978) has measured the conduction velocity of the axons of direction-selective ganglion cells in the rab-

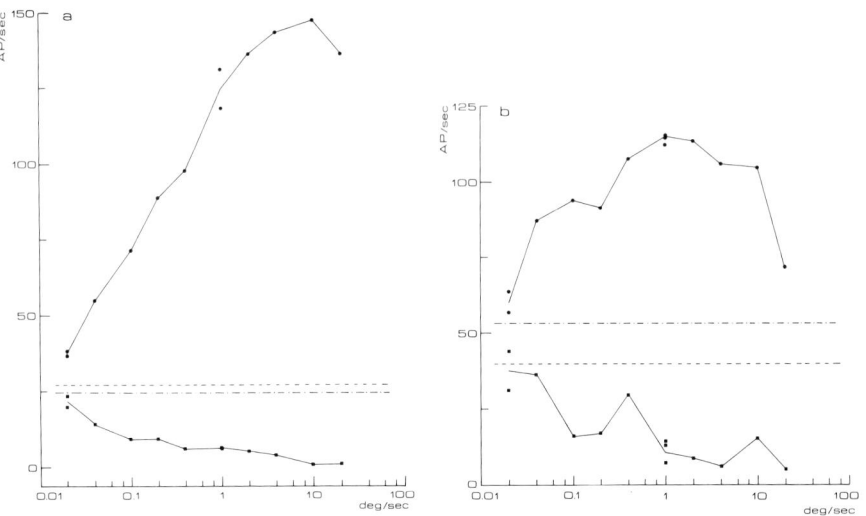

Fig. 60. A Velocity sensitivity curve of a single unit in the NOT with a preference for high velocities. *Dotted horizontal lines* range of the resting discharge during the recording period. *Round dots* excitation by anterior motion. *Squares* inhibition by posterior motion. **B** As **A**, for a unit most sensitive at intermediate velocities (about 1°/s)

bit retina by antidromic excitation and found a range of 8-20 m/s, which is in good agreement with our estimate.

Histological reconstruction of the recording sites (Fig. 61) based on microlesions made at the end of the recordings shows that all units of the direction-selective type as described were confined to the area of the NOT. No units of the same type were found outside this area.

These findings in the rabbit have been almost exactly duplicated for the NOT in the cat (Hoffmann and Schoppmann, 1975). These results are best explained by a massive convergence of retinal direction-selective units upon the NOT neurons. The neuroanatomical studies available (see also Fig. 51) clearly show a dense termination of optic nerve fibers in the contralateral NOT. Since retinal direction-selective receptive fields are about 3° in diameter (Barlow et al., 1964), a heavy convergence and strong synaptic connections are indicated. NOT units have a high resting discharge; practically all are excited by forward motion and inhibited by backward motion. Since inhibition in the null direction is not a very prominent feature of retinal direction-selective units (Barlow et al., 1964), this suggests that NOT units are in general excited by retinal units coded for anterior motion and inhibited by units reacting to backward movement. Levick et al. (1969) have proposed a similar mechanism for direction-selective units in the rabbit's lateral geniculate nucleus. Since many NOT units responded to a large range of velocities (0.01°-20°/s), it seems likely that both retinal on and on-off type units converge on NOT units.

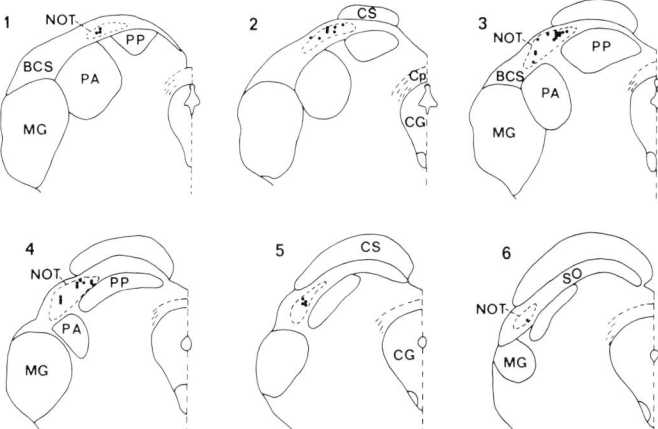

Fig. 61. Localization of 39 DS units (*dots*) according to microlesions. Sections are frontal (parallel to electrode tracks) and in rostrocaudal order. The interval between two sections is 0.2 mm. *BCS* brachium of superior colliculus; *Cp* posterior commissure; *CS* superior colliculus; *CG* central gray; *MG* medial geniculate nucleus; *NOT* nucleus of the optic tract; *PA* anterior pretectal nucleus; *PP* posterior pretectal nucleus; *SO* stratum opticum. (Collewijn, 1975b)

Electrical stimulation of the NOT elicits a horizontal nystagmus with the slow phase to the ipsilateral side. A similar nystagmus is elicited by forward motion seen by the contralateral eye. The large majority of NOT units is excited by precisely this stimulus. The agreement between these findings supports a pathway for horizontal OKN through the NOT. The large size of the receptive fields is also perfectly suitable, since the adequate stimulus for OKN is not local but generalized motion in a wide sector of the visual field. A final point of agreement between NOT and optokinetic responses is the visual latency. For the OKN the minimal latency was estimated at 75 ms (4.3, Fig. 39 C), while NOT units had a latency for excitation by movement of 60 ± 10 ms. Practically all of this must be due to retinal processing, since electrical stimulation of the chiasm excited the NOT after 2.2 ms. This would leave about 15 ms for central processing of NOT signals into motor commands and for neuromuscular activation time.

5.4 Direction-Selectivity in the Posterior Accessory Optic System

The NOT is tuned to horizontal motion and it seemed likely that vertical motion information and OKN would be mediated by another system. This is supported by the recent recordings by Simpson et al. (1979) in the nuclei of the posterior accessory system. The posterior accessory optic tract descends from the main optic tract between the superior colliculus and the medial geniculate nucleus at the lateral surface of the brain. It has terminations in the tiny dorsal terminal nucleus (close to the NOT) and the more ventrally situated lateral terminal nucleus but mainly in the medial terminal nucleus (MTN) (Fig. 51), also called the nucleus of the transpeduncular tract. The anatomy of this system has been described for the rabbit (Giolli, 1961; Giolli et al., 1968). Walley (1967) first reported that over half of the neurons in the nucleus of the transpeduncular tract in the rabbit were direction-selective for vertically moving stimuli. Recordings by Westheimer and Blair (1974) in the monkey also indicated direction selectivity of this nucleus in the vertical (but also horizontal) direction. The properties of cells in the medial terminal nucleus as described by Simpson et al. (1979) are highly similar to those of the NOT (Collewijn, 1975b) except for the preferred directions and velocities. The background activity is 25-50 spikes/s, the latency to electrical stimulation of the optic chiasm is 2-2.5 ms. The only effective visual stimulus is motion of large (20° x 20°), slowly moving, textured patterns. Receptive fields are large, averaging about 40° vertical by 60° horizontal. Best modulation occurs at speeds in the range 0.1°-1°/s; the total sensitive range extends from about 0.01° to 5°/s. Preferred directions are vertical with a posterior component. Two thirds of the cells were best excited by upward and slightly posterior movement. These cells were most profoundly inhibited by a movement not exactly in the opposite direction, but downward with a slight posterior component as well. The remaining one third of the cells were excited by downward and slightly posterior movement. All cells were direction-selective but also showed some on-response with steady illumination. The direction and velocity preferences of these cells agree perfectly with those of the on-type direction-selective cells in the retina (Oyster, 1968; Oyster et al., 1972), in particular the upward and downward component of the three-lobed distribution of preferred directions, which have a distinct inclination in the posterior direction. Apparently, cells in the medial terminal nucleus are excited by one of these vertically sensitive groups and inhibited by the other, possibly through an interneuron. In contrast to the NOT, the medial terminal nucleus is not excited by velocities of 10°/s or higher, thus is apparently not innervated by on-off type direction selective ganglion cells. This restriction to low velocities is also found for vertical OKN (Chap. 4.5) and it seems most likely that the medial terminal nucleus mediates vertical optokinetic responses.

The retrograde transport of horseradish peroxidase (HRP) by the optic nerve fibers terminating in the NOT or MTN seems to offer a unique opportunity to identify the direction-selective ganglion cells in the retina. The NOT is not very suitable for this experiment, as all surrounding optic tract fibers, when lesioned, would also transport the marker. However, the MTN is removed from any optic nerve fibers which do not terminate there, and the HRP injection experiment has been carried out successfully by Takahashi et al. (1979). After complete injection of the MTN, about 2000 large ganglion cells were labeled in the contralateral eye. The density of these cells (presumably of the "on" direction-selective type) was highest in the visual streak. Unlike the situation in pigeons (Karten et al., 1977), none of the ganglion cells was displaced (Dogiel's cells).

The cells in the lateral terminal nucleus are also vertically direction-selective, with a preference for down and posterior. In the dorsal terminal nucleus, cells were horizontally direction-selective with a preference for anterior motion, similar to the neurons of the immediately adjacent NOT (Simpson et al., 1979).

Simpson and Hess (1977) and Simpson et al. (1979) have proposed that the three preferred directions in visual space described by the on-direction-selective ganglion cells (and relayed to the NOT and accessory optic tract nuclei and further projections) are related to and derived from the three principal axes of the semi-circular canals, allowing for dynamic visual vestibular interaction in one basic coordinate system.

5.5 Efferent Connections from the Nucleus of the Optic Tract

In an attempt to further elucidate the optokinetic pathways, we recently traced the efferent fibers from the NOT using the anterograde axonal transport of radioactively labeled amino acids (Holstege and Collewijn, in press). Double-barreled micropipettes were used to first localize the NOT on the basis of its direction-selective properties and then inject it with ^{3}H leucine (about 25 μCi contained in 1 μl). After a survival time of two weeks the brains were processed for autoradiography with an exposure time of three months. The neurons of the NOT had taken up a massive amount of labeled leucine in four rabbits, while the injection site extended very little beyond the NOT area. Efferent fibers, as well as terminal projections from the NOT, were well defined in these preparations and the following connections were consistently found (Fig. 62 I-III). In the thalamus, strong ipsilateral projections were found to the dorsal and vertral lateral geniculate and lateral posterior (pulvinar) nuclei, as well as to the dorsal part of the medial geniculate nucleus. The ipsilateral superior colliculus received strong projections. Crossing fibers were observed in the posterior commissure and seemed to project to the contralateral pretectum and superior colliculus, but only sparsely to the contralateral NOT. Further strong projections at the midbrain level were found to the ipsilateral medial terminal nucleus, lateral tegmentum and parabigeminal nucleus. The ipsilateral dorsal and lateral pontine nuclei also received a heavy projection. More caudally, the descending fibers could be traced to the ipsilateral prepositus hypoglossi nucleus, the dorsal medial medullary reticular formation, the abducens nucleus (weakly), and the contralateral facial nucleus (m. orbicularis oculi part). Practically all more caudally descending fibers seemed to terminate in the caudal part of the dorsal cap of the inferior olive ipsilaterally (massively) and contralaterally (weak-

Fig. 62. I, II. Darkfield photomicrographs of sections processed for radioautography after injection of ^{3}H leucine in the nucleus of the optic tract. The injection site is visible in D-F. Rostrally, projections are visible in the dorsal and ventral lateral geniculate and the lateral posterior nucleus (*A-C*). The superior colliculus is labeled extensively. The dorsal part of the medial geniculate (*E, arrow*) was always labeled, as well as the medial terminal nucleus (*F, arrow*). Crossing fibers pass through the posterior commissure (*D, E*) to the contralateral pretectum. Fiber tracts descend through the midbrain tegmentum to terminate in the lateral tegmental field (*H*), the parabigeminal nucleus (*I, arrow*) and the pontine nuclei (*I-K*). More caudally descending fibers are seen dorsally and ventrally (*L, arrows*) which terminate in the prepositus hypoglossi nucleus (*M, N, upper black arrows*), the dorsal medial medullary reticular formation (*M, left white arrow*), the contralateral facial nucleus (*M, right white arrow*) and the dorsal cap of the inferior olive (*O, white arrow*). The descending fibers in the ventral brainstem are indicated by *black arrows* in *M-O*. *Sp V* spinal trigeminal complex; *VII* facial nucleus; *IO* inferior olive; *XII* hypoglossal nucleus. (Holstege and Collewijn, in press)

Efferent Connections from the Nucleus of the Optic Tract

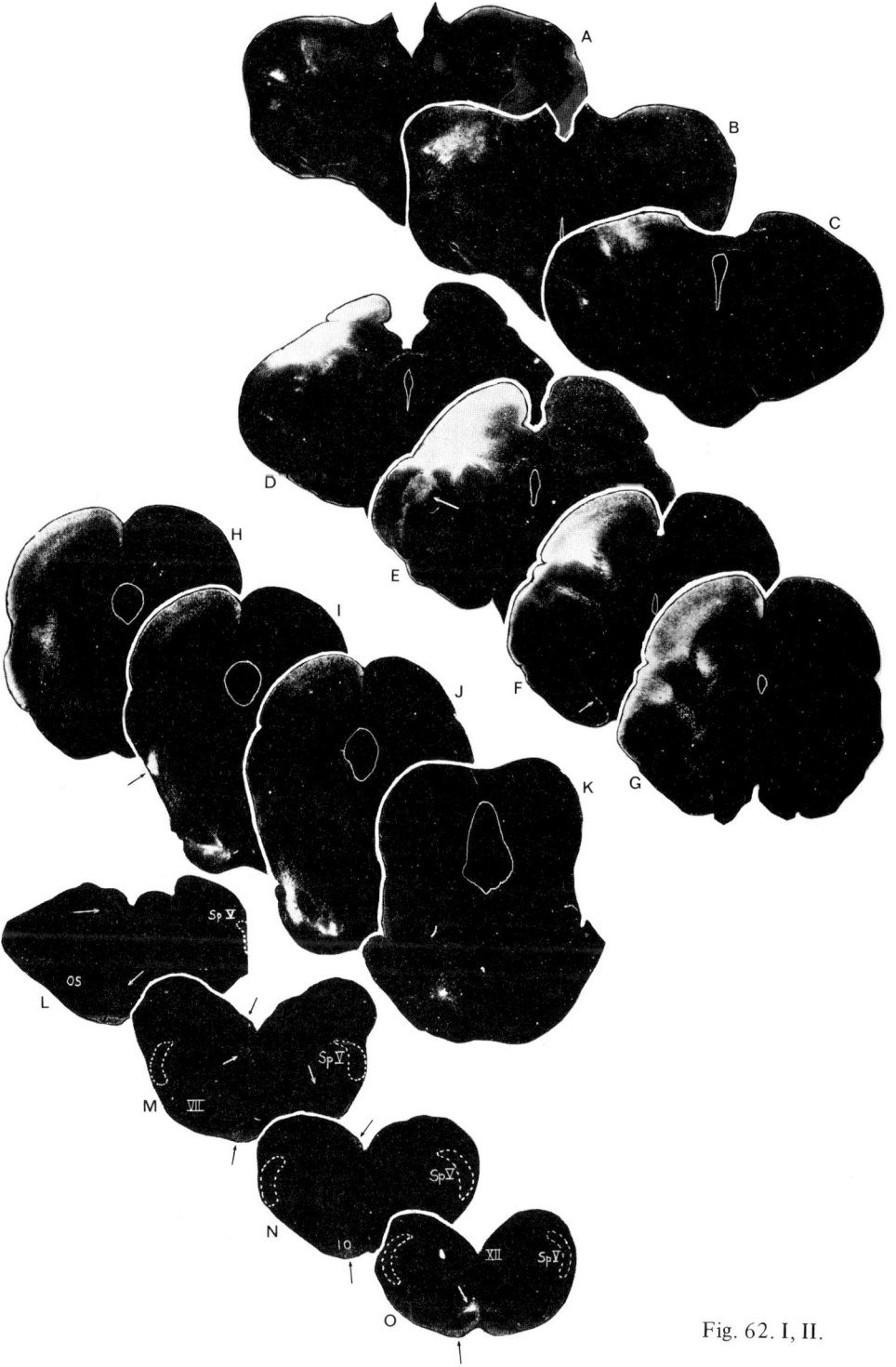

Fig. 62. I, II.

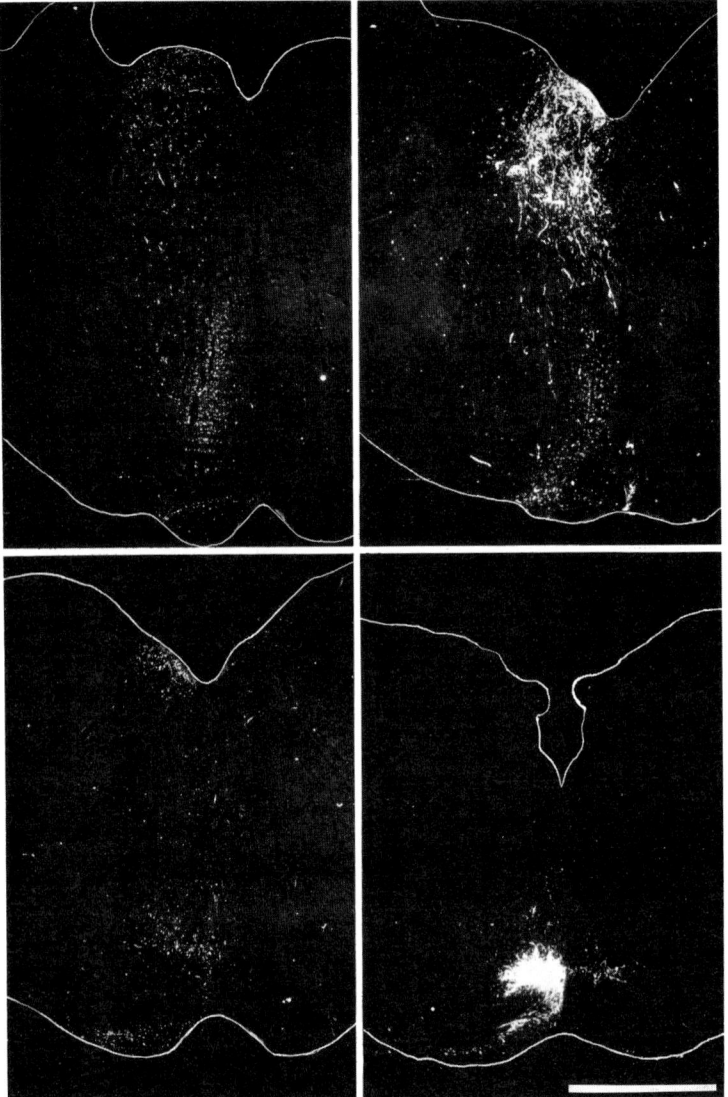

Fig. 62. III Autoradiographs (*dark field*) of NOT projections in the caudal brainstem. *Upper left* descending fibers at the level of the superior olive. *Upper right* termination in ipsilateral prepositus hypoglossi nucleus and dorsal medial medullary reticular formation. *Lower left* endings in prepositus hypoglossi nucleus and descending fibers in the ventral brainstem. *Lower right* massive projection to ipsilateral dorsal cap and weak to contralateral dorsal cap of inferior olive. Also projection to part of ipsilateral principal olive. Calibration 2 mm

ly). Since all labeled axons could be clearly traced, we are confident that no other projections of any significance exist. In particular, no significant projections of the NOT were found to the oculomotor or trochlear nucleus, the interstitial or Darkschewitsch nuclei, the reticular tegmenti pontis nucleus, or any of the vestibular nuclei. Likewise, no direct fiber pathway to the cerebellum was observed, but it is clear that the cerebellum receives a very heavy indirect projection from the NOT through the dorsal cap of the inferior olive (climbing fibers, the pontine nuclei (mossy fibers) and possibly the prepositus hypoglossi nucleus.

Efferent projections from the pretectum have been investigated before, mainly in the cat (Berman, 1977; Itoh, 1977), but none of these studies addressed itself particularly to the efferents of the NOT. The latter were studied specifically in the rat by Terasawa et al. (1979) with the Nauta-Gygax technique. After small lesions in the NOT they found terminal degeneration in the contralateral pretectum, the pontine nuclei and the dorsal cap, which we confirm for the rabbit. We do not find a projection to the nucleus tegmenti pontis as they described for the rat. The NOT-dorsal cap connection was identified previously by Mizuno et al. (1973, 1974) and Takeda and Maekawa (1976), while the projection of the dorsal cap to the flocculus was shown by Alley et al. (1975) and by Hoddevik and Brodal (1977). A similar pathway originating in the dorsal terminal nucleus of the accessory optic tract (which is functionally and anatomically closely related to the NOT) was physiologically traced by Maekawa and Simpson (1972, 1973) and Maekawa and Takeda (1976). The direction selectivity of the NOT-dorsal cap-flocculus pathway was demonstrated by Simpson and Alley (1974) at the climbing fiber level and by Barmack (1977) and Barmack and Hess (1980a) in the dorsal cap. The main pathway is from one eye to the contralateral NOT, then to the contralateral dorsal cap and with a second decussation to the flocculus ipsilateral to the eye (Fig. 63). However, climbing fiber excitation in the flocculus through the contralateral eye has also been described (Maekawa and Takeda, 1976). The latter may be mediated by the small projection we found from the NOT to the contralateral dorsal cap. Mossy fiber responses in the rabbit's flocculus (bilateral) have also been obtained by electrical stimulation of the optic pathway (Maekawa and Takeda, 1975, 1976). A modulation of "simple" spikes in the rabbit's flocculus (mediated through mossy fibers) by moving visual stimuli was first described by Ghelarducci et al. (1975). The effect was small, but this may be related to the use of an inadequate visual stimulus (a single light slit). The effect was later found to be larger with slower movement of the slit (Ito, 1977), and Barmack (1979) obtained very clear simple spike modulation by using large patterns. Hoddevik (1977) has described a bilateral projection from the pontine nuclei to the flocculus in the rabbit; our finding (Holstege and Collewijn, in press) that the NOT projects to the pontine nuclei completes the route for a direction-selective mossy fiber input to the flocculus. A pontine projection to a part of the flocculus was also found by Yamamoto (1979). On the other hand the pontine area labeled in our experiments may project to the vermis, as it resembles the zone which is connected to vermal lobules VII and VIII in the cat (Hoddevik et al., 1977).

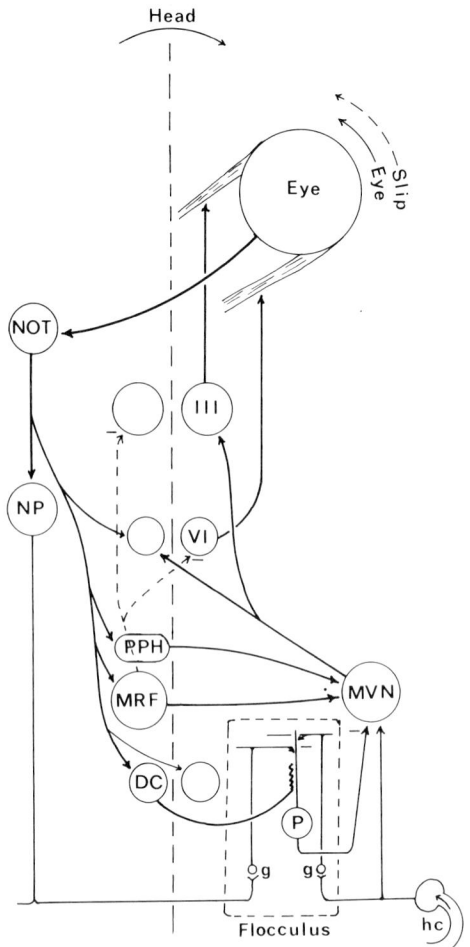

Fig. 63. Diagram of some of the connections related to OKN and VOR, as discussed in the text. Connections known to be inhibitory are marked with a *negative sign*. Head rotation to the right will excite the left NOT and right horizontal canal and cause a compensatory eye movement to the left. *NOT* nucleus of the optic tract; *NP* pontine nuclei; *III* oculomotor nucleus; *VI* abducens nucleus; *PPH* prepositus hypoglossi nucleus; *MRF* medullary reticular formation; *DC* dorsal cap of inferior olive; *MVN* medial vestibular nucleus; *P* Purkinje cell in flocculus; *g* granule cells in flocculus; *hc* right horizontal canal

Of the noncerebellar projections, the most likely ones to be involved in the OKN are those to the lateral midbrain tegmentum, the medial terminal nucleus, the prepositus hypoglossi and abducens nuclei and the dorsal medial medullary reticular formation. Future physiological investigations will have to elucidate the role of these areas in the OKN. The intimate connection of the prepositus hypoglossi nucleus with oculomotor functions has been recognized in recent years (Graybiel and Hartwieg, 1974; Baker et al., 1976; Lopez-Barneo et al., 1979), although its precise function has still to be defined. It is known to project to the vestibular nuclei (Pompeiano et al., 1978; McCrea et al., 1979). The medial dorsal medullary reticular formation (dorsal med RF), situated ventral to the prepositus hypoglossi nucleus, has been strongly implicated in eye movements (see Büttner-Ennever, 1979). In the rabbit, Duensing and Schaefer (1957) recorded eye movement-related units in this area. The dorsal med RF projects to the contralateral medial vestibular nucleus in the cat (Graybiel, 1977b; Pompeiano et al., 1978; Corvaja et al., 1979). It also projects to the medial rectus division of the ipsilateral oculomotor nucleus (Graybiel, 1977a; Büttner-Ennever, 1979) and to the contralateral abducens nucleus (Graybiel, 1977b). The latter connection appears to be inhibitory (Hikosaka and Kawakami, 1977). If the projection from the dorsal med RF to the oculomotor nucleus is also inhibitory, this zone might inhibit eye muscles which execute horizontal conjugate eye movements to the contralateral side (Büttner-Ennever, 1979). On the other hand, the connection to the contralateral medial vestibular nucleus would, if it is excitatory, produce conjugate eye movements to the side ipsilateral to the dorsal med RF. Graybiel (1977b) has found a projection from the area of the dorsal med RF to the NOT in the cat; if this also exists in the rabbit, the connections between NOT and dorsal med RF would be reciprocal.

The projections of the NOT to the prepositus hypoglossi nucleus and the dorsal med RF are highly interesting, as they provide a pathway for visual direction selective information to the vestibular nuclei.

A strong convergence of visual direction-selective and vestibular motion signals upon single cells in the vestibular nuclei has been demonstrated in the goldfish (Dichgans et al., 1973b; Allum et al., 1976), the rabbit (Dichgans and Brandt, 1972), the cat (Keller and Precht, 1978), the pigmented rat (Precht and Cazin, 1979), and the monkey (Henn et al., 1974). The vestibular nuclear activity has been recorded in the monkey during OKN (Waespe and Henn, 1977a) and OKAN (Waespe and Henn, 1977b). A close parallel between the time course of OK(A)N slow phase velocity and vestibular nuclear single unit discharge frequency was found. During OKN in the monkey (Waespe and Henn, 1977a) the discharge frequency was built up slowly and saturated for a slow phase velocity of about $60°/s$. This may indicate that the visually induced vestibular nuclear activity reflects the basic optokinetic reflex (as found in the rabbit) without an extra contribution by smooth pursuit.

The pathway for the visual information to the vestibular nuclei has been unclear so far, although several possibilities have been excluded. Primary vestibular afferents (which could be influenced theoretically through the efferent vestibular system) are not modulated by optokinetic stimuli in the alert monkey (Keller, 1976) or cat (Blanks and Precht, 1978). The pathway through the cerebellum, as such certainly present, is also unessential for the visual control of vestibular activity, as this is preserved after complete cerebellectomy in the cat (Keller and Precht, 1978). Precht and Strata (1979) have suggested a link through the nucleus reticularis tegmenti pontis, to which we find no projection from the NOT. A pathway through the prepositus hypoglossi nucleus and the dorsal med RF seems plausible. An alternative pathway through the subparafascicular region has been suggested by Barmack et al. (1979). A diagram of some of the proposed pathways for OKN and its interaction with the VOR is shown in Fig. 63.

5.6 Effects of Bilateral Labyrinthectomy

The finding of a visual modulation of vestibular nuclei by optokinetic stimuli supports the concept of OKN as a postural reflex and its tight functional relationship with the VOR. This relationship is further supported by the finding that OK(A)N is strongly affected or even abolished by bilateral destruction of the labyrinth in the monkey (Cohen et al., 1973), man (Zee et al., 1976b) and rabbit (Gutman et al., 1964; Baarsma and Collewijn, 1974; Collewijn, 1976).

The effects of labyrinthectomy on OKN elicited by a drum rotating at a constant velocity are shown in Fig. 64. First, the normal reactions to stimulus velocities of 1°/s (immediate) and 30°/s (slow build-up) are shown. After bilateral labyrinthectomy (1 and 3 days postoperatively) the OKN elicited by a stimulus of 1°/s is normal, but the reactions to a stimulus of 30°/s are severely deficient. The usual gradual increase in slow-phase velocity is absent and slow-phase velocities do not consistently exceed a few °/s, even after a long period of stimulation. When the lights are turned off, no optokinetic afternystagmus is ever seen. These findings in the rabbit agree with those for monkey and man. OKN elicited in open-loop conditions or nystagmus due to electrical stimulation of the NOT also never reached slow phase velocities faster than a few °/s, and the response never outlasted the stimulus (Collewijn, 1976). Figure 65 shows the OKN responses to sinusoidal stimulation, recorded 1 month after bilateral labyrinthectomy, which should be compared to the normal results in Fig. 34 A. The gain after labyrinthectomy is definitely subnormal. The rate of decline of gain at higher stimulus speeds is normal, but starts already for stimulus speeds much below 1°/s. Gutman et al. (1964) reported a marked decrease in the frequency of OKN beats in labyrinthectomized rabbits for all stimulus velocities tested (about 1°-100°/s), while the general shape of the response as a function of stimulus velocity was unchanged.

It must be concluded that OKN is severely disturbed by vestibular deafferentiation, and it seems likely that this is due to disorganization of the visuo-vestibular interaction in the vestibular nuclei. Labyrinthectomy is known to profoundly depress the resting discharge level in the vestibular nuclei, and although recovery of the activity level within days to weeks has

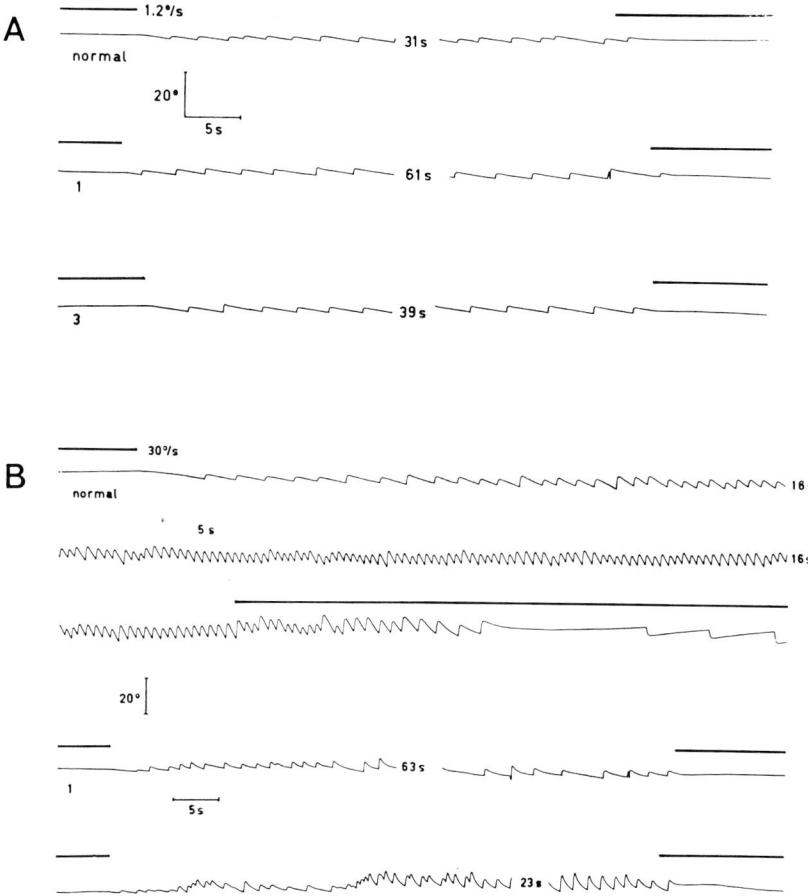

Fig. 64. Optokinetic nystagmus elicited by drum rotation at 1.2°/s (**A**) and 30°/s (**B**). *Upper traces* reactions of normal rabbit. *Middle* and *lower traces* reactions 1 and 3 days after labyrinthectomy. *Horizontal bars* indicate periods of darkness. *Numbers* in the traces indicate duration (s) of the part of the recording not shown. (Collewijn, 1976)

been reported (Precht et al., 1966; Precht, 1974; Ryu and McGabe, 1976), there may be an irreversible change in the processing of visual information, as most of the OKN defects appear to be permanent.

The effect of labyrinthectomy on OKN is probably due to the withdrawal of the tonic effect of the vestibular afferents (which have a resting activity of the order of 100 action potentials per second) and not to the absence of the vestibular motion information which is carried as a modulation on the resting discharge. Presumably OK(A)N will be unaffected if canals are plugged, a procedure which eliminates the modulation but not the resting discharge, but such an experiment has not been published.

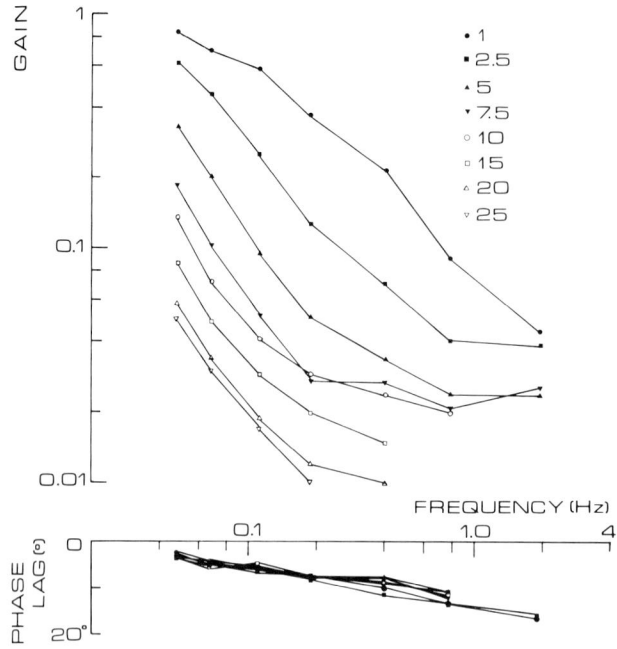

Fig. 65. Gain and phase for OKN elicited by sinusoidal drum movement, 1 month after bilateral labyrinthectomy. Averaged results of five rabbits. (Baarsma and Collewijn, 1974)

5.7 The Effect of Cerebellectomy on OKN

The statements made regarding labyrinthectomy are also valid for cerebellectomy or in general for any ablation study: it is impossible to separate the informational content from the tonic effects when a structure is removed which has important connections with oculomotor or any other circuits. Since the discharge rate of cerebellar Purkinje cells is of the same order as of vestibular afferents, and the cerebellum projects massively to the vestibular nuclei, as well as to many other centers involved in eye movements, it should come as no surprise that cerebellar lesions disrupt the delicate processing in oculomotor circuits. The significance of the information processing in the cerebello-oculomotor loops has been investigated in a great number of experiments in the past few years. The enormous growth in this field has been stimulated by the relatively advanced understanding of the oculomotor system in comparison to other motor systems. The vestibulo-cerebellum (particularly the flocculus) has been implicated in short- and long-term visuo-vestibular interaction, adaptation of VOR gain, smooth pursuit and suppression of the VOR and OKN. On the other hand, the vermis appears to be involved in the correct execution of saccades. A complete discussion of this field would exceed the scope of this monograph. An excellent survey of the strategies, results and problems concerning cerebellar modification of oculomotor and other reflex loops has recently been published by MacKay and Murphy (1979). Other reviews were given by Precht (1975, 1978).

Long before cerebello-oculomotor research reached its present level of sophistication, I studied the effect of complete cerebellectomy on OKN in the rabbit (Collewijn, 1970b). The cerebellum was totally removed in young rabbits (age 4-6 weeks) and optokinetic responses were tested 3-5 months later. Optokinetic responses in these animals were basically normal as long as no saccades were required. Thus, sinusoidal oscillation of a striped drum elicited normal responses with a good gain for low stimulus velocities and a rapidly decreasing gain for stimuli faster than a few degrees per second. When the drum was rotated at a constant velocity to produce regular optokinetic nystagmus, optokinetic nystagmus was initially normal but the rabbits failed to generate adequate saccades to balance the slow deviation. The saccades were too small and were generated too late to keep the eye deviation in the normal range (Fig. 66). At low drum velocities, a steady state was still often reached in which OKN was beating at a small amplitude in a very peripheral position. Eye deviations reached up to 40° from the resting position, whereas 25° is about the maximum excursion in a normal rabbit (Collewijn, 1970a, 1977a). With higher drum velocities, the insufficiency of saccades became more severe and the eye tended to become locked in an eccentric position. Once this condition was reached, the eye continued to generate a fine nystagmus with the slow phase beating to the periphery and the fast phase to the center. These directions are opposite to the ones described for gaze-paretic nystagmus after cerebellar lesions in cat (Robinson, 1974) and man (Zee et al., 1976a). It was very hard to reverse this condition by visual stimuli, but after some time the eye would return to the midposition (no vestibular stimulation was used at that time). The amplitude-velocity relationship of the saccades produced after cerebellectomy was not grossly abnormal. Obviously this experiment was very crude, but one specific conclusion can be reached: optokinetic pursuit as such is independent of cerebellar pathways. In the cat as well (Robinson, 1974), slow phase of OKN can still be produced after total cerebellectomy. For primates the situation is more complex. Absence of smooth pursuit has been reported for the monkey after complete cerebellectomy (Westheimer and Blair, 1973). OKN is retained in the cerebellectomized monkey (Takemori and Cohen, 1974), but its velocity range is reduced from 150°/s (normal) to about 50°/s.

In man, the vestibulo-cerebellar dysplasia associated with the Arnold-Chiari malformation seems to affect preferentially foveal smooth pursuit, with relative sparing of OKN elicited by large moving patterns (Zee et al.,

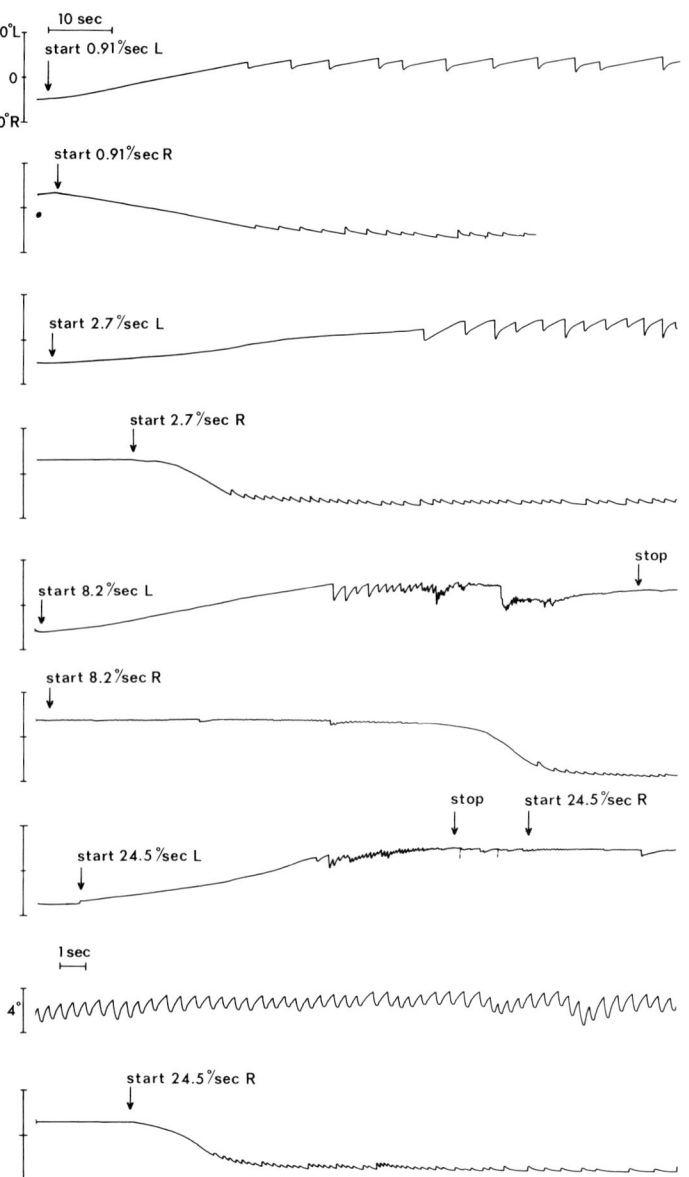

Fig. 66. Optokinetic nystagmus in a cerebellectomized rabbit induced by drum rotation at the velocities as indicated. Calibration of upper trace valid for all traces except the second from below, which is continuation of the third from below at 10 × higher sensitivity. (Collewijn, 1970b)

1974, 1976a; Dichgans et al., 1978). These lesions are often accompanied by down-beat nystagmus. Yee et al. (1979) reported that in two patients of this type OKN could be elicited by full field stimulation at 30°/s. However, the response was built up from an initial velocity of a few °/s to a maximum of about 20°/s in a period of 20-40 s. OKAN was present, but smooth pursuit was very poor. We can conclude that — apart from the spontaneous nystagmus — these patients' optokinetic eye movements had become remarkably similar to those of rabbits. Presumably, the rather selective elimination of smooth pursuit in these lesions unmasks the more primitive OKN system with its typical slow build-up, afternystagmus and saturation for low velocities. Zee et al. (1976a) have reported a similar dissociation between smooth pursuit defects and relatively intact OKN in patients with hereditary cerebellar ataxia. These findings support that OKN as found in normal human subjects is a combination of true OKN (as found in afoveate animals) and smooth pursuit.

A specific function of the flocculus is thought to be the correct modulation of the VOR by visual stimuli. Floccular lesions in man cause a characteristic inability to suppress the VOR when a subject is rotated and instructed to fixate a target rotating with the head (Zee et al., 1976a; Dichgans et al., 1978). This suggests a parallel with the smooth pursuit defect: the same patients may be unable to pursue small targets because they cannot suppress the conflicting OKN caused by the opposite movement of the background.

In the monkey, bilateral flocculus lesions also caused loss or at least a reduction of suppression of calorically induced vestibular nystagmus by vision of the stationary world. It is unclear whether this is caused simply by the defect of smooth pursuit or by a defective interaction between the OKN (which is present) and VOR.

In the rabbit, the modulation of the VOR by the cerebellum and specifically by visual signals has been extensively investigated by Ito and his colleagues.

The three-neuronal pathways (primary vestibular afferent — vestibular nuclear neuron — oculomotor neuron) have been traced for the canal-ocular reflexes in the rabbit (Highstein, 1973a, b; Highstein et al., 1971; Ito et al., 1976a, b, c). The specific neuronal connections for the control of these reflexes by the flocculus have also been worked out (Ito et al., 1973, 1977) and a differential localization of eye movements in different directions has been shown by local stimulation of the flocculus (Dufossé et al., 1977). Taking the horizontal VOR as an example, we can summarize the neuronal interaction as follows. When the head is rotated to the right, the right horizontal semicircular canal is excited, which in turn excites secondary vestibular nuclear neurons (type I in the medial vestibular nucleus on the right side). From there, motoneurons of the ipsilateral medial rectus muscle and the contralateral lateral rectus muscle are excited (Fig. 63). Complementary inhibitions are exerted at the motoneurons of the antagonistic muscles. The result is a compensatory rotation of the eyes to the left. (We know of course that this three-neuronal reflex arc can only partly explain the VOR, since such aspects as integration have to be added, presumably by secondary circuits, see (Robinson, 1975). This reflex is inhibited by electrical stimulation of the ipsilateral flocculus, which is understandable since the Purkinje cell axons project directly onto vestibular nuclear cells and are inhibitory in nature.

The interaction between the VOR and vision has been investigated in Ito's laboratory with a single light slit as the visual stimulus in the albino rabbit. The general outcome of these experiments in the normal rabbit was compatible with the findings of Baarsma and Collewijn (1974), but two problems are the choice of the visual stimulus and the type of rabbits. The single slit is a poor optokinetic stimulus (originally it was reported to have no optokinetic effect at all; Ito et al., 1974a). Moreover, the albino rabbit shows serious anomalies in optokinetic pursuit (Collewijn et al., 1978; see Chap. 6). With these stimulus conditions, it was found (Ito et al., 1974a) that unilateral floccular lesions abolished the synergic effect on the VOR of a stationary slit (seen by the ipsilateral eye) as well as the suppressive effect of a slit rotated with the animal. These experiments should be repeated with adequate full field stimulation and pigmented rabbits. Barmack (1979) has studied the effects of unilateral left flocculectomy on OKN and VOR (but not their interaction) in the rabbit. Postoperatively, all animals showed a conjugate spontaneous nystagmus with the slow phase (1°-40°/s) to the right. The VOR was affected by the rightward bias, but in the range 0.2-0.8 Hz, the gain was near normal. The OKN as well was initially biased by this drift. The bias was eventually compensated, after which the VOR was normal, but OKN showed a permanent impairment when elicited from the eye ipsilateral to the lesion. Such a decrease of OKN might cause the modulation defect observed by Ito et al. (1974a). In summary, it is not clear whether flocculectomy in the rabbits affects only OKN or specifically its interaction with the VOR.

Ghelarducci et al. (1975) in Ito's laboratory investigated the discharge rates of Purkinje cells in the rabbit's flocculus. In a large number of cells, the activity was modulated by rotation of the animal in darkness. This modulation is undoubtedly caused by the direct mossy fiber projections of collaterals of vestibular afferents to the flocculus (Brodal and Høivik, 1964). In about half of these cells, the modulation was *in-phase* with the rotation (excitation during ipsilateral motion) and in the other half it was *out-of-phase*. An *in-phase* discharge would tend to inhibit the VOR. The visual stimulus (light slit) was in itself not very effective, but in combination with head rotation caused a shift in this distribution: a stationary slit augmented the proportion of *out-of-phase* responses, a slit moving with the head produced a dominance of the *in-phase* responses. These responses agree with the changes observed in the VOR.

Later, Ito (1977) has slightly amended these findings in the sense that with a suitably slow motion of the light slit alone, simple spikes in the flocculus Purkinje cells were clearly modulated. In the floccular zone associated with horizontal eye movements, simple spikes were mostly enhanced by anterior to posterior motion seen by the ipsilateral eye. For head movements in stationary visual surroundings, this would correspond to an *out-of-phase* modulation.

For the complex spikes caused by the climbing fibers the situation is more complicated. Head rotation to the right will cause excitation of the left NOT and left dorsal cap and increase complex spikes in the right flocculus with *in-phase* responses. This in itself would inhibit the VOR instead of enhancing it. Indeed, inhibitory effects on the VOR by single shock electrical stimulation of the contralateral dorsal cap have been reported (Ito et al., 1978a). Interestingly, the caudal part of the dorsal cap, which receives a projection of the horizontally direction-selective NOT (Holstege and Collewijn, in press) influences the horizontal VOR, while the rostral part of the dorsal cap affects the vertical VOR and receives a projection from the vertically direction-selective medial terminal nucleus (Simpson, personal communication).

Probably, the net effect of climbing fiber excitation under physiological conditions will be opposite, since the excitation of the Purkinje cells by climbing fibers reduces the number of simple spikes (and thus the overall Purkinje cell output) in the successive period (Murphy and Sabah, 1970). Barmack (1979) has recorded from floccular Purkinje cells in alert rabbits during optokinetic stimulation with large patterns. Climbing fiber responses were – if present – always evoked by posterior to anterior stimulation of the ipsilateral eye, in agreement with the pathway through the NOT and dorsal cap. Simple spike responses were always modulated in an antiphasic manner, increasing their rate of discharge during anterior to posterior stimulation of the ipsilateral eye. The antiphasic modulation of simple spikes with respect to complex spikes is not necessarily only due to an inhibitory effect of complex spikes, since such a mutual relation was often not obvious in individual Purkinje cells (Barmack, 1979) and an independent direction-selective mossy fiber pathway to the flocculus probably exists (Maekawa and Takeda, 1975, 1976; Hoddevik, 1977; Holstege and Collewijn, in press).

In agreement with the disfacilitation hypothesis, Barmack and Hess (1980b) observed low-velocity conjugate eye movements in the direction of the stimulated dorsal cap when stimulus trains with a duration of several seconds were used. Apparently, this stimulation caused a disinhibition of the vestibular nuclei contralateral to the stimulated dorsal cap, with ipsilateral movement of the eyes as a result. These results support the hypothesis that retinal slip, signaled through the NOT-olivary-floccular pathway, will modulate the VOR in such a way as to reduce retinal slip, which is of course the only way for the system to make sense. In a complementary experiment, Barmack and Simpson (1980) made microlesions of the dorsal cap. This caused a mild postoperative drift ($0.1°$-$2°/s$) to the side contralateral to the lesion for a period of 2-48 h.

The VOR showed a velocity bias in the same direction. This drift is opposite to the one caused by stimulation of the dorsal cap. However, it is a short-term phenomenon and is compensated in a few days. After this compensation, optokinetic stimulation of the eye projecting to the damaged dorsal cap gave a severely defective response for posterior to anterior motion. Notice that this long-term effect of a dorsal cap lesion is identical to that caused by a contralateral flocculus lesion as described by Barmack (1979). This creates some difficulties in interpreting the results of a dorsal cap lesion in terms of an increased net Purkinje cell activity of the contralateral flocculus (Barmack and Simpson, 1980). A solution of this discrepancy is offered by the recent finding of Ito and associates (Dufossé et al., 1978; Ito et al., 1978b; Ito et al., 1979b) that destruction of the inferior olive causes synaptic depression of the innervated Purkinje cells; thus, elimination of the right dorsal cap would functionally be equivalent to destruction of the left flocculus.

Taken together, the evidence seems to indicate that visual direction-selective information is processed through both climbing and mossy fiber circuits. The cerebellar loop is connected in parallel to the three-neuronal vestibulo-ocular loop and its overall effect is to optimize the VOR (and possibly OKN) and minimize retinal slip. Direct destruction of the flocculus (or its indirect elimination through contralateral dorsal cap lesions) leaves, after compensation of initial imbalance (drift), the VOR largely intact, but decreases the possibility for visual direction-selective signals to modulate the VOR and also decreases optokinetic responses alone. It is difficult to see why such complex additional cerebellar circuits would have been developed unless they provide the system with a capability for long-term adaptation and recalibration (see Chap. 6).

5.8 Modeling of the Rabbit's Optokinetic System

The relatively advanced state of understanding of the input-output relations and functions has invited many attempts to construct partial mathematical or electronic models of the oculomotor system (e.g., Robinson,

1971, 1975, 1977a). Such models are not meant to replicate nervous circuits in hardware, nor on the other hand to simply reproduce an input-output relation by an arbitrary circuit in a black box. Rather, the intention of modeling is to improve our understanding of signal processing, and particularly to reveal what kind of processes and transformations should be searched for in the nervous system. Several years ago (Collewijn, 1972b) an analog model was developed to account for some of the input-output relations of the rabbit's OKN, particularly the gain as a function of stimulus velocity and time. The principal merit of this model (Fig. 67) was to show that the input provided by the retinal direction selective elements could be transformed to the known oculomotor output by a few linear, conceptually simple operations. The properties of the velocity detectors were simulated by two differentiating circuits, connected in parallel. One branch represented the on-off type direction-selective retinal units. Its output was proportional to the velocity (voltage change) of the input up to $10°/s$ and saturated at that level for higher velocities. The second branch mimicked the on-type direction selective units. It had a maximum output for an input between $0.1°$ and $0.5°/s$ and was entirely unresponsive to input velocities of $3.5°/s$ and higher. The outputs of the two branches were added to obtain a total velocity signal in which the contribution of the on-off units was reduced by a factor 0.3 to comply with the open-loop gain as a function of velocity (Oyster et al., 1972). Further processing consisted of two stages of integration. One of these was pure integration, needed to transform the slip-velocity signal into a position signal as found to be coded at the motoneuron level. We do not know how this neuronal integrator works or where it is exactly situated, although the paramedian pontine reticular formation seems a likely place (see Robinson, 1975). This integrator was provided with a reset mechanism as a crude analog to the generation of fast phases. A second integrating stage (with a proportional bypass) was introduced into the circuit to simulate the slow build-up of slow phase velocities larger than a few $°/s$ and also optokinetic afternystagmus. This leaky integrator had a time constant of 30 s. As a further element, a delay of 100 ms was incorporated. The optokinetic loop was closed by connecting the output of the final integrator to the input stage. If this connection was omitted, the model simulated open-loop OKN. The performance of the model for a constant velocity input in closed-loop conditions (traditional OKN) is illustrated in Fig. 68. Apart from the overall input-output relations (which are satisfactory) the total velocity signal representing the activity of the direction-selective elements is of interest. It is a nonlinear function of retinal slip velocity and may indicate the type of signals which can be expected when an attempt is made to record from velocity coded neurons (e.g., the NOT) during OKN in an alert animal. The model also correctly simulates the responses to sinusoidal motion stimuli,

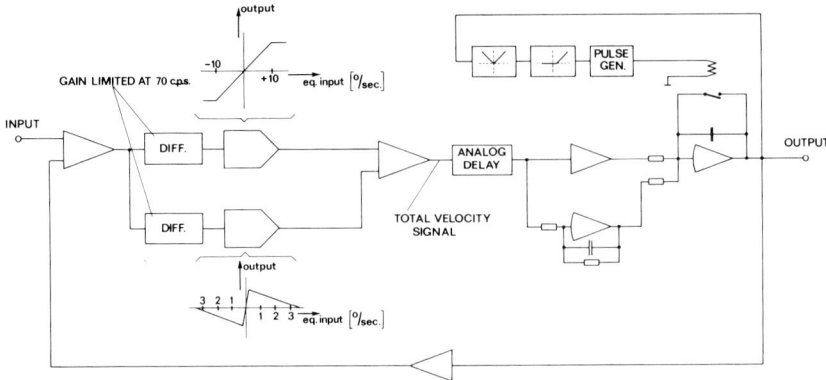

Fig. 67. A simple model to simulate the input-output relations of OKN. (Collewijn, 1972b)

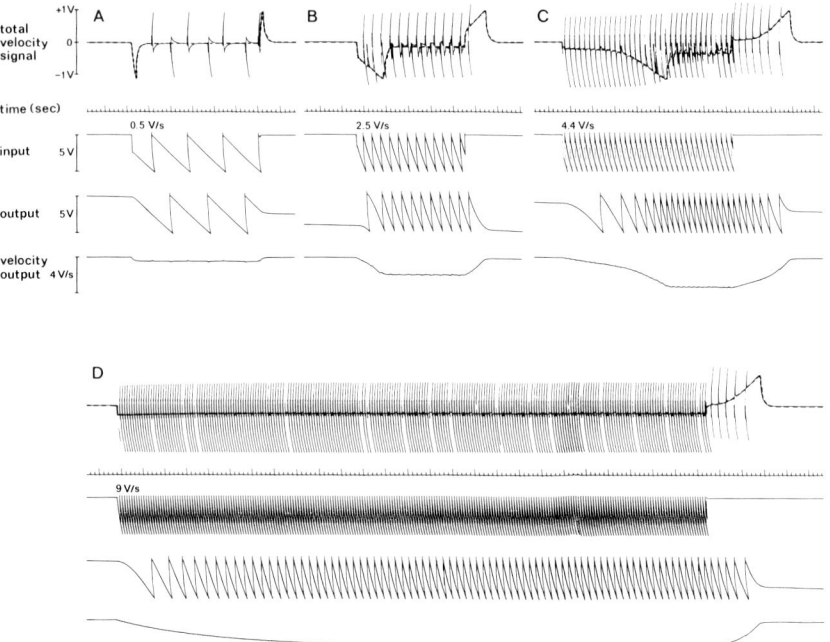

Fig. 68. Output of the model (Fig. 67) for various steady stimulus velocities. The "total velocity" signal and the velocity of the output are also shown. (Collewijn, 1972b)

specifically the rapid decrease in gain without significant changes in phase for higher frequencies and amplitudes.

Although the general form of the input-output relations for OKN is correctly simulated, the model contains one serious flaw: the high open-loop gain (which can reach 100) results in very high closed loop gains (about 0.99) for low stimulus velocities, while such a high gain is usually not found in the rabbit. This difficulty was already alluded to in the discussion of open-loop OKN (see Chap. 4.4).

A conceptually related model accounting for the build-up and afternystagmus was recently proposed by Cohen et al. (1977). Robinson (1977a) introduced a model in which OKN and VOR have been integrated. A major difference from Collewijn's (1972b) model is the replacement of the integrator with the long time constant by an internal positive feedback loop which carries an efference copy of eye velocity. This loop, which must have a gain slightly below 1.0 to prevent instability, could account for many properties of OKN, VOR, OKAN, and circularvection. Robinson (1977b) has succesfully applied his model to data of Waespe and Henn (1977a) to show a linear addition of optokinetic and vestibular signals in the vestibular nucleus.

A further flaw of the old model (Collewijn, 1972b) is the exponential decay of afternystagmus, created by the leaky integrator, which we now know to be incorrect for the rabbit (Chap. 4.6).

6. Adaptation and its Limits

A fundamental property of the nervous system is its capability to learn, i.e., to modify its responses in such a way that they are most adequate with respect to the stimuli, according to certain criteria. In the case of the oculomotor reflexes concerned with stabilization of gaze the criterion for optimal performance might well be the absence of more than a minimal amount of retinal image slip when the animal moves around. Since compensatory eye movements are controlled by several sensory systems through complex circuits, many parameters have to be correctly set for a reliable performance, just to name a few: (a) the overall system should be in balance, i.e., no systematic drift in one direction should occur, otherwise the animal will have a spontaneous nystagmus; (b) the gain and phase of the VOR should be neither too large nor too small, which could easily be the case since the VOR is a feed-forward system without direct feed-back from the eye movements to the labyrinth; (c) the gain of the OKN should be adequate to complement the VOR; (d) adequate interaction should exist between canal-ocular, maculo-ocular, optokinetic, and cervico-ocular responses.

Even if genetic planning were perfect, these systems could not function adequately throughout a lifetime if no adjustments were possible. The systems depend on the functioning of thousands of hair-cells, neurons and muscle fibers, and all of these are affected by growth, disease, trauma, and aging. In recent years, a large number of investigations have been devoted to adaptive processes in the oculomotor system. Adaptive changes in these experiments have been provoked mostly by radical changes in the input signals, or by lesions. The ontogenetic development has also been manipulated at critical stages, e.g., by light deprivation after birth. In some cases genetic defects, such as the neuronal wiring defects in albinism, offer a clue to the capacities and limits of adaptation.

We have seen that the cerebellum is connected in parallel to the essential oculomotor control circuits. The vestibulocerebellum has a major output to the vestibular nuclei and receives all the relevant inputs, among then the direction-selective retinal slip signals. The hypothesis that the cerebellum is important in optimally setting the system's parameters is very attractive and has received considerable support, but on the other hand the unraveling of the causes and effects and the nature of the changes at the neuronal and synaptic level has proven to be an enormously complex task.

As I have not directly investigated the neuronal mechanism of adaptation, I shall restrict this chapter mainly to a discussion of the phenomenology of adaptivity (and maladaptivity) as found in the rabbit's compensatory eye movements.

6.1 Unilateral Labyrinthectomy

The effects of the sudden loss of one labyrinth have been known for a century (Bechterew, 1883). They essentially consist of an imbalance in all vestibular control circuits due to the unilateral deafferentiation. These acute phenomena subside in a period of days to weeks (depending on the species) and a reasonable equilibrium is restored. This compensation is a beautiful example of functional adaptivity. Characteristics of this compensation have been reviewed by Precht (1974) and Schaefer and Meyer (1974). Compared to the extensive knowledge on the compensation of the imbalance, little is known about the dynamic performance of vestibular reflexes when the acute symptoms have disappeared. We have studied the VOR elicited by sinusoidal oscillation in the compensated stage after unilateral labyrinthectomy in the rabbit (Baarsma and Collewijn, 1975b). The left labyrinth was destroyed in seven rabbits using a lateral approach. The effects were as described by Winkler (1907) and Magnus (1924). In the acute stage there was a vigorous nystagmus (slow phase to the left), rotation of the head to the left side around both the sagittal (roll) and vertical axis, and the whole animal rolled spontaneously to the left side. The rolling and nystagmus disappeared gradually within a few days. However, the rabbits showed several permanent symptoms: (1) a spiral rotation of the body toward the left side, in particular of the head on the trunk, but also of the thorax on the pelvis; (2) hypertonic and extended right legs, hypotonic left legs; (3) tonic deviation of the eyes: right eye upward and forward, left eye downward and backward. These phenomena persisted undiminished until the final measurements, which were made 6 months after labyrinthectomy. The total persistent head rotation around the sagittal axis was usually about 90° to the left (right ear upwards). For the measurements the head was immobilized in the normal upright position. The average resting position of the right eye (which was always recorded) was displaced 20°-25° anterior to the normal resting position. These permanent biases to the left in posture of head, body, and eyes indicate that compensation is only partial in the rabbit, even in the static situation.

With the eyes covered, drift was either absent or very slow (0.05°-0.20°/s) and directed to the *right* side. Oscillation of the animals in darkness produced a VOR of a normal shape but subnormal magnitude. Gain and phase for a number of amplitudes are shown in Fig. 69 (averages for seven rabbits). For comparison, the results obtained under the same circumstances with normal rabbits are also shown (Baarsma and Collewijn, 1974). In the hemi-

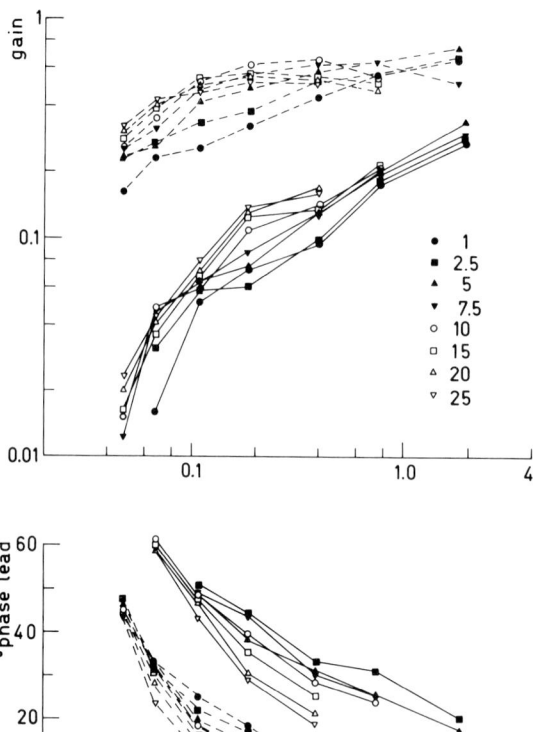

Fig. 69. Gain and phase of VOR in darkness, as a function of frequency of sinusoidal stimulus. *Solid lines* 6 months after destruction of left labyrinth (average of seven rabbits). *Interrupted lines* normal rabbits (average of 17 rabbits). (Baarsma and Collewijn, 1975b)

labyrinthectomized rabbits VOR gain was lowered throughout the frequency range; the difference with normals was highly significant ($p < 0.001$). For the operated animals the average gain varied from 0.02 at the lowest frequency (0.05 Hz) to 0.34 at the highest one (1.8 Hz); for normal rabbits the comparable values were 0.16 and 0.75. Phase was advanced at least 20° more than in normal rabbits throughout the whole frequency range, thus the eye movements showed a phase lead even at 1.8 Hz. Moran (1974) has observed similar phase shifts in hemilabyrinthectomized cats. For the lowest amplitudes and frequencies reliable measurements could not always be obtained, but no evidence for a true threshold was found. Directional asymmetry was expressed as

$$\frac{R - L}{R + L}$$

in which R is the peak-to-peak amplitude of the sinusoidal eye movement while the eye moves from the maximal left to the maximal right deviation and L is the amplitude of the smooth movement in the left direction. Any saccades were eliminated before this calculation by reconstructing the cumulative slow phase.

While normal animals show no systematic directional preference (overall asymmetry −0.01, statistically not significant) the hemilabyrinthectomized rabbits showed an average asymmetry of +0.14 to the right (healthy) side. The difference from normals was significant ($p < 0.04$).

Visuo-vestibular interaction was tested by repeating the stimulus program with the eyes open and a structured visual background. As shown in Fig. 70,

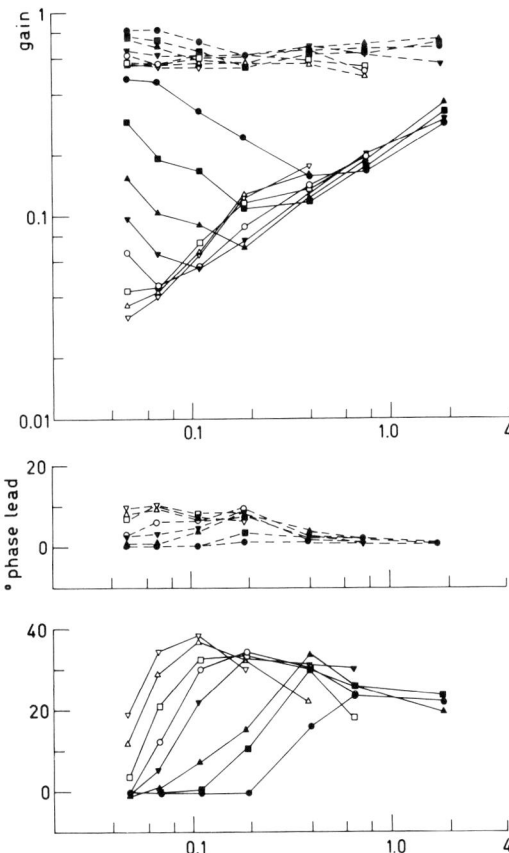

Fig. 70. Gain and phase of compensatory eye movements as a function of the frequency of the passive oscillation in stationary, illuminated surroundings. *Solid lines* 6 months after destruction of left labyrinth. *Interrupted lines* normal rabbits. Same animals as in Fig. 69. (Baarsma and Collewijn, 1975b)

the responses were only moderately improved by this procedure. For comparison, results in normal rabbits (Baarsma and Collewijn, 1974) are shown again. Only for the low frequencies and amplitudes are the synergic responses markedly better than the vestibular responses in darkness. A comparison with Fig. 34 A will show that in normal rabbits even OKN alone has a higher gain for the low frequencies than the combined VOR and OKN in labyrinthectomized animals. Although OKN was not tested in these rabbits, these results strongly suggest that not only bilateral (Chap. 5.6) but also unilateral labyrinthectomy induces an impairment of OKN.

The detrimental effect upon the VOR is unexpectedly large. The remaining VOR has a gain which is less than half the normal value, although the input has only been reduced by a factor of 2. The increase in phase as well cannot be explained by the decreased sensory input, thus there must be a dramatic change in the central processing of the vestibular (and probably visual) signals. Specifically, the function of the neuronal integrator, which transforms the vestibular velocity signal into a position signal (Skavenski and Robinson, 1973), could be disorganized by the elimination of the tonic discharge of a labyrinth. As an analogy, Robinson's (1974) finding may be quoted that the time constant of the vestibulo-ocular integrator in the cat decreases from the normal value of over 20 s to only 1.3 s after cerebellectomy. Unfortunately in our rabbits the time constant of the neuronal integrator was not tested in other situations, e.g., OKN and postrotatory nystagmus.

Labyrinthectomy is known to depress the activity of the ipsilateral vestibular nuclei. Some long-term recovery occurs, but even in the compensated stage both maintained discharge and modulation of type I neurons remain considerably below normal in the cat (Precht et al., 1966). Comparable data for the rabbit are unavailable, but in view of the persistent postural defects the situation may be worse. Compensatory mechanisms in the rabbit are barely sufficient to restore a stable posture and eye position, with considerable permanent deviation of the resting position to the defective side. In darkness as well drift is minimal. These drift and response asymmetries were to the right, i.e., opposite to the direction of the nystagmus immediately after labyrinthectomy. Clearly, no adjustment could be made to restore the dynamic response of the VOR to a normal level. This indicates that adaptation of the eye movement control systems in the rabbit is limited. In this respect unilateral loss of a labyrinth cannot be considered a highly unusual demand on the system, as this condition occurs rather frequently as a result of pathological processes. The rabbit may be exceptional in this respect and it will be important to test the input-output properties of the reflex in species which seem to recover better from a unilateral labyrinthal lesion, e.g., the cat, monkey, and man (see Schaefer and Meyer, 1974).

There are strong indications that balance control is relatively independent of the cerebellum (Schaefer and Meyer, 1974; Haddad et al., 1977) although in the rat the inferior olive has been reported to be essential for the acquisition and retention of balance after unilateral labyrinthectomy (Llinás et al., 1975).

6.2 Dark-Rearing

Compensatory eye movements are made in the interest of stable vision. In complete darkness, the VOR is elicited but it is functionally meaningless, and no visual feedback with regard to its efficacy is available. The OKN is of course absent in darkness. It is of great interest to know how the VOR and OKN develop in animals deprived of visual feedback for an extended period after birth. Dark-rearing has been a frequently used paradigm recently and is known to have profound effects on the visual system. Earlier generations of investigators have also seen this problem and observations on dark-reared rabbits were reported as early as 1924 by Nasiell. By visual inspection, he concluded that after three weeks dark-rearing, rabbits had no spontaneous nystagmus and qualitatively normal vestibulo-ocular reflexes. Mowrer (1936b) reared pigeons in darkness for 5-6 weeks. Within the limits of his recording techniques he found no adverse effects on the VOR, but a marked depression of OKN, which recovered within 3 days of normal vision.

Van Hof-Van Duin (1976a) found that the development of visually observable OKN took 5-9 days in kittnes dark-reared for 4 months and 19-27 days after dark-rearing for 7 months.

The effect of dark-rearing was recently investigated (Collewijn, 1977c) with precise measurement of eye movements. The methods for raising rabbits in darkness have been developed in our department by Dr. M.W. van Hof (Van Hof and Kobayashi, 1972), who also kindly provided the animals used in this study. Litters of pigmented Dutch rabbits were raised in absolute darkness from about 7 days after birth (before the opening of the eyes) till the age of 7 months.

As a control group eight normal rabbits (N) were raised under ordinary lighting conditions (12 h light, 12 h dark). Food, care and housing were identical to those for the dark-reared (D) rabbits.

The normally reared controls were subjected to the same tests at an age of about 10 months.

The data obtained from the eight normal animals were in close agreement with the usual findings in our laboratory as described before. Repeated measurements indicated that response characteristics differend considerably among animals but were remarkably constant for one and the same rabbit.

The responses in the dark-reared animals proved to be qualitatively similar but of subnormal magnitude. When measured for the first time, with the eyes still covered, the spontaneous eye movements of dark-reared rabbits showed no clear abnormalities. A certain amount of random, slow drift as is usual in darkness was observed. No spontaneous nystagmus was ever present, in agreement with Nasiell (1924). When the eyes were uncovered and the illumination level gradually raised, no spectacular reactions occurred. The animals remained quiet and the eyes were kept normally opened. The pupils were of normal size. Blink reflexes were elicited by a little spot light. The amount of drift was reduced and at the final illumination level of 15 cd/m^2 the eyes were rather well stabilized, though in many cases the remaining slow drift (up to 0.2°/s) was larger than in most normal rabbits.

6.2.1 Responses to Sinusoidal Movement in Darkness (VOR)

In a dark-reared animal with the eyes still covered, vestibulo-ocular responses were immediately elicited when the oscillation of the torsion swing was started. As in a normal animal (Fig. 71 N), the responses consisted of a mixture of smooth and saccadic movements (Fig. 71 D, O). The only obvious difference from normals was the small response amplitude found for all frequencies. The averaged data for gain and phase as a function of frequency for eight N and five D-rabbits at different times after light deprivation are shown in Fig. 72. In normals gain varied between about 0.6 for the lower and 0.8 for the higher frequencies, with a phase lead of about 25° for 0.1 Hz decreasing to about 0° between 1 ans 2 Hz, on the average. The responses of dark-reared rabbits before exposure to the light (marked 0) had a gain between about 0.15 and 0.35, with a similar function of frequency as in normals. In contrast to this defect in gain, phase relations were practically normal. The responses were sustained and completely repeatable; no habituation was evident.

In the subsequent period of normal exposure to light, some recovery of gain toward normal values was seen. Even after only 2 h of vision, the gain was already shifted upward (Fig. 72, 2h) and after 1 day (Fig. 72, 1d) the improvement was substantial. This trend continued at a lower rate in the following period (Fig. 71 D, 3m; Fig. 72, 3m). Values for VOR gain and phase, averaged over all animals and frequencies, as a function of time are shown in Fig. 73 (black columns). Gain was initially very low (0.25 ± 0.13 S.D.) with rapid improvement in the first few days and then a much slower one in the following months to 0.49 ± 0.16 (S.D.) on the average, in contrast to 0.73 ± 0.17 (S.D.) for the normals. Abnormalities and changes in phase, on the other hand, appear to be minor and limited to a few degrees.

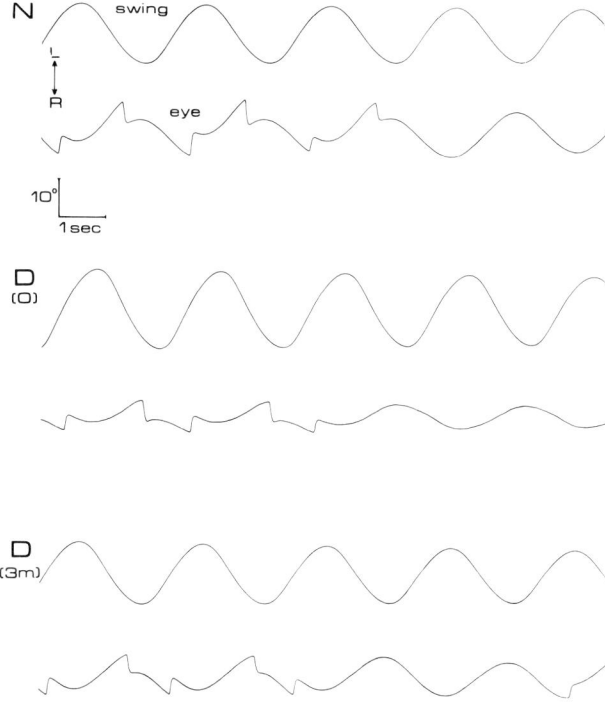

Fig. 71. VOR elicited by passive sinusoidal oscillation in darkness. Position of platform (*swing, upper traces*) and eye in head (*lower traces*) are shown. N normal rabbits; D (O) first recording after 7 months light deprivation; D (3m) same animal after 3 months in normal lighting conditions. (Collewijn, 1977c)

Analysis of variance showed that the subnormality of gain was significant ($p < 0.01$ up to 7 days, $p < 0.05$ for 1 and 3 months), as well as the improvement of gain with time ($p = 0.6 \times 10^{-5}$). The small increase in phase lead with respect to normals was not significant at time 0 and 1 h, but significant ($p < 0.01$) thereafter. In three animals in which only a smaller frequency range was examined, similar effects were observed. In these three animals values after 6 months of normal light exposure were also obtained; they were no better than after 3 months. It appears therefore that further improvement in gain after 3 months or even 1 month (Fig. 73) is negligible.

6.2.2 Responses to Sinusoidal Movement with Eyes Open (VOR and OKN)

In the normal animals, rotation of the head with vision resulted in a substantially better stabilization of the eye than by the VOR alone. Gain was

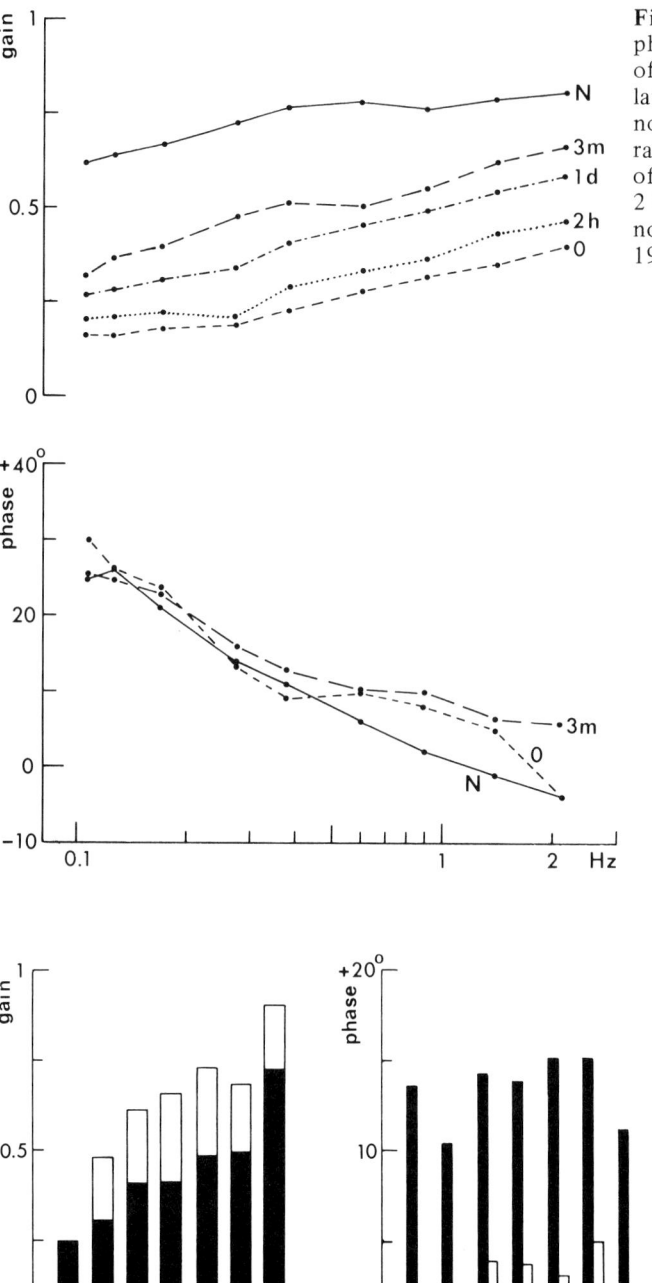

Fig. 72. Average gain and phase of VOR as a function of frequency of passive oscillation in darkness for eight normal and five dark-reared rabbits measured at the end of dark-rearing (*O*) and after 2 h, 1 day, and 3 months of normal vision. (Collewijn, 1977c)

Fig. 73. Average gain and phase of VOR in darkness (*black columns*) and in light (VOR and OKN in synergy, *open columns*). (Collewijn, 1977c)

almost flat (between about 0.75 and 0.85) over the tested frequency range and phase errors were only a few degrees (Fig. 74 N).

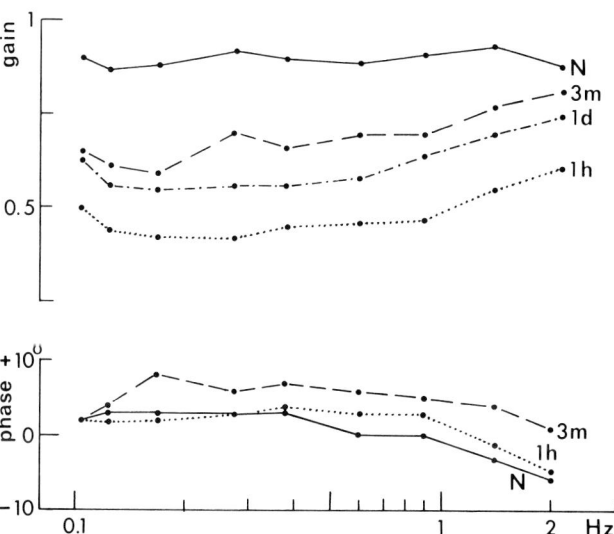

Fig. 74. Average gain and phase of vestibulo-ocular reflexes as a function of frequency, measured with eyes open in light (VOR and OKN in synergy). *Symbols* as in Fig. 72. (Collewijn, 1977c)

A similar improvement in the VOR with vision was seen in the dark-reared rabbits, but here again the response level was subnormal. The first test of this combined response, after about 1 h of normal vision, had an average gain of 0.48 ± 0.15 (S.D.) (Fig. 74, 1h; Fig. 73, open columns) and normal phase relation. In the subsequent time, especially in the first week of light exposure, the averaged gain improved to 0.73 ± 0.11 (S.D.) after 1 month (Fig. 73) with no further improvement (even some decrease) after 3 months. In the normal animals, the average gain was 0.90 ± 0.14 (S.D.). The subnormality of gain and its improvement with time were again statistically significant. The difference in gain between the conditions "eyes covered" and "eyes open" was remarkably constant for the normals and dark-reared animals at all times (average difference 0.20 ± 0.03 (S.D.); no statistically significant effect of time or group).

A small, but statistically significant ($p < 0.01$) increase in phase lead compared to normals was again present from the first day after exposure to light (Fig. 73).

6.2.3 Optokinetic Nystagmus

In all 14 dark-reared rabbits, OKN could be elicited immediately when the animals were exposed to normal illumination for the first time. Figure 75 A illustrates these first responses in one rabbit for both eyes and both

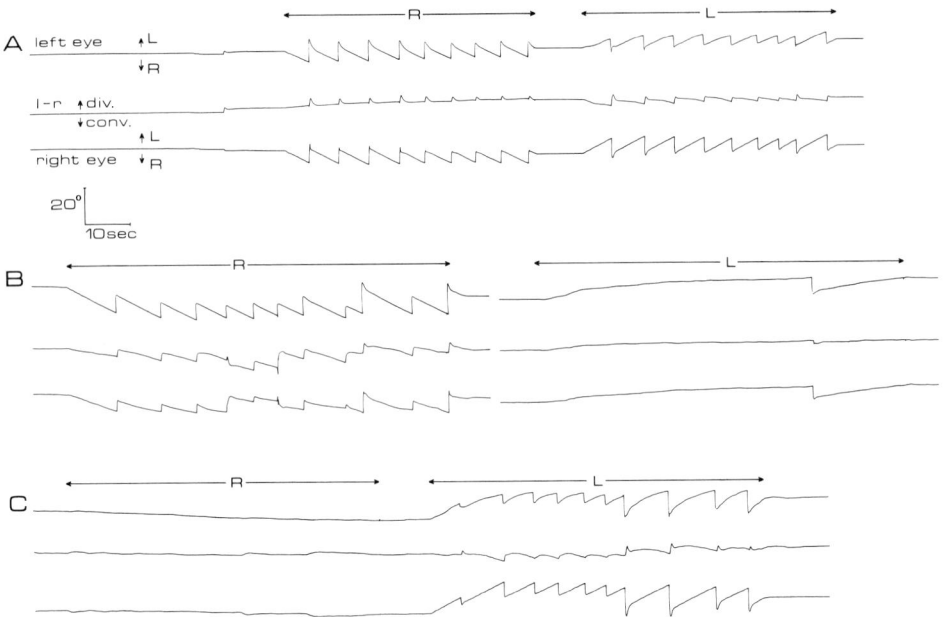

Fig. 75. First recordings of optokinetic nystagmus after dark-rearing for 7 months, immediately after first exposure to light. **A** initial responses to rotation of the drum to the right and left (as indicated by *horizontal arrows*) at 1.2°/s. Movements of left and right eye and their difference (vergence) have been recorded. Both eyes opened. Normal pattern of smooth and saccadic components. The eye which sees forward motion is usually performing slightly better than the crossed eye. **B** same animal, a few minutes later with the right eye covered. The seeing (left) eye reacts only to anterior motion. The covered eye is driven, though at a lower amplitude. **C** as **B** but with the left eye covered and the right eye free. (Collewijn, 1977c)

directions of rotation at a stimulus velocity of 1.2°/s. When the drum was started there was an immediate slow pursuit, interrupted by a normal sequence of fast phases in the opposite direction (roughly toward the midposition). Slow and fast phases were perfectly coordinated and apparently normal. The coordination between the two eyes was also normal. The reactions were sustained, also with a stimulus of long duration or high velocity; there was no evidence of habituation or abnormal fatiguability of OKN. In the normal rabbit, for each eye apart anterior movement is much more effective than posterior movement in producing OKN (Chap. 4.5). This direction preference is also present in dark-reared rabbits, as shown in Fig. 75 B and C, where the right or left eye was covered. Each eye reacted exclusively to movement in the anterior direction. The covered eye was driven by the seeing eye, but the coupling was less than perfect as revealed by the smaller movements of the driven eye and the differential trace. Thus, the eye movements were not entirely conjugate. Even with both eyes open, the most adequately stimulated eye usually showed a larger response (Fig. 75 A). However, this finding is in no way specific for dark-reared rabbits since the same phenomenon has been found in normal animals (Chap. 4.5). Gain of the OKN, averaged over eight animals and two directions of rotation as a function of stimulus velocity, is shown in Fig. 76. In the N-rabbits, optokinetic

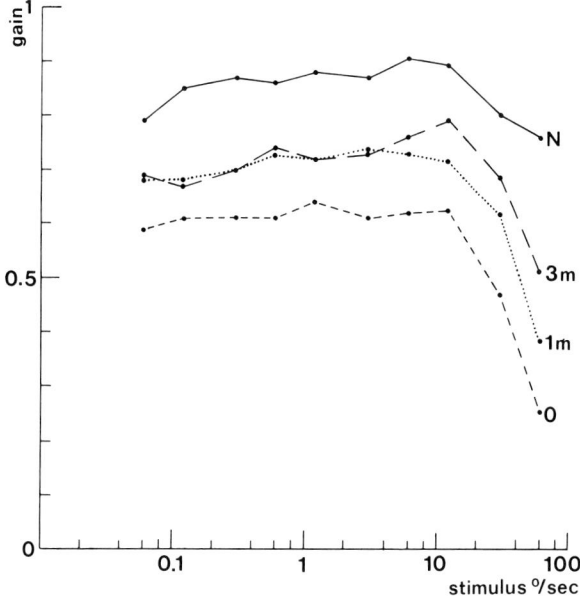

Fig. 76. Average optokinetic gain as a function of stimulus velocity for eight normal (N) and eight dark-reared rabbits immediately after first exposure to light (*O*) and after 1 and 3 months of normal vision. (Collewijn, 1977c)

gains between 0.8 and 0.9 were reached if sufficient stimulus duration was allowed, with the exception of the highest stimulus velocities (30° and 60°/s). The normal gain averaged over all animals, directions, and velocities was 0.85 ± 0.20 (S.D.). As shown in Fig. 76 (graph O), a response of essentially the same shape, but at a lower level, was obtained immediately after light deprivation. The overall average gain in these first OKN responses was 0.56 ± 0.23 (S.D.). Although there is apparently some overlap between these data and those of normals, the difference proved to be statistically highly significant ($p = 0.6 \times 10^{-3}$).

When measured again after 1 month, gain had recovered to an overall average of 0.67 ± 0.23 (S.D.). Figure 76 (1m) shows that this improvement was present at all velocities. The difference from normals was still significant ($p = 0.018$). After 3 months (Fig. 76, 3m), further improvement was slight. Average gain was now 0.70 ± 0.20 (S.D.), still significantly below normal ($p = 0.02$). The improvement of gain with time in the D-animals was also significant ($p = 0.003$). In three of the eight chronically implanted D-rabbits, OKN gain was also measured 1 week after the end of light deprivation. In these animals all improvement in gain was achieved within the first week and no further increase occurred in the next 3 months. The gradual build-up of higher slow phase velocities as well as OKN in dark-reared rabbits proved to be similar to those in normal rabbits.

These experiments reveal a limited sensitivity to light deprivation in the rabbit's oculomotor reflexes. Apparently, the presence of vision is not essential to the development of canal-ocular and optokinetic reflexes, since these were operational after dark-rearing for 7 months after birth. In many respects the reactions were entirely normal, in particular the integrated pattern of fast and smooth components, the overall shape of gain and phase as a function of velocity and frequency, the direction preference of each eye and the largely conjugate character of eye movements. Since no qualitative abnormalities were found, apparently no fundamental changes in the elements and wiring of these reflexes had occurred.

However, some quantitative defects, which were restored only in part by 3-6 months of normal visual experience, were evident. These defects were most clear in the VOR, which had an average gain about 1/3 of normal values, with an eventual recovery to about 2/3 of normal. Since the vestibulo-oculo reflex arc normally operates in a feed-forward (open loop) fashion, there being no immediate feedback from the eye movements to the labyrinth, this reflex is essentially quite vulnerable. After prolonged absence of visual feedback, as in dark-rearing, the VOR gain might take some arbitrary value, according to the bias of the system. A part of the present results may be explained in this way. However, as long as only long-term adaptation is involved, one might expect a complete normalization once the VOR becomes relevant and visually corregible. Actually, after light deprivation VOR gain is improved by a factor of 2 within a month or so, but apparently no further correction of the significant remaining defect occurs (Fig. 73). This may indicate that part of the vestibulo-ocular circuitry does not develop or is permanently lost due to light deprivation; the partial recovery could be explained by a functional restoration of connections which were not irretrievably lost and/or the normal capabilities for adaptation. Presumably the defect will be specific for the vestibulo-ocular reflex, since the other postural reflexes derived from vestibular input must be heavily used in the light-deprived condition. It would be highly interesting to measure the performance of vestibulo-spinal reflexes (e.g., stabilization of the head) in dark-reared animals. Berthoz et al. (1975) have measured a variety of vestibulo-ocular responses in visually deprived kittens. Though their use of the electro-oculogram did not allow firm quantitative conclusions, their observations (e.g., a deficit of fast phases) strongly suggested a decreased gain, in agreement with the present results.

The optokinetic reflex functions as a negative feedback (closed loop) system with an open loop gain of the order of 10 over a large part of the velocity range and is therefore inherently less vulnerable. Therefore, even a considerable loss of connections in the optokinetic circuit might not show up clearly in the closed-loop performance of the system. Actually, the results show a statistically significant decrease of OKN gain, but the deficit is much smaller than for the VOR.

In this case as well, visual experience is followed by an improvement but no complete normalization of the gain. Open-loop measurements, which might reveal larger defects of the circuit, have not as yet been made.

Vital-Durand et al. (1974) could elicit OKN in kittens immediately after dark-rearing for 15-19 weeks after birth. These animals had a sustained OKN in all directions except downward, while normal controls only displayed a few saccades at the onset of a new stimulus. Although a precise measurement of gain was not achieved in these kittens, these results, in agreement with the present findings, do not indicate a profound defect of OKN after dark-rearing such as reported by Mowrer (1936b) for pigeons. As usual, the possibility of species differences has to be considered. Such differences are also indicated by the results reported for rearing with unidirectional motion vision. Biasing of the OKN in one direction was readily achieved in the cat (Vital-Durand and Jeannerod, 1974), while in the rabbit (Daw and Wyatt, 1974) the effects on OKN were very small and the distribution of retinal direction-selective elements was not affected. This is in agreement with the present finding that in the rabbit the normal direction preference of each eye for anterior (temporal to nasal) motion is preserved after dark-rearing. As discussed before (Chap. 4.5) in the cat, a similar direction preference, which is absent in the normal animal (Braun and Gault, 1969), can be produced by monocular lid closure (Van Hof-Van Duin, 1976b) and by removal of the visual cortex (Wood et al., 1973). In the rabbit, OKN is hardly affected by cortical ablations (Ter Braak, 1936; Hobbelen and Collewijn, 1971). These findings indicate that a symmetrical optokinetic reaction of each eye as found in the cat is dependent on cortical processing of binocular visual information, which is known to be severely affected by monocular deprivation (Wiesel and Hubel, 1963). At the cortical level, biasing of the direction preference of single units by rearing in a unidirectionally moving environment has been readily achieved in the cat (Daw and Wyatt, 1976) in contrast to the negative results in the rabbit (Daw and Wyatt, 1974). Unfortunately, a monocular test of OKN in binocularly deprived or unidirectionally exposed cats has not been reported. The optokinetic responses in monocular deprived cats and in normal and binocularly deprived rabbits appear to be mediated by a similar subcortical pathway which is fairly resistant to visual deprivation.

The possibility that the decreases of VOR and OKN could be explained by some defect in the extra-ocular muscles seems remote. Firstly, it is not evident how such a muscular defect could originate without a prior nervous defect, and secondly, the normal aspect of saccadic movements and the equal distribution of the defect over the whole range of pursuit velocities argues strongly against muscular weakness as a cause.

An important question is whether the quantitative defects of ocular stabilization had any effects on the animal's behavior. Our observations in this respect are quite casual and limited to the unnatural conditions of an animal room, but a paucity of active locomotor behavior compared to normal animals was quite obvious in the first weeks of exposure to light. Van Hof and Kobayashi (1972) trained similar dark-reared rabbits in a visual discrimination task. Their rabbits needed 3-4 weeks more than normal animals to become familiar with the discrimination box and develop the necessary visuomotor dexterity. After this period, learning of pattern discrimination was normal except for a defect in visual acuity. Although decreased ocular stability (with partial recovery) could be a causative factor in these defects, it seems more likely that visuomotor coordination in general is not functioning at a normal level of performance in dark-reared animals. It must be concluded that dark-rearing does have deleterious effects on later capabilities to use visual information, even in the simplest ocular stabilization reflexes.

6.3 Long-Term Adaptation of VOR and OKN

As we have seen, the VOR and OKN each has its own working range within the total range of head movement frequencies and velocities, but the two systems show a complementary action when functioning in synergy. The result is a fairly constant gain and small phase error through the physiological frequency range. This immediate interaction has been approximated by a linear, vectorial addition of the responses of the two systems (Batini et al., 1979).

In addition to this direct interaction, a long-term modulation of the VOR by visual slip signals has been postulated. Ito (1972) pointed out the need for such an adjustment. The VOR in its simplest form is a feed-forward system, in which the sense organ (the labyrinth) is not informed about the output (the eye movements). It seems unlikely that such a system could operate optimally under all circumstances, since external disturbances and changes in the parameters of the control system will occur.

A common reason for recalibration in man is the wearing of corrective glasses. These reduce or magnify the world and also the eye movements needed to compensate correctly for a head movement. The need for recalibration of the VOR when refraction is corrected was already clearly pointed out by Rönne in 1923. Ito (1972) specifically postulated that the parameters of the VOR are corrected by the cerebellar flocculus, which receives vestibular and visual input and projects to the vestibular nuclei (Chap. 5). These circuits would not only be involved in immediate interaction, but also in a long-term learning process. As a consequence the input-output properties of the VOR alone, operating in darkness, would reflect the effects of the previous history of the system in terms of visual slip.

The existence of this type of long-term modification has been supported by a variety of experiments in several species, although the neuronal processes involved are still somewhat elusive.

It appears fairly likely that the flocculus and its connections are involved (Ito et al., 1974b; Ito and Miyashita, 1975; Ito, 1977; Robinson, 1976). There may also be good reasons for extending the hypothesis. Since the VOR and OKN operate as an integrated system, the OKN loop may also show adaptivity. The effect of long-term visual stimulation alone (without simultaneous head movements) on OKN and/or VOR has hardly been investigated. It is also insufficiently known whether adaptation is generalized or somehow specific for the conditioning motion stimulus.

However, before we even try to visually modify the VOR, we should know what the effects of long-term stimulation of the VOR alone are, as we have to establish a baseline for evaluating possible visually induced modifications.

6.3.1 Adaptive Phenomena in the VOR

For a long time it has been known that repeated testing of the VOR by certain types of stimuli may lead to a response decline. A progressive decrease in the duration and amplitude of nystagmus induced by repeated unidirectional rotation (velocity steps) was already noticed by early investigators (Abels, 1906; Griffith, 1920; Dodge, 1923). Collins (1964) found a 30% decline in slow phase velocity in postrotatory nystagmus in man after

200 unidirectional rotations in the dark. These changes have been confirmed for man (Guedry, 1965; Dix and Hood, 1969), cat (Crampton, 1962; Collins and Updegraff, 1966) and dog (Collins and Updegraff, 1966). More recently, it has been shown that the time constant of postrotatory nystagmus in the monkey is progressively shortened by repeated velocity steps (Blair and Gavin, 1979). On first glance these observations are somewhat puzzling, as we know that the VOR continues to operate throughout life and a progressive decline of gain to repeated head movements should result in virtual elimination of the VOR. However, these results were obtained for velocity steps in the dark, which are presumably very unphysiological stimuli. All natural head movements consist of brief rotations with successive accelerations in two opposite directions. It is more likely that outside the laboratory, stimulus patterns associated with post-rotatory nystagmus would be due to pathology (unreliable signals of hair cells) rather than to a head movement. Therefore, the gradual elimination of responses to such stimuli may represent a useful mechanism. A different situation occurs when an animal or human subject is rotated at a constant velocity and stopped *with vision* in stationary surroundings. Although such a stimulus is not very common, it is coped with by ballet dancers and ice skaters in self-generated spins. The suppression of postrotatory nystagmus in such situations seems highly useful and indeed it has been found that visual fixation of the stationary world can suppress the unwanted effects of postrotational vestibular excitation (Collins, 1964, 1966, 1968; Guedry, 1965; Dix and Hood, 1969). These reactions are of course perfectly understandable in terms of gaze stabilization and, as already discussed, postrotatory nystagmus after rotation in the light is practically absent, even when the light is turned off simultaneously with the arrest of rotation (Chap. 4.6), due to the cancelling effect between postrotatory vestibular nystagmus and optokinetic afternystagmus.

In the rabbit, a response decline due to repeated rotation has been described (Hood and Pfaltz, 1954) but these experiments were apparently done in the presence of vision, while part of the surroundings was rotating with the animal.

A different question is whether the VOR elicited in darkness adapts to sinusoidal stimulation *in the physiological range*. For rotatory stimuli, this is apparently not the case. Kleinschmidt and Collewijn (1975) and Collewijn and Kleinschmidt (1975) did not find a systematic change of gain or phase at a frequency of 0.17 Hz with an amplitude of 1 or 10°. Ito et al. (1974b, 1979a) also failed to find progressive changes in the rabbit's VOR during long-term oscillation in darkness. Gonshor and Melvill Jones (1976a) found no response decline in human subjects with repeated oscillation in darkness at 1/6 Hz with a velocity amplitude of 60°/s.

However, the case may be different for rotation at very low frequencies, which are on the border of the VOR working range. For the rabbit, considerable response decline by oscillation in darkness at 0.05 Hz has been reported (Sunay et al., 1976). Recent observations in the monkey (Jäger and Henn, pers. comm. 1980) show a considerable decrease in the apparent time constant of the VOR with a similar stimulus, although such a change was absent in the light.

It is probably safe to conclude that continued stimulation of the canal-ocular reflex *in its physiological working range* in the absence of visual feedback does not lead to systematic changes in the response.

For the maculo-ocular reflex, elicited by linear oscillation (Chap. 3.4) the situation seems to be different. Kleinschmidt and Collewijn (1975) oscillated rabbits continuously in the transverse direction in darkness on a parallel swing for 24 h at a frequency of 0.35 Hz and an amplitude of 20 cm. This movement caused, in combination with gravity, a tilt of the total linear vector over 5.68° in each direction. The averaged results for eight rabbits are shown in Fig. 77. During the first swinging periods, the average ampli-

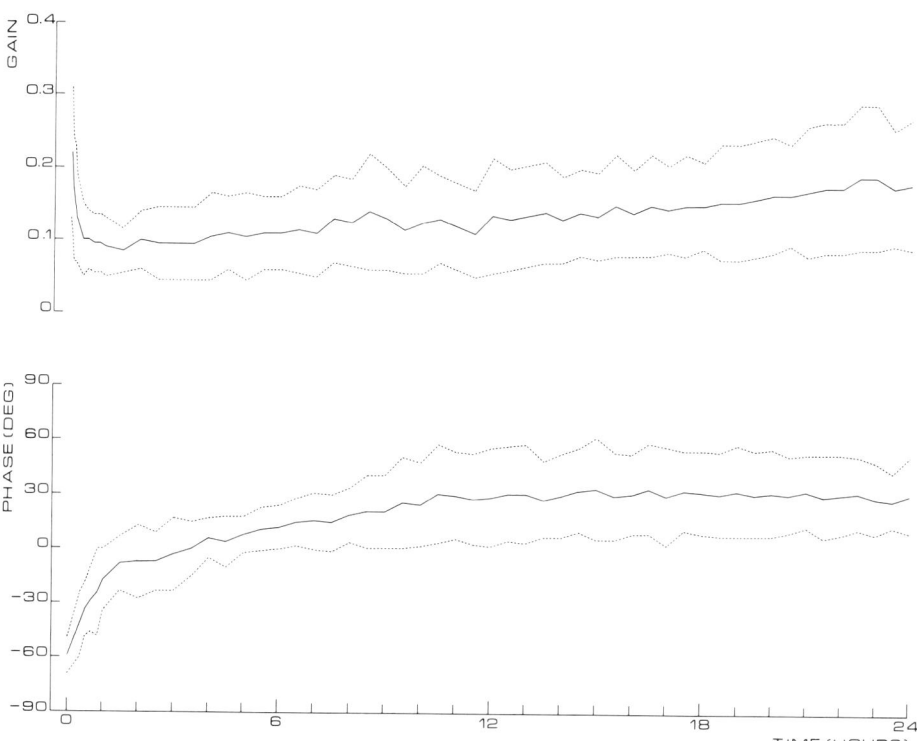

Fig. 77. Average gain and phase (*solid lines*) of maculo-ocular reflexes elicited in eight rabbits by continuous linear oscillation (0.35 Hz, amplitude 20 cm) as a function of time. The *dotted lines* indicate 1 standard deviation. (Kleinschmidt and Collewijn, 1975)

tude of the vertical eye movement was 1.25°, thus the gain was 0.22; the average phase lag was 59°. After 9 min of swinging, gain had declined to 0.13°, with a further decrease to 0.08° (about a third of the initial value) after 90 min. Thereafter, some very gradual restoration of gain was usually seen. In addition, the phase changed gradually from the initial lag of 59° to a lead of 31°, which is a total shift of 90° more lead, achieved in about 10 h. The change in phase was slower than the decline of gain, but once developed it did not recover even if the gain did (Fig. 77). In four additional rabbits, frequency specificity of these changes was tested. Continuous oscillation was done again at 0.35 Hz (for 17 h) but responses were also tested at frequencies from 0.12 to 0.62 Hz before and after this period. The changes in gain and phase proved not to be specific for the continuously applied frequency (Fig. 78). Gain had declined in the whole range tested without a clear minimum for the conditioning frequency. Phase was advanced for all frequencies; the shift was about 90° for the frequency of continuous stimu-

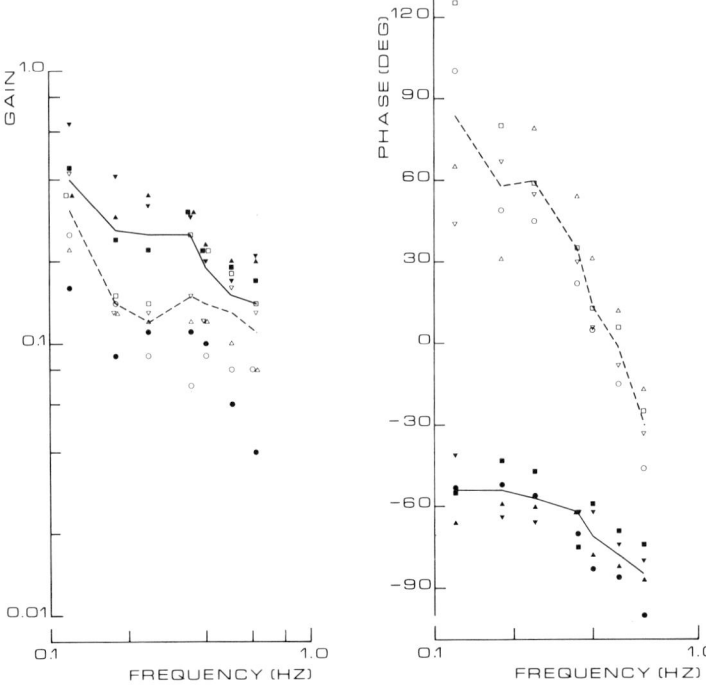

Fig. 78. Gain and phase of maculo-ocular reflexes for various stimulus frequencies before (*solid lines* and *symbols*) and after (*interrupted lines* and *open symbols*) 17 h continuous linear oscillation at 0.35 Hz (amplitude 20 cm). (Kleinschmidt and Collewijn, 1975)

lation. It was larger for lower frequencies and smaller for higher frequencies. All these changes were effected in the absence of visual feedback. Unfortunately the maculo-ocular responses to tilt in static conditions were not tested.

These changes in maculo-ocular reflexes may reflect a subtle mechanism for the elimination of undesirable eye movements. Maculo-ocular reflexes are adequate when the otolith organs are excited by tilting of the head, not when they are stimulated by linear accelerations as in running.

A forward acceleration of the head would displace the otoliths backward, which is equivalent to an upward pitch of the nose, with as a result counterrolling of both eyes (upper pole moving anterior). When the head is tilted in the frequency range as used in our experiments (0.35 Hz), the canals will be excited along with the otolith organs. Therefore, a modulation of the otolith afferents in this frequency range which is not accompanied by a concordant signal from the canal afferents should ideally be rejected by the vestibuloocular circuits. Only at extremely low frequencies (down to the static case) where the canals are insensitive should a macular excitation be translated into a compensatory eye movement. It seems possible that the fast adaptation of the maculo-ocular reflex, along with the steep decline of gain with the increase of frequency (Chap. 3.4) reflects the elimination of meaningless, even harmful oculomotor reflexes. One might even speculate that in a freely living rabbit the pure maculo-ocular responses to all but very low frequencies may be suppressed entirely and that the significant maculo-ocular responses obtained in nonadapted rabbits are related to the fact that our rabbits lived in cages and had therefore very limited locomotor experience.

If this interpretation of the response decline as a useful adaptation is accepted, then a remarkable fact is that it occurred without visual feedback. This would indicate that adaptive circuits can use extraretinal signals (e.g., corollary motor discharge) in addition to visual slip.

6.3.2 Conditions for Visual Adaptation of the VOR

As we are now satisfied that the canal-ocular reflexes in the physiological frequency range are not systematically adapted by prolonged stimulation without visual feedback, we are in a position to study the long-term effects of vision.

To examine some important factors in visual adaptation, let us consider the normal condition, in which the head is moving in a stationary world (Fig. 79 A). If the compensatory eye movements are too small for total stability (gain < 1, as usually found), gaze will be displaced in the same direction as the head but at a much smaller velocity. The slip (movement of visual surroundings with respect to gaze) will be in the same direction as

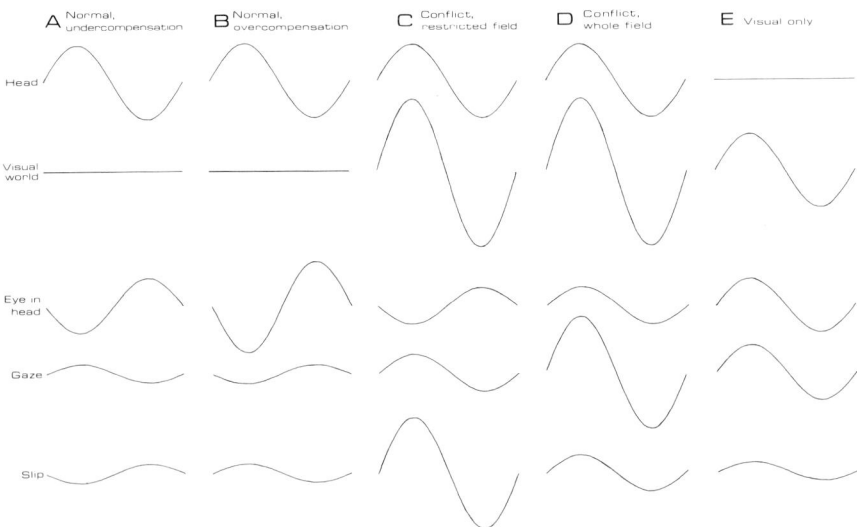

Fig. 79. Idealized, schematic stimulus-response relations of OKN and VOR under various experimental conditions. **A** Normal head movement in a stationary visual world. Compensatory eye movements are too small for complete stability. The gaze wanders with the head and the visual world slips with respect to the eye in the same direction as the eye moves in the head. This situation would require an increase in the amplitude of the eye movements. **B** Normal situation as in **A**, but with too large an amplitude of the eye movements. Slip and eye movements now have opposite directions. **C** The visual world is moved in phase with the head, at twice the amplitude (inverted motion vision); the visual field is restricted to a sector of 90°. The eye movement is still in the direction of the VOR; the slip is in opposite direction from **B**, which results in a decrease of the VOR gain. **D** Inverted motion vision as in **C**, but in the whole visual field. This visual input is so powerful that the VOR is overruled and eye movement has the same direction as the slip, as in **A**, which results in an increase of the VOR gain. **E** Rotation of the visual world alone, with the head stationary. Optokinetic eye movements are too small for complete stability. Slip is in the same direction as the eye movement (as in **A**) and the result is an increase in gain of OKN and VOR.

Gaze head + eye in head; *Slip* visual world – gaze.
(Collewijn and Grootendorst, 1979)

the movement of the eye in the head. Functionally meaningful adaptation in this condition would require an increase in the amplitude of the eye movements to reduce slip. On the other hand, if compensatory eye movements are larger than the head movements (gain > 1), slip will be opposite in sign to the eye movements in the head (Fig. 79 B). Of course, this condition would require a decrease in eye movements. Thus, it can be argued that visually detected slip should be compared to the combined output of the VOR and OKN systems to determine the desirable direction of adaptation.

The most physiological test of this system would be to change the magnitude of the slip signal. This has been done in monkey (Miles and Fuller,

1974) and man (Gauthier and Robinson, 1975) by fitting subjects with telescopic magnifying or reducing spectacles. A substantial increase or decrease in the VOR was indeed induced by these conditions, which simulate under- and over-compensation.

In most other experiments on adaptation, visual motion information has been altered more drastically by right-left inversion. Although such conditions may seem quite artificial, they have resulted in a strong decrease in the magnitude and sometimes even inversion of the VOR in man (Gonshor and Melvill Jones, 1976a, b) and cat (Robinson, 1976; Melvill Jones and Davies, 1976).

The species mentioned so far possess central or foveal vision, which may account for the effectiveness of the used optical devices, notwithstanding the small field of vision which they allow. In the rabbit, which has a panoramic and visual-streak type of visual field, strong restriction of the visual field seems undesirable and other strategies to modify visual slip have been designed. An inverted retinal slip signal can also be created by introducing movements of the visual surroundings in correlation with the head movements. If the head is oscillated at an amplitude A and the surroundings are moved in phase with the head but at an amplitude 2A, the relative motion between head and surroundings is opposite to the usual one in a stationary world. Ito et al. (1974b, 1979a) have applied this method to the rabbit, using a single vertical light slit positioned near the optical axis of the eyes in albino rabbits. The results of several stimulus combinations, applied over 8-12 h, were as follows. Vestibular stimulation alone (oscillation in darkness at 0.1 Hz, amplitude 5° peak-to-peak) did not significantly modify the VOR. Visual stimulation alone with the slit moving around the stationary animal at 0.1 Hz (amplitude 2.5° or 5° peak-to-peak) induced an optokinetic response with a gain of about 0.4. Neither this optokinetic nor the vestibulo-ocular gain changed during 8 h of continuous visual stimulation. When the animal was oscillated for 8 h with the light slit on, but stationary, there was a tendency for the synergic gain (in the light) as well as the VOR gain (measured in darkness) to significantly increase to about 140% of the initial values during the first few hours of the experiment. Finally, rabbits were oscillated at 0.1 Hz and an amplitude of 5° while the light slit was moved in phase but at an amplitude of 10°. Under these conditions of conflicting visual and vestibular information, a gradual decrease in the gain of compensatory eye movements was seen both with the light slit on and in darkness. With the light on, gain decreased from 0.23 to 0.17 in 2.5 h, while the VOR gain in darkness decreased in the same period from 0.39 to 0.28 (about 70% of the initial value). An important point is that although the moving slit reduced the compensatory eye movements, its effect was usually not powerful enough to actually reverse the eye movements. This means that the direction of the eye movements remained in harmony with the vestibular, not with the visual stimulus. No evidence for a frequency specificity of these effects was found (Ito et al., 1979a).

These experiments by Ito et al. (1974b, 1979a) have been repeated in our laboratory (Collewijn and Grootendorst, 1978). Applying oscillation at 0.17 Hz with an amplitude of 10° peak-to-peak, we were unable to obtain similar results in Dutch pigmented rabbits. In the control group (oscillated in darkness) a slight decrease in VOR gain was found in this series, in contrast to earlier findings (Chap. 6.3.1). With the stationary light slit on, a slight gain decrease was also found, while with the slit light moving in phase, no significant trend in the VOR gain could be demonstrated (Fig. 80). When

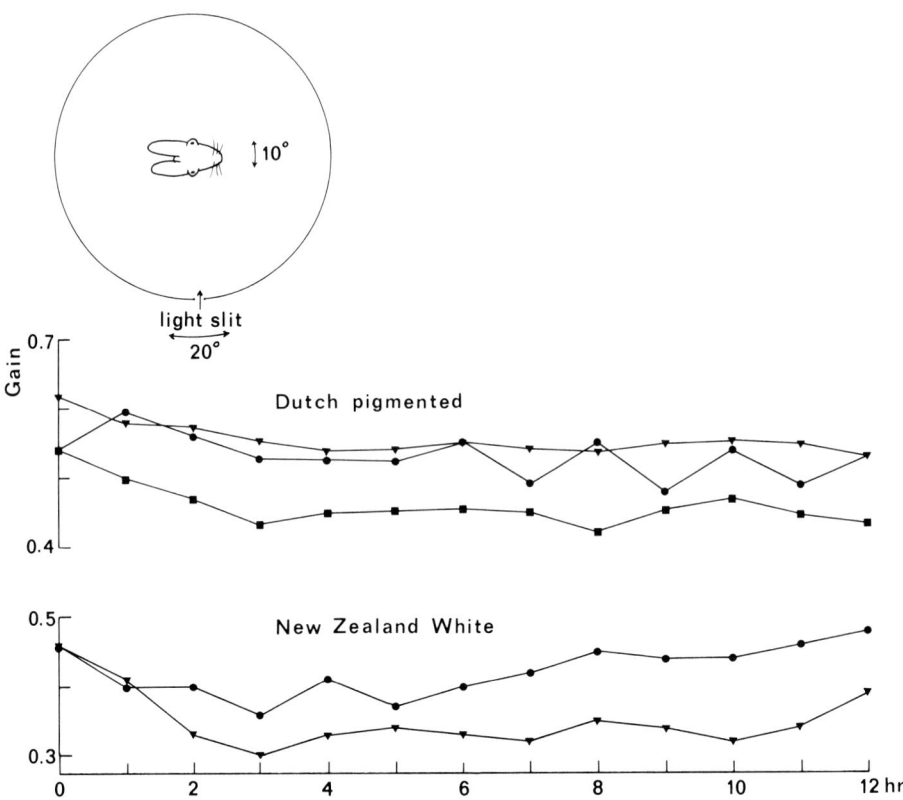

Fig. 80. Gain of the vestibulo-ocular reflex (measured in short, hourly intervals of darkness) under different conditions with a single visual slit as the only visual stimulus. *Circles* stationary slit (synergic condition); *triangles* slit moving in phase (as indicated in inset on top, conflict condition); *squares* complete darkness (no visual stimulus control). Average values for eight Dutch (*above*) and eight albino (*below*) rabbits. (Collewijn and Grootendorst, 1978)

we repeated the experiment with New Zealand White albino rabbits, we were able to confirm the trend of Ito's findings. In these animals the moving slit condition resulted in a systematically lower VOR gain than the stationary slit. However, the actual changes in gain were very small and we felt that the experimental situation with a single light slit was only marginally effective due to the extremely reduced behavioral and visual conditions.

Therefore, we decided to test the effect of a more normal visual stimulus. Dutch pigmented rabbits were mounted in a black box, which left only an anterior sector of 90° of the visual field free. A mirror could be attached to this frontal opening. The whole assembly could be oscillated with the same motion as used before (0.17 Hz, 10° peak-to-peak). Each rabbit was subjected to this continuous oscillation for 8 h in a normal laboratory room on two occasions: once without the mirror (normal condition) and once with the mirror (inverted motion vision). This experimental paradigm, which resembles one of the first conditions tested in man by Gonshor and Melvill Jones (1973, 1976a), proved to be highly effective. The averaged results in eight rabbits are shown in Fig. 81.

With the mirror, a prompt decrease of VOR gain was achieved in all rabbits. Most of this change occurred in the first 3 h of stimulation, although in the later hours there was still a tendency to further decrease. The effect was statistically highly significant ($p < 0.001$). The combined optokinetic and vestibulo-ocular reflex, measured with the light on, showed a similar effect and, as expected, the overall level of this combined reflex is lower than that of the VOR alone (Fig. 81), but the eye movements remained in the direction of the vestibular stimulus and were out of phase with the drum. Without the mirror, the VOR gain and the combined optokinetic- and VOR gain showed a tendency to increase slightly (statistically not significant).

It may be concluded that vision of a normal environment with a visual field of 90° is a much more potent stimulus than a single light slit in eliciting adaptive changes in the VOR. With this arrangement, adaptation is readily obtained in pigmented Dutch rabbits, in which the slit was entirely ineffective.

When we finally attempted to also expose albino rabbits to the condition of a 90° anterior visual field, we discovered a profound anomaly in the albino rabbit's optokinetic reactions. Horizontal optokinetic responses in the anterior 90°-180° of the visual field proved to be inverted in albino rabbits: in this sector the direction of pursuit was opposite to that of the stimulus. These findings, which will be discussed later (Chap. 6.4), indicate a profound abnormality in the processing of visual motion information in albino rabbits. Ito's findings are probably not affected by this anomaly, as the stimulus in his experiments was situated laterally and not frontally in the visual field.

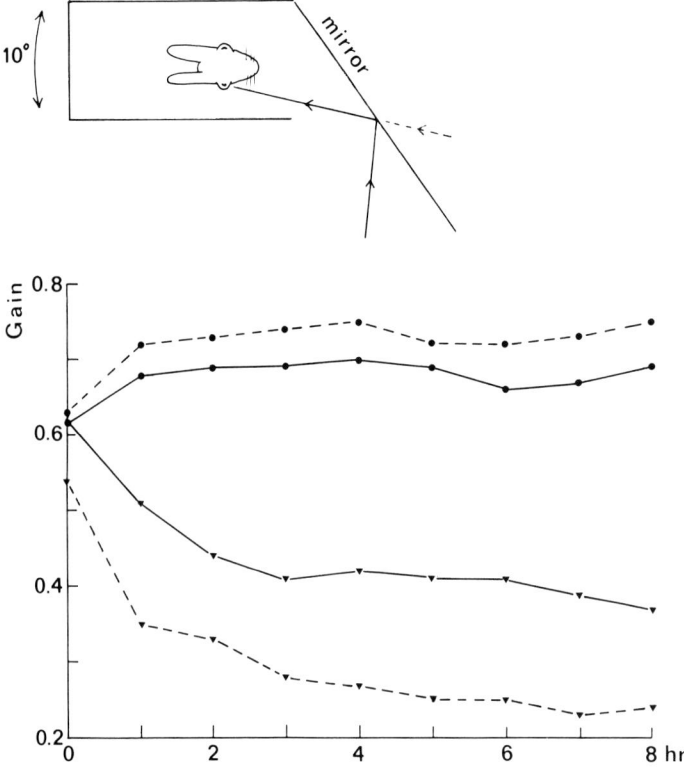

Fig. 81. Gain of the vestibulo-ocular reflex as a function of time when the visual field was restricted to an anterior sector of 90°, which was viewed via a mirror (*triangles*, see *inset on top*) or without a mirror (*circles*). *Solid lines* VOR gain measured in darkness (in short hourly intervals); *interrupted lines* VOR gain with lights on. (Collewijn and Grootendorst, 1978)

The findings (Fig. 81) of Collewijn and Grootendorst suggest that a relatively large visual field (90°) is more effective in modulating the VOR than a single light slit. On the other hand, an earlier attempt to adapt the VOR by a similar experiment with a whole drum (360° around) as the stimulus had been unsuccessful (Collewijn and Kleinschmidt, 1975). In those experiments rabbits were oscillated at a frequency of 0.17 Hz (amplitude 2° peak-to-peak) and a stripped drum was moved in phase but at an amplitude of 4° peak-to-peak. This conditioning stimulus was briefly interrupted each half hour to measure the responses to a pure vestibular, a pure optokinetic or a combined (synergic) stimulus. In this case the visual stimulus was so powerful that in the in-phase (conflict) condition the eyes followed the visual instead of the vestibular stimulus. During 24 h of stimulation, this optokinetic tracking of the drum in the conflict condition improved considerably (Fig. 82).

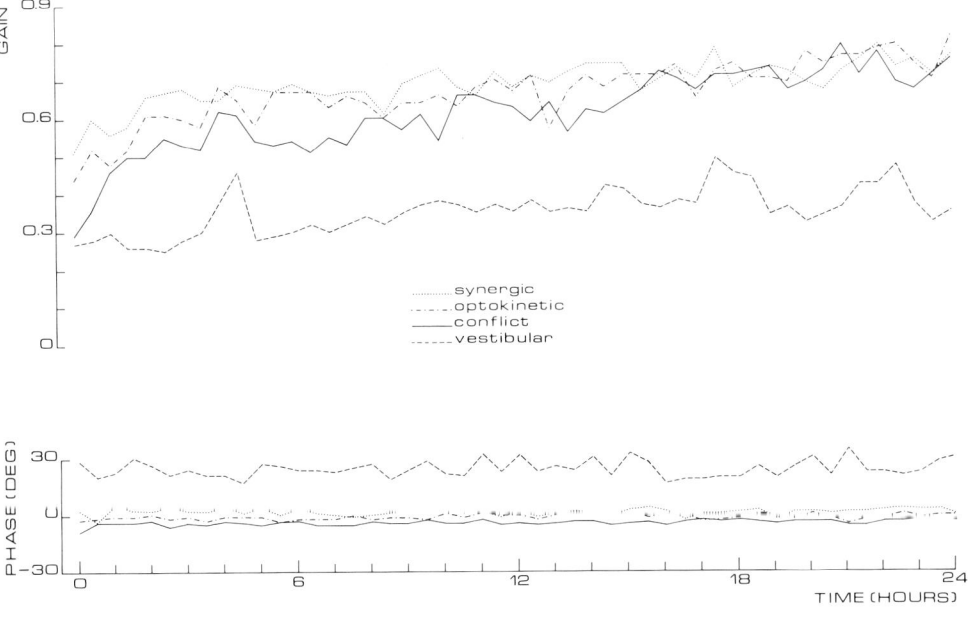

Fig. 82. Gain and phase (as a function of time) of compensatory eye movements elicited by passive oscillation in darkness (vestibular), in stationary lighted surroundings (synergic), with visual surroundings moving in phase at the double amplitude (conflict), and by oscillation of an optokinetic drum (optokinetic). Oscillation frequency 0.17 Hz, amplitude 2° peak-to-peak. The continuous condition was in phase oscillation (conflict), the other conditions were measured briefly every 30 min. (Collewijn and Kleinschmidt, 1975)

The gain of optokinetic and synergic responses also improved. These effects showed a considerable adaptation of the system since the stability of the visual image on the retina was greatly improved. However, the gain of the VOR tested in darkness remained totally unaffected (Fig. 82). There was no decrease, maybe even a small increase in the VOR gain, and no change in phase.

Recently (Collewijn and Grootendorst, 1979) we performed a new series of measurements to resolve the apparent conflicts in our results. Dutch belted rabbits were surrounded by a large optokinetic drum and oscillated at 0.17 Hz, with an amplitude of 10° peak-to-peak. The drum was either stationary or moved in phase at the double amplitude (20° peak-to-peak). Alternatively, the drum could be oscillated around the stationary rabbit. The drum filled the entire visual field, but in a first series of experiments the visual field was restricted to a total angle of 90° anterior by a black screen around the rabbit.

6.3.3 Adaptation to Inverted Motion Vision, Restricted Visual Field

Optically, this condition is equivalent to that with the mirror used by Collewijn and Grootendorst (1978), except that the visual stimulus now consisted of a random-dot pattern instead of the experimental room.

The results (average of seven rabbits) are shown in Fig. 83. As expected, the amplitude of the VOR and the response to the conflict condition de-

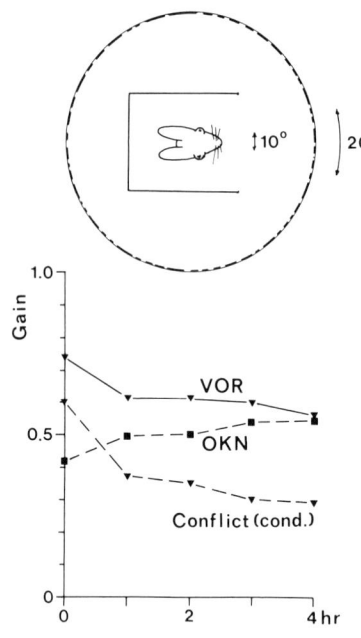

Fig. 83. Gain as a function of time for OKN, VOR, and conflicting stimulation. The conflicting stimulus consisted of an optokinetic drum, moving in phase with the platform, with the visual field restricted to the anterior 90°. This condition was the continuous one, the others were briefly tested every hour (average of seven rabbits). Platform frequency 0.17 Hz, amplitude 10° peak-to-peak. (Collewijn and Grootendorst, 1979)

creased, as in the previous experiments (Collewijn and Grootendorst, 1978). With the visual stimulus present, the gain of compensatory eye movements decreased from 0.60 ± 0.11 (SD) at 0 h to 0.29 ± 0.10 (SD) at 4 h. The gain of the VOR in the dark decreased from 0.74 ± 0.07 (SD) to 0.56 ± 0.07 (SD). Both of these changes were highly significant (t-test: $p < 0.0005$). The gain for the conflict condition is expressed in terms of VOR gain, thus the decrease indicates that the eye movements were progressively less determined by the vestibular and more by the visual input. However, the sign of the responses remained positive, thus no inversion occurred even in the presence of the inverted visual stimulus. Quite remarkably, the responses to visual stimulation alone (OKN) significantly increased ($p < 0.025$) from 0.42 ± 0.13 to 0.54 ± 0.16 (SD), while the VOR decreased. Both trends would of course favor the stability of the retinal image and the decrease in slip.

The relations are further clarified in Fig. 79 C. The eye movement is out of phase with the head, but the slip signal (difference between visual surroundings and gaze) is in phase with the head. Thus, slip is out of phase with the eye movement. This situation would normally occur if the compensatory eye movements were too large, and therefore the decrease of the VOR is physiologically meaningful. Since the OKN is a negative feedback system, an increase in gain is always a meaningful response to increased slip. During the adaptation of the VOR, a directional preponderance often occurred, which could result in strongly asymmetrical reactions. Gonshor and Melvill Jones (1976b) made a similar observation in man and attributed it to a temporary inequality of the adapting processes on both sides of the brain.

6.3.4 Adaptation to Inverted Motion Vision, Whole Visual Field

The next step was to repeat these experiments with an unobstructed visual field, analogous to the experiments of Collewijn and Kleinschmidt (1975). Six rabbits were oscillated at 1/6 Hz, 10° p.p., and the drum was moved in phase at 20° p.p. for a period of 8 h. The whole drum proved to be a much more powerful visual stimulus than the 90° field, and the response to the conflicting stimulus showed a strong adaptation toward visual stability, as shown in Fig. 84.

At the start of the conditioning, the eye movements were still in the direction of a VOR (in counterphase with head and drum), but within 1 h the sign of the responses was inverted and the eye was tracking the visual pattern with a gain which gradually increased. The total change in the gain with the visual stimulus present was from 0.10 ± 0.21 (SD) at 0 h to -0.70 ± 0.24 (SD) at 8 h (t-test: $p < 0.0005$). This improvement in visual tracking was also reflected in the optokinetic gain. This went from 0.60 ± 0.23 (SD) up to 0.85 ± 0.13 (SD) for a stimulus of 1/6 Hz, 10° p.p. and from 0.37 ± 0.17 (SD) to 0.66 ± 0.19 (SD) for a stimulus of 1/6 Hz, 20° p.p. (t-test: $p < 0.01$).

Paradoxically, however, the VOR gain showed no decrease, but an increase from 0.59 ± 0.07 (SD) to 0.79 ± 0.18 (t-test: $p < 0.025$). Actually, the changes in the VOR gain showed two varieties in the individual animals. In four out of the six rabbits, the VOR decreased in the first hour and increased later. In these same animals, the eye moved in the sense of a vestibular response at the beginning of the conditioning and in the direction of the optokinetic stimulus after 1 h. Representative recordings from such an animal are shown in Fig. 85. In two other animals the response to the

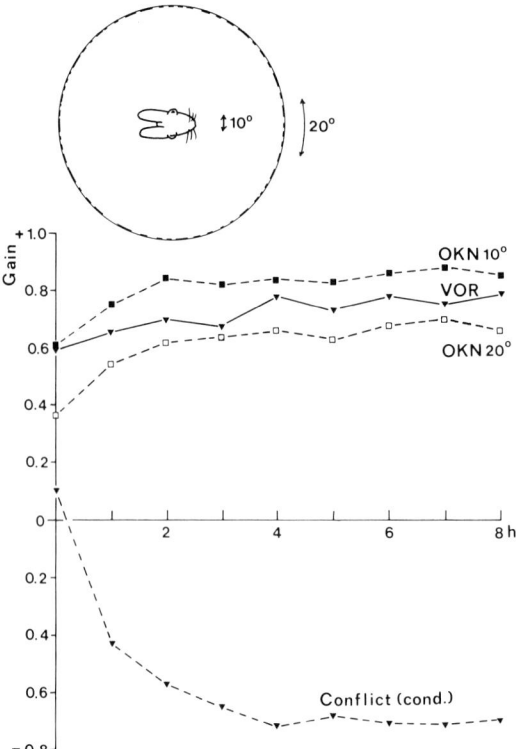

Fig. 84. Gain as a function of time for OKN (stimulus amplitude 10° and 20° peak-to-peak), VOR and conflict, as Fig. 83, but with full visual field exposed to drum. Averages of six rabbits. (Collewijn and Grootendorst, 1979)

conflict stimulus was in the direction of the optokinetic stimulus immediately from the start of the experiment. In these same rabbits the VOR gain showed an increase from the very beginning. These findings offer a clue to the paradoxical increase of the VOR: the direction of VOR change appears to be related to the actual direction of the compensatory eye movements. This relation is further clarified in Fig. 79 D, which shows idealized responses for whole field conflict stimulation at a time when the eye is following the visual and not the vestibular stimulus. In this condition, the slip and the eye movement in the head have the same direction, which is normally the case when compensatory eye movements are too small (Fig. 79 A). Thus, our findings suggest that the adaptation of the VOR is a function of slip and eye movement, not of slip and head movement.

6.3.5 Adaptation by Visual Stimulation Only

In a third experiment, six rabbits were mounted on the stationary platform and only the drum was oscillated at 1/6 Hz, 20° p.p. for a period of

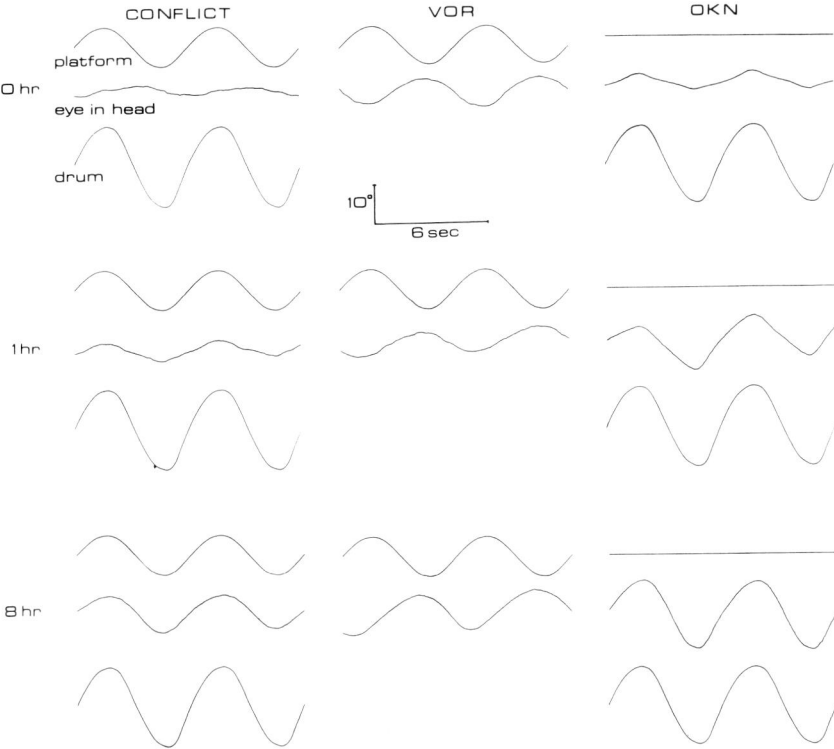

Fig. 85. Representative recordings from one rabbit conditioned with inverted motion vision in the whole visual field. At the start of the experiment (0 h) VOR (in darkness) and OKN are normal; the response to the combined stimulus (conflict) is still dominated by the VOR. After 1 h the eye is tracking the drum (eye movements in phase with the head) under the combined stimulus, as in Fig. 79 D. The VOR has slightly decreased, the OKN is increased. After 8 h, the eye is tracking the drum almost perfectly in conflict and OKN conditions; the VOR gain has paradoxically been increased. (Collewijn and Grootendorst, 1979)

4 h. This movement is rather fast for the rabbit's optokinetic system and the gain of the compensatory eye movements was substantially below 1.0.

The VOR was tested briefly at hourly intervals in complete darkness: the head was never moved with the lights on. As illustrated in Fig. 79 E, the slip of the surroundings will be in phase with the eye movements. Head movement is of course absent. The averaged results are shown in Fig. 86. The OKN gain increased from 0.29 ± 0.18 (SD) at 0 h to 0.56 ± 0.28 (t-test: $p < 0.001$). At the same time, the gain of the VOR increased from 0.50 ± 0.17 (SD) to 0.82 ± 0.42 (t-test: $p = 0.025$). Both trends consistently occurred in all rabbits tested. These results confirm the findings of Collewijn and Kleinschmidt (1975) who used a similar condition but a ten times smaller stimulus amplitude (2° peak-to-peak). Their results for visual stimulation

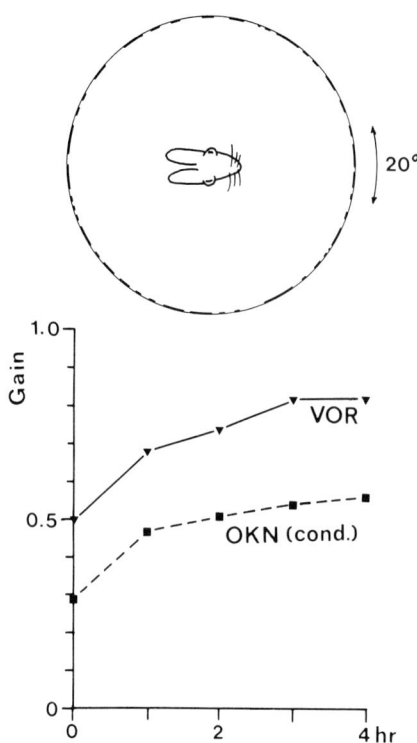

Fig. 86. Gain and phase of VOR and OKN as a function of time, with continuous optokinetic stimulation alone (0.17 Hz, amplitude 20° peak-to-peak)

alone are shown in Fig. 87. Thus, visual slip alone can modify both OKN and VOR, in the absence of any combined visuo-vestibular stimulation.

In none of the three conditioning regimes described were the changes in gain accompanied by any significant changes in phase relations. The VOR was always almost in counterphase with the head movement and optokinetic pursuit was nearly in phase with the drum.

6.3.6 Frequency Specificity of Adaptation

To investigate whether the adaptations described were generalized for all movements or somehow specific for the conditioned frequency (which was always 1/6 Hz), the VOR and OKN were tested in a frequency range around 1/6 Hz immediately before and after the total period of conditioning (4 or 8 h). Some evidence for specificity was indeed found. Figure 88 illustrates this for a rabbit conditioned with visual stimulation only. Graphs a, b, and c show the VOR before and after conditioning. The increase at 1/6 Hz is remarkable, but the response at 1/12 and 1/3 Hz show only minor changes. Figure 88 d, e and f shows the same for the OKN responses. The enhance-

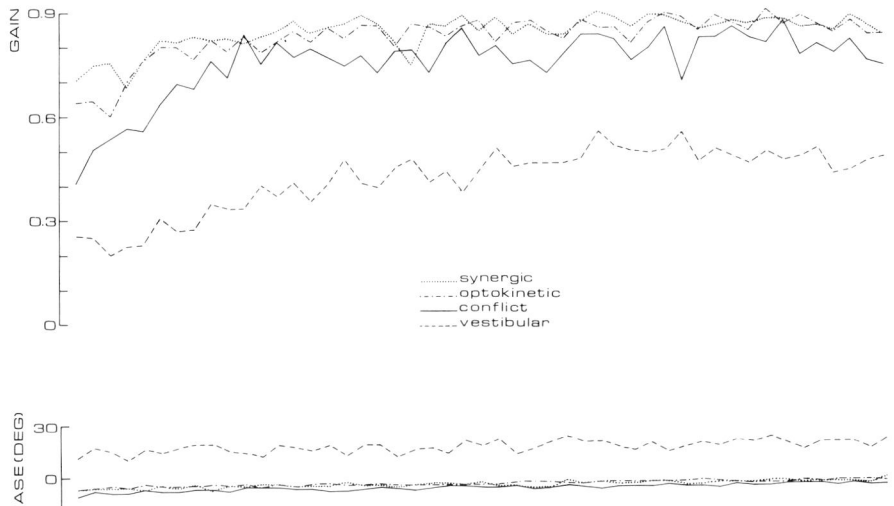

Fig. 87. As Fig. 82, with optokinetic stimulation (0.17 Hz, amplitude 2° peak-to-peak) as the continuous stimulus. Gain increases for all stimulus situations. (Collewijn and Kleinschmidt, 1975)

ment at 1/6 Hz is very large; the reactions at the other stimulus frequencies were unchanged (1/3 Hz) or even distinctly smaller (1/12 Hz).

The averaged frequency responses before and after the three types of conditioning used are shown in Fig. 89. Under all conditions, the changes in VOR as well as OKN were largest at 1/6 Hz, the conditioned frequency. For the conflict stimulus with the whole visual field (Fig. 89 A) the VOR was markedly increased at 1/6 Hz, less so at 1/3 Hz and not (on the average) at 1/12, 5/6 and 10/6 Hz. The OKN was also mostly enhanced at 1/6 Hz, less at 1/3 and 1/12 Hz and even decreased at 1/30 Hz.

With the conflict stimulus limited to a 90° sector of the visual field (Fig. 89 B), the VOR decreased most stongly at 1/6 Hz, less so at the other frequencies and even increased at 10/6 Hz. The OKN gain showed its largest increase at 1/6 Hz, with an average decrease at 1/30 Hz.

With visual stimulation only (Fig. 89 C), the frequency specificity of the changes in VOR and OKN gain was even more distinct than in the other conditions.

A further argument for the specific adaptation to the conditioned stimulus was found in the occasional occurrence of aftereffects. Figure 90 A illustrates such a phenomenon in a rabbit which had been conditioned for 6 h with visual stimulation (1/6 Hz, 20° p.p.) only. When the VOR was tested in darkness at 1/12 Hz, the responses were strongly interfered with by the

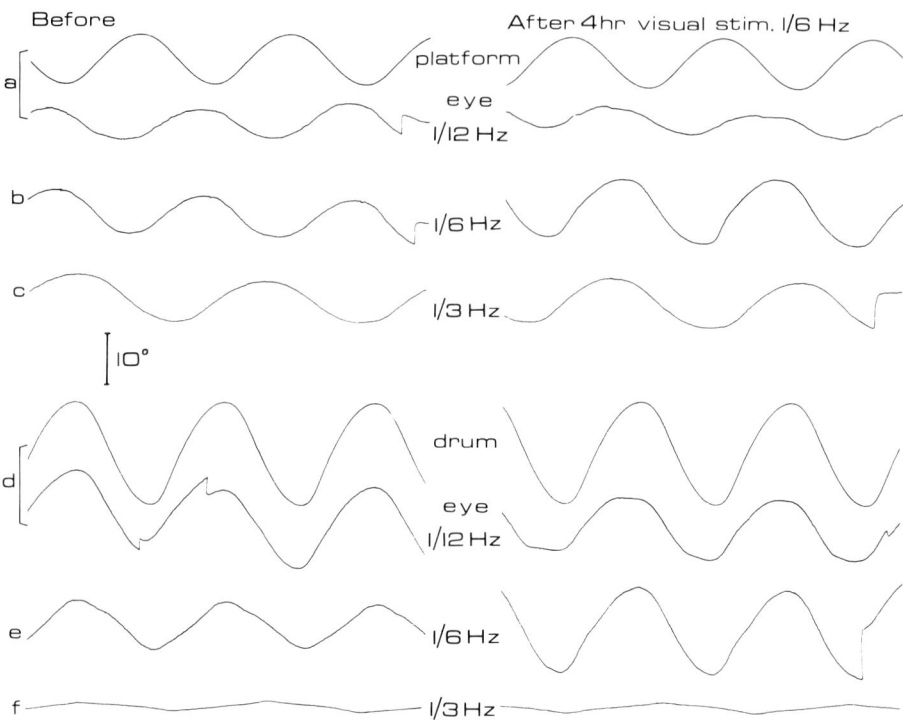

Fig. 88. Response of OKN and VOR to different frequencies before and after conditioning with visual motion alone (1/6 Hz, 20° p.p., 4 h). *a, b, c* VOR tested in the dark. The platform motion (stimulus) is shown only for *a* and gives no phase information for *b* and *c*. Optokinetic responses shown in *d* (with the stimulus motion), *e* and *f*. Both VOR and OKN show an increased amplitude at 1/6 Hz but little changes at 1/12 and 1/3 Hz. (Collewijn and Grootendorst, 1979)

spontaneous generation of sinusoidal eye movements at 1/6 Hz. The platform was stopped, and in the absence of any stimulation the eyes continued to oscillate at exactly 1/6 Hz for several minutes. Another such event is shown in Fig. 90 B. The rabbit had been conditioned for 2 h with the drum moving in phase with the head (conflict, whole visual field) at 1/6 Hz. The VOR was tested in darkness at this moment and when the platform was stopped the eyes continued to move spontaneously with a nearly perfect sine wave at exactly 1/6 Hz. These oscillations gradually damped down, but were reinstated several times after the occurrence of spontaneous saccades (Fig. 90 B). These findings strongly suggest that the conditioned slip pattern was stored in the nervous system, although it should be emphasized that this spontaneous reproduction was only seen in a few rabbits.

A further test for the generality or specificity of adaptation consisted of the optokinetic responses to steady drum rotation at velocities from 1°-

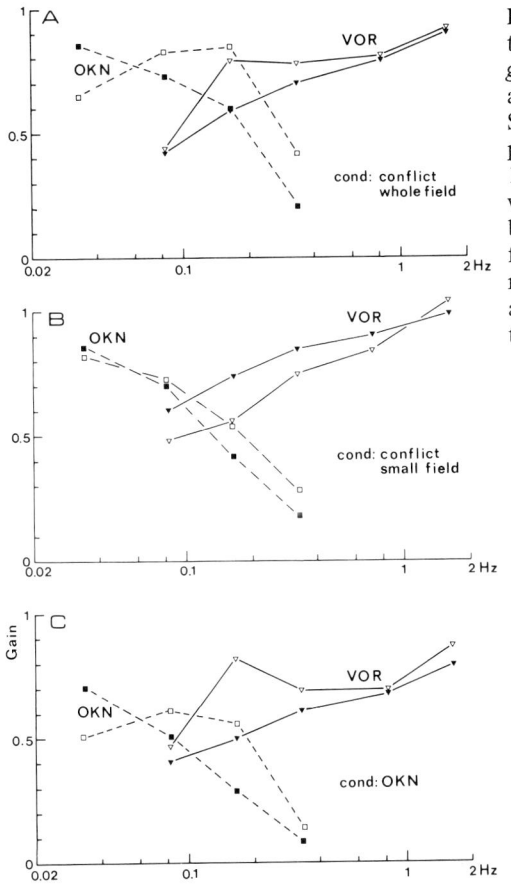

Fig. 89. Frequency specificity of adaptation of OKN (*squares*) and VOR (*triangles*) before conditioning (*solid symbols*) and after conditioning (*open symbols*). Stimulus amplitudes were 10° peak-to-peak, except at 5/6 Hz (5° p.p.) and 10/6 Hz (2.5° p.p.). **A** inverted motion vision, whole field (average of six rabbits), **B** inverted motion vision, visual field restricted to 90° (average of seven rabbits). **C** visual stimulation only (average of six rabbits). (Collewijn and Grootendorst, 1979)

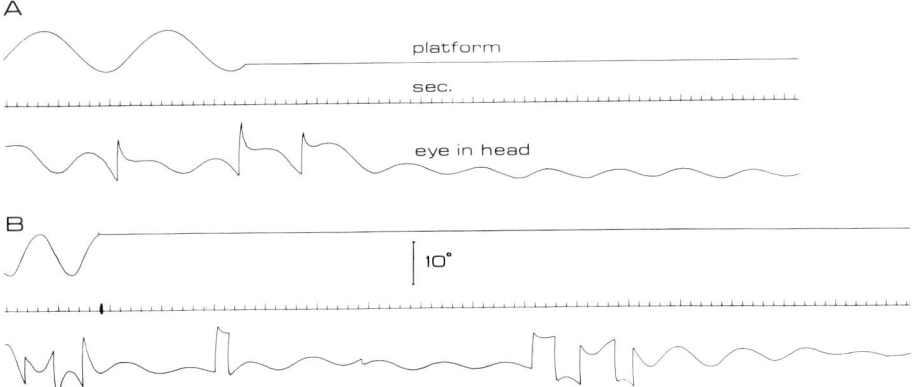

Fig. 90. Spontaneous post-oscillatory eye movements as after-effect of conditioning. **A** spontaneous oscillation of the eye at 1/6 Hz during and after test of the VOR at 1/12 Hz. The animal had been conditioned 6 h with visual motion only at 1/6 Hz, 20° p.p.. **B** similar effect after test of the VOR at 1/6 Hz. The animal had been conditioned for 2 h in a conflict (whole field) situation. (Collewijn and Grootendorst, 1979)

100°/s, which were recorded before and after the conditioning with sinusoidal motion of the drum alone (1/6 Hz, 20° p.p.). Responses were measured after sufficient time for the pursuit velocities to become maximal. Although the responses to the conditioned frequency had markedly increased, the gain of the OKN at all steady velocities had decreased, particularly in the higher velocity range. This again demonstrates that the adaptive changes are not generalized, but fairly specific for the motion pattern conditioned.

The existence of a storage system for patterns of motion (a "pattern center") has been postulated before, notably in connection with the occurrence of motion sickness, habituation and aftereffects due to unfamiliar patterns of motion (Groen, 1957). The aftereffects of sinusoidal vestibular stimulation in darkness seem to be rather weak. Some spontaneous postoscillatory sinusoidal eye movements have been described in man (Festen and Clemens, 1970). In all rabbits oscillated for 24 h (1/6 Hz, 20° p.p.) in the dark, Kleinschmidt (1974) found some spontaneous oscillatory eye movements as aftereffects, but the shape was quite irregular and the frequency was variable and unrelated to the stimulus frequency (Fig. 91).

6.3.7 Adaptation in Synergic Operation of VOR and OKN

In normal life the head will rotate in stationary visual surroundings and this is the only condition for which adaptation should be optimal (Fig. 79 A, B). Strangely enough, this condition has rarely been investigated, but Collewijn and Kleinschmidt (1975) included it in their stimulus program. Figure 92 shows the average results for five rabbits oscillated for 24 h in stationary visual surroundings at 0.17 Hz (amplitude 2° peak-to-peak). In addition the gain to pure optokinetic, vestibular and conflict (in phase) stimuli was tested every 30 min. The synergic gain increased from 0.65 to 0.85 within 10 h. Optokinetic gain increased from about 0.5 to about 0.7. Vestibular gain remained practically unchanged at about 0.3. For the conflict situation the eye followed the drum, but the gain remained low (about 0.4), in contrast to the improvement when the in-phase visual stimulus was continuously applied (Fig. 82). These results show that the absolute values of gain as obtained in passive oscillation experiments (Chap. 3) should be interpreted with some caution, since these values tend to increase when stimulation is extended over a long period. The animal may be optimally adapted to its habitual movement pattern, which in our animals may be somewhat restricted due to their living in cages.

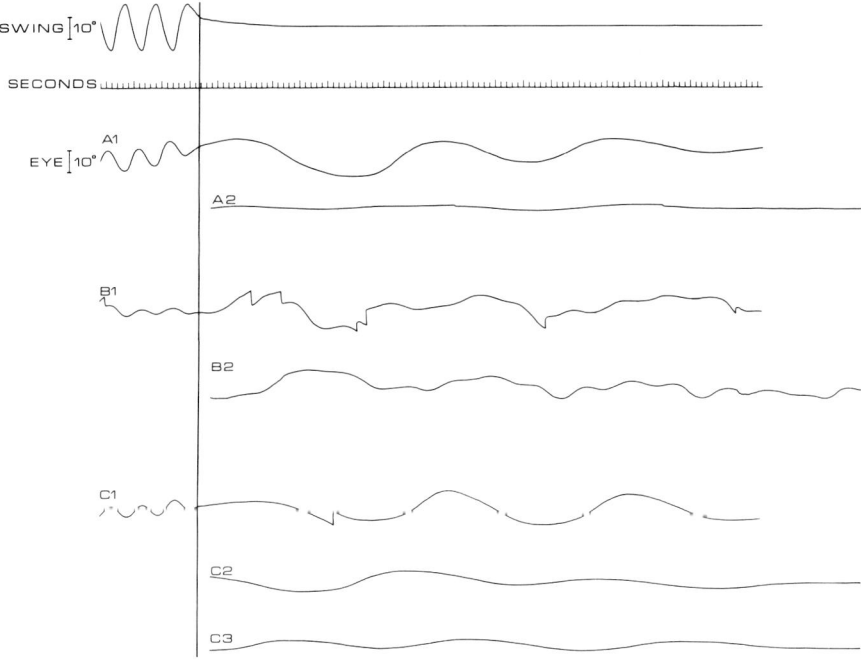

Fig. 91. Examples of after-effects after continuous passive oscillation in darkness (0.17 Hz, amplitude 10° p.p.) for 24 h. The *vertical line* marks the moment at which oscillation is stopped. Three rabbits are shown (*A-C*). Recordings *A 1-2* continuous. Between *B1* and *2* an interval of 1 min. Interval of 3.5 min between *C1* and *2*; 4 min between *C2* and *3*. Variable after-effects at unspecific frequencies are seen. (Kleinschmidt, 1974)

6.3.8 Conclusions on Adaptation

The present experiments show that adaptive plasticity in the rabbit's compensatory eye movements is not limited to the VOR, but is also clearly present in the OKN. They also show that the VOR can be adapted, without being activated, by visual stimulation alone. Both of these facts were already noticed by Collewijn and Kleinschmidt (1975), who also failed to obtain a decrease of VOR gain by inverted whole field optokinetic stimulation. The present findings suggest that this apparent controversy with the earlier results of Ito et al. (1974b) and the recent ones by Collewijn and Grootendorst (1978) can be solved if the actual relationship between visual slip and eye movements is taken into account. It now appears that visual slip in the same direction as the eye movements in the head will increase the gain of both the VOR and the OKN, while slip in the direction opposite to that of the eye movements will also increase the gain of the OKN, but decrease that

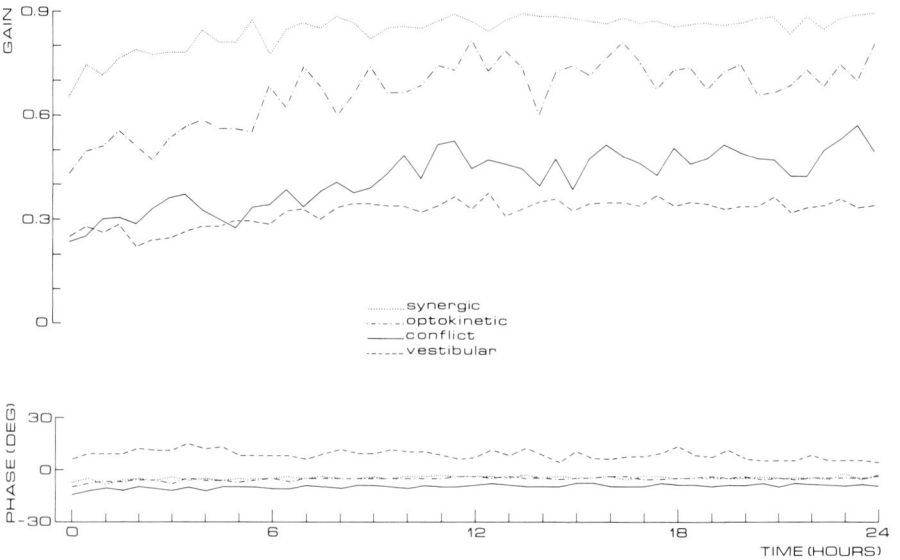

Fig. 92. As Fig. 82, with synergic stimulation (passive oscillation in stationary, lighted surroundings) as the continuous stimulus. Gradual improvement of synergic, optokinetic (also in conflict) gain. (Collewijn and Kleinschmidt, 1975)

of the VOR. Thus, slip and eye movements seem to be relevant signals for the adaptation of the rabbits visuo-vestibular oculomotor reflexes, as illustrated in Fig. 79.

A further finding is the specificity of the adaptation as documented in the frequency response relations of OKN and VOR (Fig. 89) and the occasional manifestation of highly specific aftereffects (Fig. 90). A similar aftereffect has been recorded by Kleinschmidt (1974) in conflict experiments of the same type. Apparently, the oculomotor control system has the possibility of storing a consistent slip pattern. It appears legitimate, then, to postulate that the adaptation of compensatory eye movements involves the storage and retrieval of a specific movement pattern, which is derived from the visual slip.

Adaptation of compensatory eye movements could then work roughly as follows: A consistent pattern of slip occurring over a period of hours is stored in the nervous system. The relation of the slip to the eye movements is also recorded somehow. The stored pattern interacts with the eye movements whenever the same motion pattern occurs. In the integrated visuo-vestibular response the interaction is always such as to decrease visual slip. When the OKN alone is elicited the pattern interacts in an enhancing way if slip and eye movements have been in phase during the previous storage period; if they have been in counterphase (opposite direction), then the pattern interacts with the VOR to decrease its gain.

The resultant compensatory eye movements are then a function of visual and vestibular inputs and of any stored patterns similar to the stimulus patterns. The retrieval of the pattern may occur by an input or output sufficiently similar to the one used to form it. Precise terms with regard to the nature of the interactions are avoided, since they have not been investigated and may be nonlinear. It is apparent that any interaction by stored patterns will make it impossible to predict the integrated visuo-vestibular response from the visual and vestibular components alone. Baarsma and Collewijn (1974) and Collewijn and Kleinschmidt (1975) already noticed discrepancies between the VOR and OKN tested alone and their integrated response in a synergistic or conflicting condition.

The current hypothesis obviously differs from earlier theories, which mainly assume a teaching function of the visual slip on the gain of the feedforward VOR loop (Ito, 1972; Robinson, 1976; Gonshor and Melvill Jones, 1976b). Although it may have some validity for other species, the hypothesis is only founded on the rabbit data at present. The relations in foveate species might be more complex, due for instance to the capability of foveate animals to suppress the VOR during visual pursuit.

The marked learning effect in optokinetic tracking of periodic stimuli has not been noted so far in other species; Gonshor and Melvill Jones (1976a) deny its occurrence in the human experiments with reversed vision. An improvement in optokinetic responses by repeated stimulation with a moving stripe pattern was described by Miyoshi et al. (1973).

In another type of experiment on visuo-vestibular interaction (Young and Henn, 1974, 1976), a period of OKN elicited in one direction was found to have a decreasing effect on the VOR with slow phase in the same direction, elicited by velocity steps. Although these results were obtained with different stimuli and species (man and monkey), essentially their tendency is in opposition to that of the present rabbit data. Thus, care in extrapolating the latter is due.

6.4 Optokinetic Anomalies in Albino Rabbits

Albinism can be due to a variety of congenital defects which prevent the synthesis of melanin (Witkop et al., 1973). In man it is accompanied by profound disturbances of visual function such as low visual acuity, photophobia, strabismus, and nystagmus (Duke-Elder, 1964). A special form is the variety in which melanin can by synthesized at the reduced temperatures in the extremities but not at the core temperature (37°-38°) of the body. This type of albinism is found in Siamese cats and Himalayan rabbits, which have pigmented ears, feet, and noses but albino eyes.

6.4.1 Inverted OKN in Albino Rabbits

The nystagmus and strabismus in albinos may be caused in part by the poor optical quality of the unpigmented eye, in which the iris does not function as an effective diaphragm and the unpigmented chorioid and retinal pigment epithelium are unable to absorb photons not caught on first passage through be photoreceptors. However, a more fundamental cause may be the systematic aberrant course of optic nerve fibers which has been discovered in recent years in albinos. A large proportion of optic nerve fibers originating in the temporal retina, which normally do not decussate, are misrouted and terminate contralaterally. This anomaly has been investigated in great detail for the geniculo-cortical pathway. At this level it has been described for the Siamese cat (Guillery and Kaas, 1971; Hubel and Wiesel, 1971; Elekessy et al., 1973), the albino rabbit (Sanderson, 1975), the albino ferret (Guillery, 1971), the albino mouse (Guillery et al., 1973), the white tiger (Guillery and Kaas, 1973), minks with reduced retinal pigment (Sanderson et al., 1974), albino rats (Giolli and Creel, 1974), and albino humans (Creel et al., 1974; Guillery et al., 1975; Creel et al., 1978; Coleman et al., 1979). However, a paucity of ipsilateral projections to the pretectum and superior colliculus has also been described specifically for albino rats (Lund, 1965), Siamese cats (Kalil et al., 1971; Berman and Cynader, 1972; Lane et al., 1974; Weber et al., 1978) and albino guinea pigs (Giolli and Creel, 1973).

If direction-selective optic nerve fibers projected to the wrong side of the brain, they could activate the wrong nucleus of the optic tract and further optokinetic pathways, with optokinetic eye movements in the wrong direction as a result. Serendipitously, we discovered such an anomaly in the albino rabbit when, in the course of adaptation experiments (Chap. 6.3.2), the visual field of some New Zealand White rabbits was restricted to an anterior angle of 90°. Without exception, a vigorous spontaneous horizontal nystagmus developed immediately. It was abolished by darkness. This observation suggested a sign error in the optokinetic circuit related to the posterior part of the retina. We then systematically investigated OKN in New Zealand White rabbits and Polish albino rabbits, and later in Himalayan rabbits. In all of them the same defect was found (Collewijn et al., 1978).

With a full visual field the OKN of albino rabbits is relatively normal (Fig. 93 A). The eye was stable in a stationary drum, and rotation induced OKN

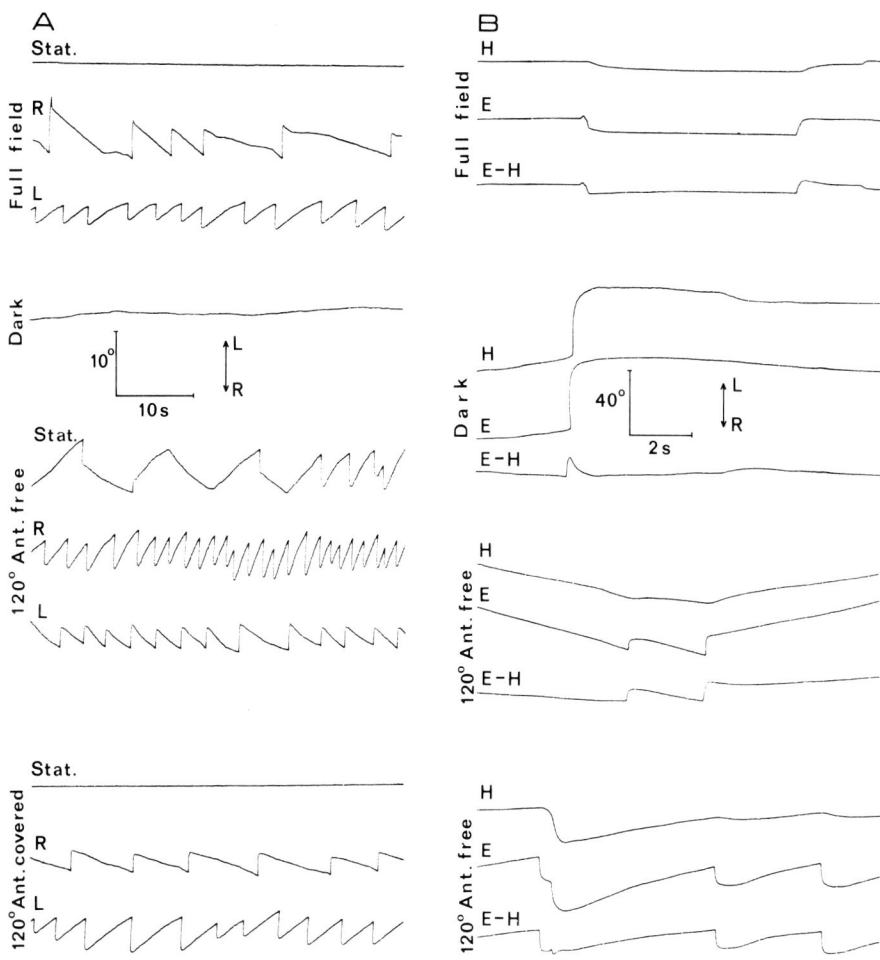

Fig. 93. Typical eye and head movements of Polish rabbits. **A** angular eye position in optokinetic drum with full visual field (*Full field*), 120° anterior sector visible (*120° Ant. free*), and 120° anterior sector covered and posterior field visible (*120° Ant. covered*) to a stationary drum (*Stat.*), to rotation of the drum to the right (*R*) and left (*L*) at 1.2°/s, and in darkness (*Dark*). **B** angular position of the head in space (*H*), eye in space (*E*), and eye in the head (*E-H*) in freely moving but quiet animals with full visual field (*Full field*), in darkness (*Dark*), and when 120° anterior sector was free (*120° Ant. free*). The rabbit's cubicle (80 x 80 cm) was draped with black and white gingham (elements 1 cm). (Collewijn et al., 1978; Copyright of the American Association for the Advancement of Science, 1978)

in the normal direction. The gain was rather poor, particularly when rotation was in the posterior direction for the measured eye (both eyes were stimulated). In darkness some drift occurred (about 0.4°/s) which was in the normal range. Restriction of contrast to an anterior sector of 120°

(60° on each side of the sagittal plane) resulted in permanent, severe instability. The spontaneous movements were smooth but frequently interrupted by saccades.

The velocity of these spontaneous movements was about 3°/s, with peak velocities up to 18°/s. The anterior visual field sector producing instability was about 120° in the Polish albino rabbits, 30°-180° in New Zealand Whites and about 90° in Himalayan rabbits. In pigmented rabbits exposure of a part of the visual field never induced more instability than darkness. Occasionally the smooth movement would change direction, often immediately after a saccade. This instability was always abolished by darkness. When darkness was replaced by a moving drum, visible only in the anterior sector, a smooth movement was always induced in the direction *opposite* to the drum movement.

The gain of the OKN was compared for a number of New Zealand White, Polish albino and Dutch pigmented rabbits. The results for a full visual field are shown in Fig. 94 A. For the pigmented rabbits, the results were as usual (steady-state gain is shown). Performance was poorer in both albino strains, particularly the Polish rabbits in which the unstable zone was very large. To show that this poor OKN was due to the inverted reflexes mediated by the posterior retina, we screened the *anterior* visual zone in both albino and pigmented rabbits. An overall increase of gain in albinos and a decrease in pigmented rabbits was found. The performance of the two groups became comparable (Fig. 94 B).

To investigate the local properties of the retina more precisely, the visual field was systematically probed with small stimuli which were stabilized on the retina in an optically created open-loop situation (Dubois and Collewijn, 1979a).

Within a stabilized frame of 20° horizontal by 40° vertical a random-dot pattern was moved at 1.2°/s in the four principal directions. The results are summarized in Fig. 95 for the Polish albino rabbits, which showed little individual differences. When the stimulus was positioned in the posterior visual field or along the interocular axis, the eye was stable with a stationary pattern and slightly unstable when the pattern was locked to the retina (open-loop situation). Motion of the pattern caused eye movements in the same direction. Open-loop gain of these rabbits was comparable to that of pigmented rabbits. Anterior and posterior pursuit could be elicited but, as in normal rabbits, the response was much better to anterior motion. When the stimulus was positioned 30° or more anterior to the interocular axis, a stationary stimulus elicited horizontal instability similar to that seen in the drum with anterior vision only. Vertically the eye was stable. Horizontal drift velocities with a stable pattern, indicated in Fig. 95, were maximal (3.5°/s) for a pattern 60° anterior to the interocular axis. This spontaneous

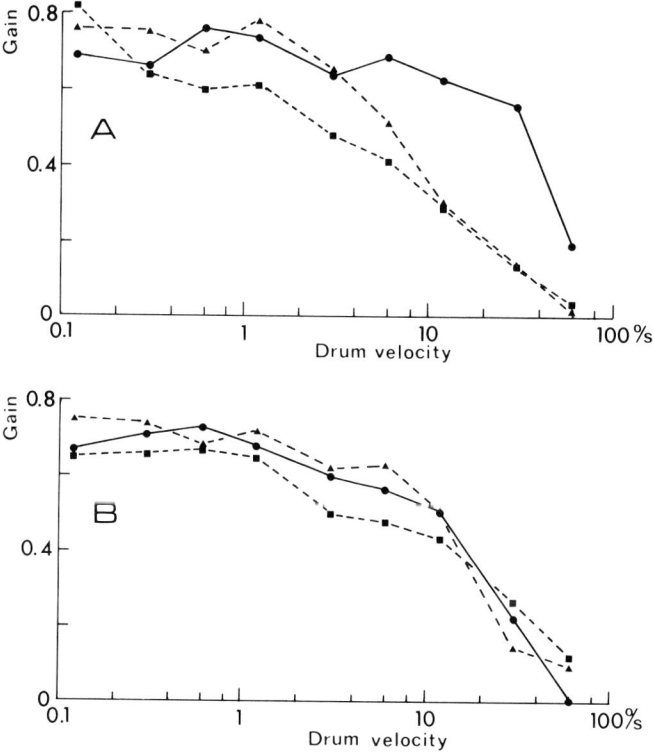

Fig. 94. A Optokinetic pursuit gain was obtained with a fully visible drum for two strains of albino rabbits — New Zealand White (*triangles*) and Polish type (*squares*) — and pigmented Dutch rabbits (*circles*). Both eyes were open. Gain was averaged over left and right rotation and over rabbits. **B** Optokinetic pursuit gain was obtained with the anterior anomalous visual field (90° to 180°) masked for the albinos and 90° of the anterior sector masked for pigmented rabbits (*symbols* same as in **A**). Both eyes were open. Gain was averaged over left and right rotation and over rabbits. (Collewijn et al., 1978 Copyright of the American Association for the Advancement of Science, 1978)

drift was abolished not only by darkness but also by locking the stimulus to the retina. The instability is therefore due to the motion of the retinal image and not to the presence of the pattern as such. Horizontal motion of the pattern in this anterior zone again caused inverted pursuit and thus a negative open-loop gain. Posterior movement was more effective in this zone than anterior movement, which means that in general the eye had a preference to rotate in the anterior direction. Vertical motion of the pattern elicited pursuit in the correct direction, even in the anterior anomalous zone.

In the New Zealand White rabbits, the boundary of the anomalous zone was more variable than in the Polish albinos and was found 30° (two animals), 60° (two animals), and 75° (one animal) anterior to the interior axis. For comparison, Fig. 95 also shows the result obtained in a similar series of

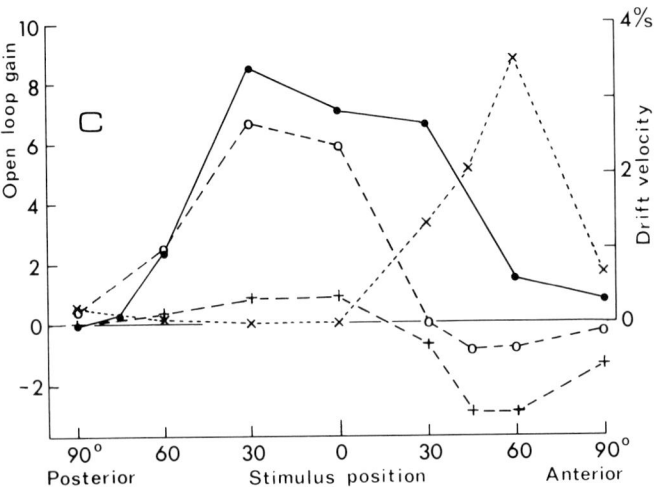

Fig. 95. Open-loop optokinetic pursuit gain was obtained with stimulation from positions along the horizontal meridian for the right eye of pigmented rabbits to anterior motion (*filled circles*) and of Polish albino rabbits to anterior motion (*open circles*) and to posterior motion (*plus signs*). Gain was averaged over rabbits. The *crosses* show average maximum drift velocity for a stationary stimulus not stabilized on the retina. (Collewijn et al., 1978 Copyright of the American Association for the Advancement of Science, 1978)

experiments on pigmented Dutch rabbits; in these gain was always positive. The magnitude depended upon retinal position. No stimulus position induced instability.

Finally, the spontaneous rotations of eye and head were measured in freely moving animals. The animals were provided with spectacles masking different parts of the visual field.

In pigmented rabbits, the eye position in space was very stable between saccades, even for very long intersaccadic intervals.

Figure 93 B illustrates typical findings for the albino rabbits. With an unrestricted visual field, the eyes were about as stable as in pigmented rabbits. Typical drift velocities were smaller than 0.2°/s. In darkness, drift velocities were higher and averaged about 0.7°/s, but, when vision was restricted to an anterior sector of 120°, stability was entirely lost. The eye and head usually drifted together, with typical average velocities of about 4°/s and 3°/s, respectively. Spontaneous reversals of direction occured at irregular intervals, usually after a saccade. In pigmented rabbits, restriction of the visual field to the anterior sector did not noticeably affect stability.

These experiments clearly prove that in albino rabbits optokinetic reactions are inverted in the anterior part of the visual field. With this part of the field selectively exposed, even a stationary pattern will induce spontaneous nystagmus since the slightest spontaneous eye movement will excite the OKN, which in this zone has been converted into an inappropriate, positive feedback system. Some defects in OKN in albino rabbits were also reported recently by Hahnenberger (1977) and intermittent inversion (with full field stimulation) was noticed. The inverted zone can be very extensive (even 180°) in some rabbits and under these circumstances, instability and inverted OKN may be expected, even without any screening of the visual field. Indeed one can observe spontaneous head oscillation and nystagmus in some freely moving albino rabbits, and we have noticed the same phenomenon in certain albino rats. The OKN defects in albino rats may be even more severe than in rabbits, as Precht and Cazin (1979) were unable to elicit OKN in albino rats or to find any visual modulation of single unit activity in the vestibular nuclei, although these phenomena were easily elicited in brown rats. Selective exposure of parts of the visual field was not attempted. Possibly, the spontaneous nystagmus of human albinos could be related to inversion of OKN, which has been observed in a number of cases with full field stimulation (Wildberger and Meyer, 1978).

Figure 96 shows a diagram of the hypothetical connections which might cause the inverted OKN. The optic tract in the pigmented rabbit contains

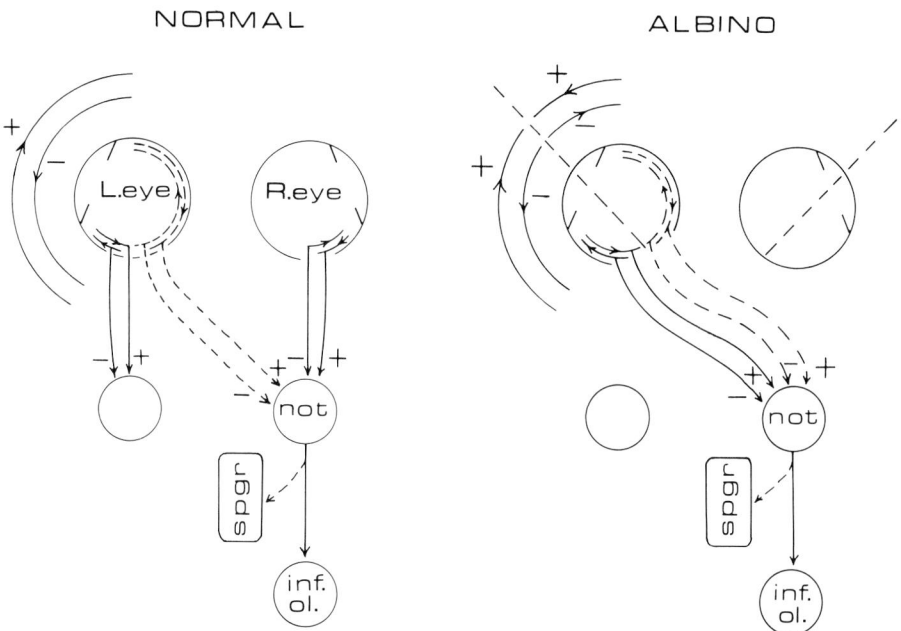

Fig. 96. Hypothetical connections of the retina to the nucleus of the optic tract (NOT) through uncrossed and crossed fibers in normal (pigmented) and albino rabbits. *inf.ol.* inferior olive; *spgr* generators of smooth eye movements to the right side. (Collewijn et al., 1980a)

about 10% ipsilateral optic nerve fibers and an ipsilateral projection to the NOT has been anatomically traced by some investigators (Giolli and Guthrie, 1969; Takahashi et al., 1977), although it was not found by Scalia (1972). If the ipsilateral fibers, which probably originate largely from the posterior retina, do aberrantly cross in albinos, the posterior part of the retina would be connected to the wrong optokinetic circuit and therefore elicit misdirected OKN. The determination of the ipsilaterality of retinofugal connections may have its basis in a left-right exchange of material at a very early embryonic stage, as found by Jacobson and Hirose (1978) in *Xenopus*. A defect in this exchange might be the fundamental reason for the abnormal right-left distribution of optic fibers in the adult albino rabbits. In this respect it is remarkable that vertical OKN in albino rabbits was completely normal.

The diagram of Fig. 96 may be too simplistic. One problem is that the ipsilateral projection to the NOT in pigmented rabbits seems to be extremely sparse, if present at all, in our own material in which the projections were traced by injection of HRP in one eye. Neurophysiologically, an ipsilateral projection to the NOT has been insufficiently investigated so far. If the basis of the defect is a faulty exchange of embryonic material, it is also conceivable that direction-selective elements have already developed abnormally at the retinal stage.

6.4.2 Anomalous Receptive Fields in the Nucleus of the Optic Tract in Albino Rabbits

Possible abnormalities of direction-selective retinal ganglion cells in albinos have not been investigated, but a clear abnormality has been found in the NOT of albino rabbits (Winterson and Collewijn, 1979 and in press). The properties of NOT units in normal rabbits have been described (Chap. 5.3). In many respects the NOT cells in albino rabbits resembled those in pigmented rabbits. They could be excited with short latencies (2.2 ± 0.4 ms) by electrical stimulation of the optic chiasm. They had large receptive fields confined to the projection of the visual streak. All units showed direction selectivity in the horizontal direction. Most units were preferentially excited by low stimulus velocities ($< 1°/s$), whereas in pigmented rabbits many cells were maximally excited by velocities of $10°/s$. A clear parallel with inverted OKN was found in the distribution of preferred directions within the receptive fields. Four types of receptive fields were encountered, which are summarized in Fig. 97. The most frequent (64%) type of unit had receptive fields with two regions of direction selectivity (Fig. 97, upper left). The preferred direction was anterior in the part of the receptive field projecting into

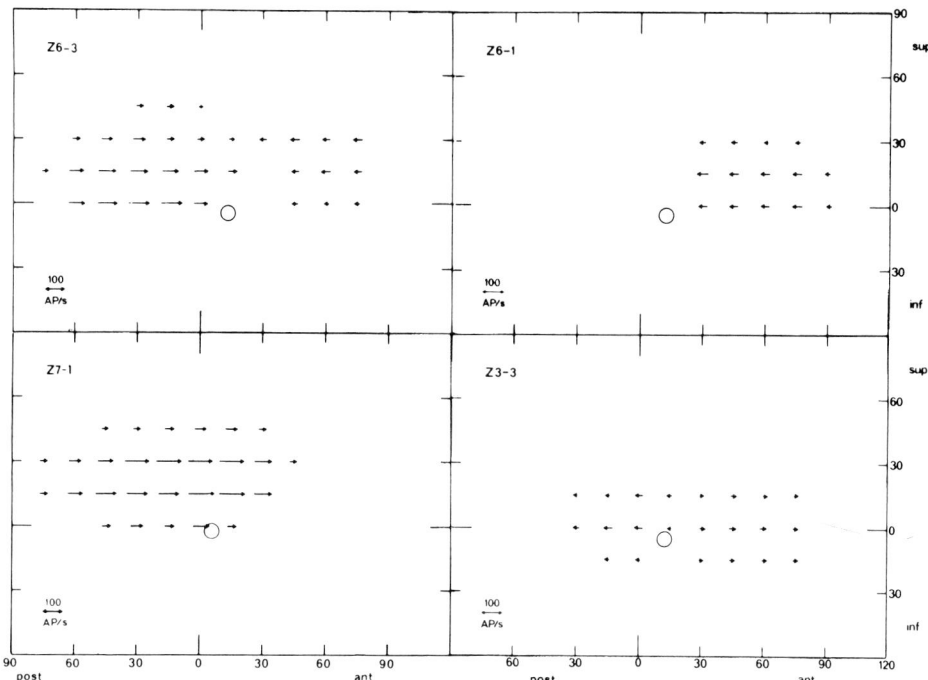

Fig. 97. Summary of direction selectivity in the receptive fields of four units which are representative of the four categories described. The *abscissa* indicates stimulus position on the horizontal meridian in degrees in the superior (sup) and inferior (inf) fields. The *open circle* represents the projection of the optic nerve. The *direction of the arrow* represents the preferred direction of the unit and its length represents response amplitude. Stimulus velocity was 1°/s. (Winterson and Collewijn, in press)

the lateral and posterior visual field and was posterior in the part of the receptive field projecting into the anterior part of the visual field.

Thus, both direction preferences were present within the receptive field of one unit and the preferred direction only depended upon the part of the retina from where the unit was excited. We assume of course that a large number of retinal direction-selective elements converge on each NOT cell. The mean position of the border between the two zones was 29.4° (S.D. = 16.2°, n = 30) anterior to the transverse axis. This is in good agreement with the border of the OKN anomaly (Fig. 95).

The second most common type (13%) of NOT units had a preference for posterior motion (Fig. 97, upper right). The receptive fields of these units projected largely into the anterior visual field. The mean posterior border of the receptive fields was 39.8° anterior, the mean anterior border was 95.8° anterior. A complementary type (11%, Fig. 97, lower left) had a direction preference for anterior motion (normal) in the whole receptive field.

All of these receptive fields projected into the lateral and posterior parts of the visual field. Their mean anterior border was 33.8° anterior. Finally a fourth, rare type was encountered (7%, Fig. 97, lower right) with receptive fields in which direction selectivity was anterior in the anterior visual field and posterior in the posterior visual field. They are complementary to the most common cells (Fig. 97, upper left). The border between the two zones was 45°-60° anterior.

These findings show that the anomaly of OKN in albino rabbits can be fully accounted for by the neurophysiological signals at the level of the NOT. Whether the origin of the abnormal receptive fields in the NOT is misrouting of optic nerve fibers or abnormal direction selectivity in the retina remains to be established.

6.4.3 Adaptation Experiments in Albino Rabbits

We have seen that a dissociation between head movements and eye movements induced by mirrors, reversing prisms or in-phase motion of the surroundings (Chap. 6.3) can cause adaptive changes in the VOR and OKN. In the albino rabbit we have a spontaneous situation in which visual motion signals are inverted. This condition can be isolated by selective exposure of the anterior visual field. The partial inversion of OKN persists apparently through adulthood without correction or suppression of the inverted parts. The dominance of the larger, normally functioning part with full visual field vision might leave insufficient pressure for such a modification. The question then arises whether a correction of the inverted OKN will be effected in albino rabbits in which the anterior visual field is exclusively used, and secondly, whether the inverted visual motion signals will result in a decrease or even inversion of the VOR. These questions have been investigated recently in albino rabbits in which the posterior (normal) parts of the visual field were permanently masked by spectacles with a narrow anterior opening of about 90° for the two eyes together (Collewijn et al., 1980a).

The most consistent effects were obtained in Himalayan rabbits. The average gain of the VOR for a stimulus frequency of $1/6$ Hz (amplitude 10° peak-to-peak) is shown in Fig. 98 for four Himalayan rabbits which had the masks on for 15 days. In this period the gain was reduced from 0.58 ± 0.12 (SD) to 0.25 ± 0.10 (SD), with a recovery to 0.41 ± 0.20 (SD) in the week after removal of the occluding spectacles. One Polish albino rabbit also showed a very marked response, with a reduction of the VOR gain from 0.64 to 0.13 in 23 days. No further decrease was seen up until 40 days, but then increase to 0.27 occurred in the remaining period up to 80 days. At day 80 the occluder was removed and a partial recovery of the gain (to 0.42) was observed in the next 7 days. In these same animals, the average drift speed of the spontaneous nystagmus induced by the masking was measured. Typically, an increase in this drift velocity was seen in the first few days, followed by a gradual decrease in the days following (Fig. 98). However, the spontaneous nystagmus was not abolished in any of the rabbits even after 80 days of selective exposure. Four other Polish rabbits showed similar, but smaller changes.

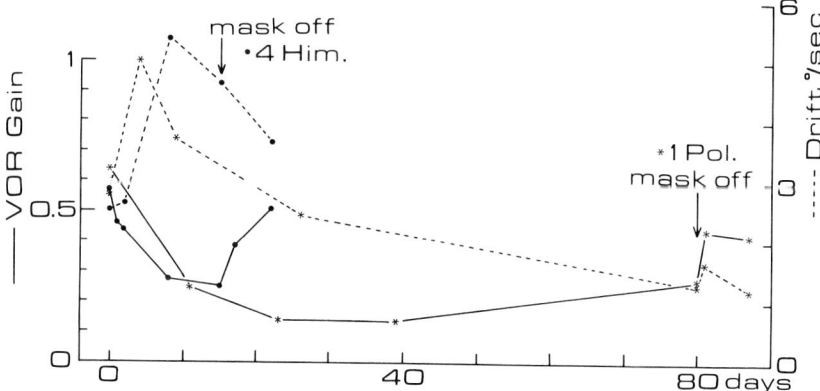

Fig. 98. Average slow phase velocity of spontaneous nystagmus (*interrupted lines*) and VOR gain (*continuous lines*) as a function of time in four Himalayan (*dots*) and one Polish (*stars*) rabbit in which the visual field was restricted to an anterior sector of 90° for a period of 15 and 80 days, respectively. (Collewijn et al., 1980a)

Gain and phase as a function of stimulus frequency are shown in Fig. 99. For the Dutch pigmented rabbits the usual relations were found at day 0, before the masking. After 15 days of selective exposure of the anterior 90° of the visual field, gain was slightly (statistically not significant) lower, but phase was significantly advanced at lower frequencies. At day 22, one week after removal of the occluding mask, gain was practically identical to that at day 0, and in addition the phase advance had partially recovered.

For Himalayan rabbits, the average gain at day 0 was lower than that in the pigmented rabbits. After 15 days of occlusion, gain had decreased to about 60% at all frequencies ($p < 0.005$). The masks were then removed and a week later (day 22) gain had mostly recovered to the original level. Phase changed as in the Dutch rabbits, with little recovery. The individual animals showed large differences. In about half of them gain was strongly reduced with only insignificant changes in phase, while in others the change in phase was larger than 90°. However, such large phase shifts were seen only at the lowest frequencies. As the change in phase due to visual inversion has been described as a slow process in man (Gonshor and Melvill Jones, 1976b) and cat (Melvill Jones and Davies, 1976) it is of interest that the Polish rabbit (Fig. 98) occluded for 80 days showed a strong reduction of gain but no change at all in phase (Fig. 99). Thus, the changes in phase were not very consistent and not specific for albino rabbits.

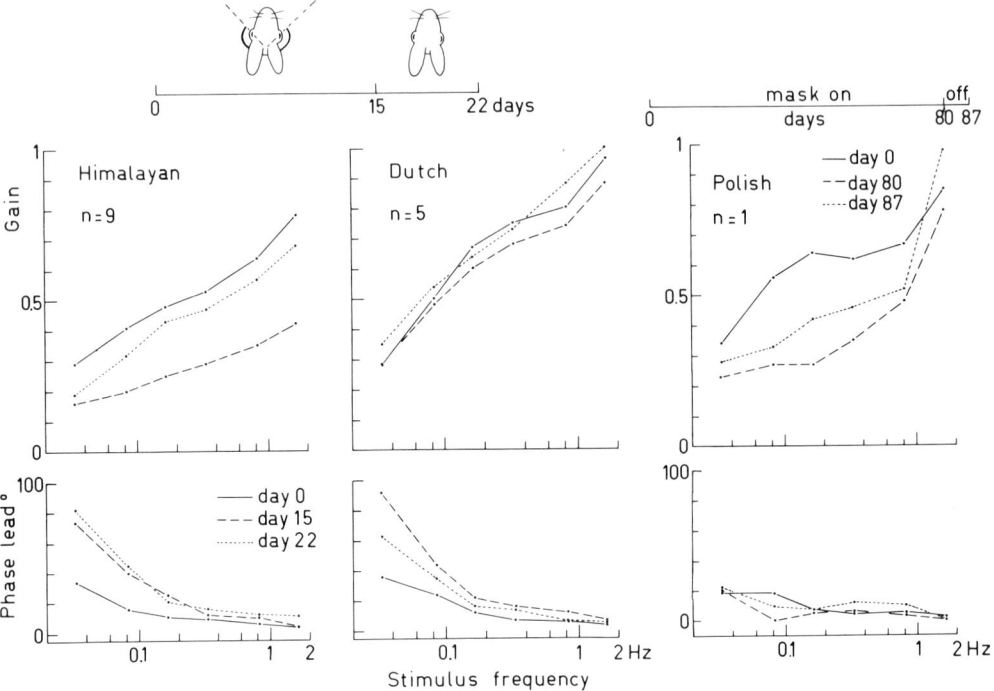

Fig. 99. Gain and phase of vestibulo-ocular responses (measured in darkness) as a function of stimulus frequency in nine Himalayan and five Dutch rabbits masked for 15 days and one Polish rabbit masked for 80 days. (Collewijn et al., 1980a)

The changes in gain were in the expected direction, but they were small. Since this conceivably could be due to a strategy of limited movement, the animals were also subjected to continuous passive oscillation for 4 h (1/6 Hz, amplitude 10° peak-to-peak). VOR gain decreased but the changes once again were small. The most interesting change was again observed in the synergic responses (oscillation in the light). In Dutch rabbits the visual field limitation reduced the synergic gain from 0.91 ± 0.17 (full field) to 0.76 ± 0.20. During 4 h of forced oscillation in the light gain was restored to 0.94 ± 0.14, a significant adaptation ($p < 0.05$). In the Himalayan rabbits the synergic gain with full field vision was 0.82 ± 0.11. Selective exposure of the anterior (inverted) field reduced this to 0.55 ± 0.12. During 4 h of forced oscillation this gain was not improved. When the same animals were oscillated with an unrestricted visual field, the synergic gain in the Dutch rabbits improved from 0.91 ± 0.17 to 1.02 ± 0.04 ($p < 0.10$), in agreement with the results mentioned in Chapter 6.3.7. In the Himalayans synergic gain rose from 0.82 ± 0.11 to 0.94 ± 0.04 ($p < 0.025$).

The same experiments with forced oscillation were also done with the anterior sector of the visual field screened, but no systematic changes were detected in this situation, from which theoretically albino rabbits should have benefited.

These results show that the anomalous processing of part of the visual motion signals in the albino, manifest in inverted OKN, is also expressed in long-term changes in the gain of the VOR. These changes are maladaptive, because they diminish rather than improve gaze stability. This maladaptivity is a consequence of the site of the inversion. In the albino, there is a discrepancy between the processing of visual direction-selective signals and the rotation of the eye with respect to the stationary world. When vision is inverted by a mirror or prism, there is a discrepancy between the direction of head movements and visually perceived slip, but the motion signals due to eye movements have the correct sign and adaptation will improve gaze stability. As prolonged exposure of the inverted retina in free animals did not lead to correction of the optokinetic inversion, the inappropriate feedback loop is apparently unable to correct itself.

6.5 Conclusions

A certain amount of adaptation can be demonstrated in the compensatory eye movement circuits of the rabbit, in agreement with findings in other animals, but the range of the adaptation has been small under all our experimental conditions.

The most pertinent changes were seen with head movements in a stationary, illuminated world. This condition always led to gradual improvement of the combined vestibulo-ocular and optokinetic gain to values close to 1. Visual stimulation alone also has a similar (but somewhat smaller) effect. Other, more artificial conditions such as visual inversion elicit changes in the expected direction but the effects are not very large. It seems likely that adaptation is controlled by a comparative evaluation of the directions of the eye movements made and of the visual slip experienced.

Loss of one labyrinth, dark-rearing and genetic (partial) wiring defects introduce serious malfunctioning of gaze stabilization which is only incompletely compensated by adaptive processes even in periods of several months. In view of these limited capabilities the rabbit is probably not a very suitable animal for the study of adaptive processes in the nervous system.

References

Abels H (1906) Über Nachempfindung im Gebiete des kinästhetischen und statischen Sinnes. Ein Beitrag zur Lehre vom Bewegungschwindel (Drehschwindel). Z Psychol Physiol Sinnesorg 43:268-269, 374-422

Alley K, Baker R, Simpson JI (1975) Afferents to the vestibulo-cerebellum and the origin of the visual climbing fibers in the rabbit. Brain Res 98:582-589

Allum JHJ, Graf W, Dichgans J, Schmidt CL (1976) Visual-vestibular interactions in the vestibular nuclei of the goldfish. Exp Brain Res 26:463-485

Alpern M (1962) Movements of the eyes. In: Davson H (ed) The eye, vol 3, pp 3-187. Academic Press, London New York

Arimoto K (1958) Superior colliculus as center of nystagmus. Wakayama Med Rep 4: 1-35

Atkinson J (1979) Development of optokinetic nystagmus in the human infant and infant monkey: an analogue to development in kittens. In: Freeman RH (ed) Developmental neurobiology of vision. Plenum Press, New York (NATO Advanced Study Institute Series A, Life Sciences: vol 27, pp 277-287)

Baarsma EA, Collewijn H (1974) Vestibulo-ocular and optokinetic reactions to rotation and their interaction in the rabbit. J Physiol 238:603-625

Baarsma EA, Collewijn H (1975a) Eye movements due to linear accelerations in the rabbit. J Physiol 245:227-247

Baarsma EA, Collewijn H (1975b) Changes in compensatory eye movements after unilateral labyrinthectomy in the rabbit. Arch Oto-Rhino-Laryng 211:219-230

Baker R, Berthoz A (eds) (1977) Control of gaze by brain stem neurons. Elsevier, Amsterdam New York (Developments in Neuroscience, vol 1)

Baker R, Gresty M, Berthoz A (1976) Neuronal activity in the prepositus hypoglossi nucleus correlated with vertical and horizontal eye movement in the cat. Brain Res 101:366-371

Baloh RW, Sills AW, Kumley WE, Honrubia V (1975) Quantitative measurements of saccade amplitude, duration and velocity. Neurology 25:1065-1070

Baloh RW, Yee RD, Honrubia V (1980) Optokinetic asymmetry in patients with maldeveloped foveas. Brain Res 186:211-216

Bárány R (1908) Die Untersuchungen der optischen und vestibulären reflektorischen Augenbewegungen in einem Falle von einseitigen Blicklähmung. Monatsschr Ohrenheilkd 42:109-113

Barlow HB, Hill RM (1963) Selective sensitivity to direction of movement in ganglion cells of the rabbit retina. Science 139:412-414

Barlow HB, Levick WR (1965) The mechanism of directionally selective units in rabbit's retina. J Physiol 178:477-504

Barlow HB, Hill RM, Levick WR (1964) Retinal ganglion cells responding selectively to direction and speed of image motion in the rabbit. J Physiol 173:377-407

Barmack NH (1976) Measurements of stiffness of extraocular muscles of the rabbit. J Neurophysiol 39:1009-1019

Barmack NH (1977) Visually evoked activity of neurons in the dorsal cap of the inferior olive and its relationship to the control of eye movements. In: Baker R, Berthoz A (eds) Control of gaze by brain stem neurons. Elsevier, Amsterdam New York (Developments in Neuroscience vol 1, pp 361-370)

Barmack NH (1979) Immediate and sustained influences of visual olivocerebellar activity on eye movement. In: Talbott RE, Humphrey DR (eds) pp 123-168. Posture and movement. Raven Press, New York

Barmack NH (in press) A comparison of the horizontal and vertical vestibulo-ocular reflexes of the rabbit.

Barmack NH, Hess DT (1980a) Multiple-unit activity evoked in dorsal cap of inferior olive of the rabbit by visual stimulation. J Neurophysiol 43:151-164

Barmack NH, Hess DT (1980b) Eye movements evoked by microstimulation of dorsal cap of inferior olive in the rabbit. J Neurophysiol 43:165-181

Barmack NH, Simpson JI (1980) Effects of microlesions of dorsal cap of inferior olive of rabbits on optokinetic and vestibulo-ocular reflexes. J Neurophysiol 43:182-206

Barmack NH, Heukel CK, Pettorossi VE (1979) A subparafascicular projection of the medial vestibular nucleus of the rabbit. Brain Res 172:339-343

Barmack NH, Pettorossi VE, Nastos MA (in press) The horizontal and vertical cervico-ocular reflexes of the rabbit.

Barnes GR (1979) Vestibulo-ocular function during coordinated head and eye movements to acquire visual targets. J Physiol 287:127-147

Barr CC, Schultheis LW, Robinson DA (1976) Voluntary, nonvisual control of the human vestibulo-ocular reflex. Acta Otolaryngol 81:365-375

Bartels M (1931) Vergleichendes über Augenbewegungen. In: Bethe A, Bergmann von G, Embden G, Ellinger A (eds) Handbuch der normalen und pathologischen Physiologie, pp 1113-165. Springer, Berlin Heidelberg New York

Bartz AE (1966) Eye and head movements in peripheral vision: nature of compensatory eye movements. Science 152:1644-1645

Batini C, Ito M, Kado RT, Jastreboff PJ, Miyashita Y (1979) Interaction between the horizontal vestibulo-ocular reflex and optokinetic response in rabbits. Exp Brain Res 37:1-15

Bechterew W (1883) Ergebnisse der Durchschneidung des N. acusticus, nebst Erörterung der Bedeutung der semicirculären Kanäle für das Körpergleichgewicht. Pflügers Arch Ges Physiol 30:312-347

Berman N (1977) Connections of the pretectum in the cat. J Comp Neurol 174:227-254

Berman N, Cynader M (1972) Comparison of receptive-field organization of the superior colliculus in Siamese and normal cats. J Physiol 224:363-389

Berthoz A, Jeannerod M, Vital-Durand F, Oliveras JL (1975) Development of vestibulo-ocular responses in visually deprived kittens. Exp Brain Res 23:425-442

Bizzi E, Kalil RE, Morasso P (1972) Two modes of active eye-head coordination in monkeys. Brain Res 40:45-48

Blair S, Gavin M (1979) Response of the vestibulo-ocular reflex to differing programs of acceleration. Invest Ophthalmol 18:1086-1090

Blanks RHI, Precht W (1978) Response properties of vestibular afferents in alert cats during optokinetic and vestibular stimulation. Neurosci Lett 10:225-229

Blanks RHI, Estes MS, Markham CH (1975) Physiological characteristics of vestibular first-order canal neurons in the cat. II. Response to constant angular acceleration. J Neurophysiol 38:1250-1268

Blohmke A (1929) Über den durch elektrische Reizung des Hirnstammes auslösbaren Nystagmus beim Kaninchen. Z Hals Nasen Ohrenheilk 23:213-241

Boghen D, Troost BT, Daroff RB, Dell'Osso LF, Birkett JE (1974) Velocity characteristics of normal human saccades. Invest Ophthalmol 13:619-623

Brandt Th, Dichgans J, Büchele W (1974) Motion habituation: inverted self-motion perception and optokinetic after-nystagmus. Exp Brain Res 21:337-352

Braun JJ, Gault FP (1969) Monocular and binocular control of horizontal optokinetic nystagmus in cats and rabbits. J Comp Physiol Psychol 69:12-16

Brecher GA (1936) Optisch ausgelöste Augen- und Körperreflexe am Kaninchen. Z Vergl Physiol 23:374-390

Brindley GS, Janota I (1975) Observations on cortical blindness and on vascular lesions that cause loss of recent memory. J Neurol Neurosurg Psychiatr 38:459-464

Brindley GS, Gautier-Smith PC, Lewin W (1969) Cortical blindness and the functions of the non-geniculate fibres of the optic tracts. J Neurol Neurosurg Psychiatr 32:259-264

Brodal A, Høivik B (1964) Site and mode of termination of primary vestibulocerebellar fibres in the cat. Arch Ital Biol 102:1-21

Brouwer B (1923) Experimentell-anatomische Untersuchungen über die Projektion der Retina auf die primären Opticuszentren. Schweiz Arch Neurol Psychiatr 13:118-137

Buettner UW, Büttner U, Henn V (1978) Transfer characteristics of neurons in vestibular nuclei of the alert monkey. J Neurophysiol 41:1614-1628

Bureš J, Buresová O, Krivanek J (1974) The mechanism and application of Leao's spreading depression of electroencephalographic activity. Academic Press, London New York

Busch F, Grüsser OJ, Nikolay H (1979) Additivity of sigma- and phi-optokinetic nystagmus in rabbits. Pflügers Arch Ges Physiol Suppl 382:R 45

Büttner U, Waespe W, Henn V (1976) Duration and direction of optokinetic afternystagmus as a function of stimulus exposure time in the monkey. Arch Psychiatr Nervenkr 222:281-291

Büttner Ennever JA (1979) Organization of reticular projections onto oculomotor neurons. In: Granit R, Pompeiano O (eds) Reflex control of posture and movement. Elsevier, Amsterdam New York Oxford (Progress in Brain Research, vol 50, pp 619-630)

Chievitz JH (1891) Ueber das Vorkommen der Area centralis retinae in den vier höheren Wirbeltierklassen. Arch Anat Entwicklungsgesch Suppl 139:311-334

Chow KL, Masland RH, Stewart DL (1971) Receptive field characteristics of striate cortical neurons in the rabbit. Brain Res 33:337-352

Clark MR, Stark L (1974) Control of human eye movements: III. Dynamic characteristics of the eye tracking mechanism. Mathem Biosci 20:239-265

Cleland BG, Levick WR (1974) Properties of rarely encountered types of ganglion cells in the cat's retina and an overall classification. J Physiol 240:457-492

Cohen B, Uemura T, Takemori S (1973) Effects of labyrinthectomy on optokinetic nystagmus (OKN) and optokinetic afternystagmus (OKAN). Equilibrium Res 3:88-93

Cohen B, Matsuo V, Raphan T (1977) Quantitative analysis of the velocity characteristics of optokinetic nystagmus and optokinetic afternystagmus. J Physiol 270:321-344

Coleman J, Sydnor CF, Wolbahrst ML, Bessler M (1979) Abnormal visual pathways in human albinos studied with visually evoked potentials. Exp Neurol 65:667-679

Colenbrander A (1964) Eye and otoliths. A centrifuge study on the ocular response to otolith stimulation. Thesis, University of Utrecht

Collewijn H (1969) Optokinetic eye movements in the rabbit: input-output relations. Vision Res 9:117-132

Collewijn H (1970a) The normal range of horizontal eye movements in the rabbit. Exp Neurol 28:132-143

Collewijn H (1970b) Dysmetria of fast phase of optokinetic nystagmus in cerebellectomized rabbits. Exp Neurol 28:144-154

Collewijn H (1972a) Latency and gain of the rabbit's optokinetic reactions to small movements. Brain Res: 59-70

Collewijn H (1972b) An analog model of the rabbit's optokinetic system. Brain Res 36:71-88

Collewijn H (1975a) Oculomotor areas in the rabbit's midbrain and pretectum. J Neurobiol 6:3-22

Collewijn H (1975b) Direction-selective units in the rabbit's nucleus of the optic tract. Brain Res 100:489-508

Collewijn H (1976) Impairment of optokinetic (after-)nystagmus by labyrinthectomy in the rabbit. Exp Neurol 52:146-156

Collewijn H (1977a) Eye- and head movements in freely moving rabbits. J Physiol 266: 471-498
Collewijn H (1977b) Gaze in freely moving subjects. In: Baker R, Berthoz A (eds) Control of gaze by brain stem neurons. Elsevier, Amsterdam New York (Developments in Neuroscience vol 1, pp 13-22)
Collewijn H (1977c) Optokinetic and vestibulo-ocular reflexes in dark-reared rabbits. Exp Brain Res 27:287-300
Collewijn H, Grootendorst AF (1978) Adaptation of the rabbit's vestibulo-ocular reflex to modified visual input: importance of stimulus conditions. Arch Ital Biol 116:273-280
Collewijn H, Grootendorst AF (1979) Adaptation of optokinetic and vestibulo-ocular reflexes to modified visual input in the rabbit. In: Granit R, Pompeiano O (eds) Reflex control of posture and movement. Elsevier, Amsterdam New York (Progress in Brain Research vol 50, pp 771-781)
Collewijn H, Kleinschmidt HJ (1975) Vestibulo-ocular and optokinetic reactions in the rabbit: changes during 24 hours of normal and abnormal interaction. In: Lennerstrand G, Bach-Y-Rita P (eds) Basic mechanisms of ocular motility and their clinical implications, pp 477-483. Pergamon, Oxford New York
Collewijn H, Noorduin H (1972a) Vertical and torsional optokinetic eye movements in the rabbit. Pflügers Arch Ges Physiol 332:87-95
Collewijn H, Noorduin H (1972b) Conjugate and disjunctive optokinetic eye movements in the rabbit, evoked by rotatory and translatory motion. Pflügers Arch Ges Physiol 335:173-185
Collewijn H, Van der Mark F (1972) Ocular stability in variable visual feedback conditions in the rabbit. Brain Res 36:47-57
Collewijn H, Van der Mark F, Jansen TC (1975) Precise recording of human eye movements. Vision Res 15:447-450
Collewijn H, Verhagen AM, Grootendorst AF (1980a) Adaptation of the vestibulo-ocular reflex in albino rabbits by selective exposure of the anterior sector of the visual field. Brain Res 192:305-312
Collewijn H, Winterson BJ, Van der Steen J (1980b) Post-rotatory nystagmus and optokinetic afternystagmus in the rabbit: linear rather than exponential decay. Exp Brain Res 40:330-338
Collewijn H, Winterson BJ, Dubois MFW (1978) Optokinetic eye movements in albino rabbits: inversion in anterior visual field. Science 199:1351-1353
Collins WE (1964) Task control of arousal and the effects of repeated unidirectional angular acceleration on human vestibular responses. Acta Otolaryngol Suppl 190: 1-34
Collins WE (1966) Vestibular responses from figure skaters. Aerospace Med 37:1098-1104
Collins WE (1968) Special effects of brief periods of visual fixation on nystagmus and sensations of turning. Aerospace Med 39:257-266
Collins WE, Updegraff BP (1966) A comparison of nystagmus habituation in the cat and dog. Acta Otolaryngol 62:19-26
Collins WE, Schroeder DJ, Rice N, Mertens RA, Kranz G (1970) Some characteristics of optokinetic eye movement patterns: a comparative study. Aerospace Med 41:1251-1262
Corvaja N, Mergner T, Pompeiano O (1979) Organization of reticular projections to the vestibular nuclei in the cat. In: Granit R, Pompeiano O (eds) Reflex control of posture and movement. Elsevier, Amsterdam New York Oxford (Progress in Brain Research, vol 50, pp 631-644)
Costin A, Chaimovitz M, Bergmann F (1965) Nystagmus evoked by intermittent photic stimulation of the rabbit's eye. Experientia 21:167-168
Crampton GH (1962) Directional imbalance of vestibular nystagmus in cat following repeated unidirectional angular acceleration. Acta Otolaryngol 55:41-48

Creel D, Witkop CJ, King RA (1974) Asymmetric visually evoked potentials in human albinos: evidence for visual system anomalies. Invest Ophthalmol 13:430-440

Creel D, O'Donnel FE, Witkop CJ (1978) Visual system anomalies in human ocular albinos. Science 201:931-933

Daw NW, Wyatt HJ (1974) Raising rabbits in a moving visual environment: an attempt to modify directional sensitivity in the retina. J Physiol 240:309-330

Daw NH, Wyatt HJ (1976) Kittens reared in a unidirectional environment: evidence for a critical period. J Physiol 257:155-170

De Graauw JG, Van Hof MW (1978) Relation between behavior and eye-refraction in the rabbit. Physiol Behav 21:257-259

De Kleijn A, Magnus R (1921) Labyrinth-reflexe auf Progressivbewegungen. Pflügers Arch Ges Physiol 186:39-60

Dichgans J, Brandt T (1972) Visual-vestibular interaction and motion perception. In: Dichgans J, Bizzi E (eds) Cerebral control of eye movements and motion perception. Karger, Basel (Bibliotheca Ophthalmologica vol 82, pp 327-338)

Dichgans J, Bizzi E, Morasso P, Tagliasco V (1973a) Mechanisms underlying recovery of an eye-head coordination following bilateral labyrinthectomy in monkeys. Exp Brain Res 18:548-562

Dichgans J, Schmidt CL, Graf W (1973b) Visual input improves the speedometer function of the vestibular nuclei in the goldfish. Exp Brain Res 18:319-322

Dichgans J, Von Reutern GM, Römmelt U (1978) Impaired suppression of vestibular nystagmus by fixation in cerebellar and non-cerebellar patients. Arch Psychiatr Nervenkr 226:183-199

Dix MR, Hood JD (1969) Observations upon the nervous mechanism of vestibular habituation. Acta Otolaryngol 67:310-318

Dodge R (1903) Five types of eye movement in the horizontal meridian plane of the field of regard. Am J Physiol 8:307-329

Dodge R (1923) Habituation to rotation. J Exp Psychol 6:1-35

Dubois MFW (1978) Optokinetische oogbewegingen tijdens selective retinale stimulatie bij konijn en mens. Thesis, Erasmus University Rotterdam

Dubois MFW, Collewijn H (1979a) The optokinetic reactions of the rabbit: relation to the visual streak. Vision Res 19:9-17

Dubois MFW, Collewijn H (1979b) Optokinetic reactions in man elicited by localized retinal motion stimuli. Vision Res 19:1105-1115

Duensing F, Schaefer KP (1957) Die Neuronenaktivität in der Formatio reticularis des Rhombencephalons beim vestibulären Nystagmus. Arch Psychiatr Nervenkr 196: 265-290

Dufossé M, Ito M, Miyashita Y (1977) Functional localization in the rabbit's cerebellar flocculus determined in relationship with eye movements. Neurosci Lett 5:273-277

Dufossé M, Ito M, Miyashita Y (1978) Diminution and reversal of eye movements induced by local stimulation of the rabbit cerebellar flocculus after partial destruction of the inferior olive. Exp Brain Res 33:139-141

Duke-Elder S (1964) System of ophthalmology. Vol 3 Normal and abnormal development, part 2 Congenital deformities. pp 803-813. Kimpton, London

Elekessy EJ, Campion JE, Henry GH (1973) Differences between the visual fields of Siamese and common cats. Vision Res 13:2533-2543

Erickson RG, Barmack NH (1980) A comparison of the horizontal and vertical optokinetic reflexes of the rabbit. Exp Brain Res 40:448-456

Evinger C, Fuchs AF (1978) Saccadic, smooth pursuit, and optokinetic eye movements of the trained cat. J Physiol 285:209-229

Fernandez C, Goldberg JM (1971) Physiology of peripheral neurons innervating semicircular canals of the squirrel monkey. II. Response to sinusoidal stimulation and dynamics of peripheral vestibular system. J Neurophysiol 34:661-675

Fernandez C, Goldberg JM (1976a) Physiology of peripheral neurons innervating otolith organs of the squirrel monkey. Response to static tilts and to long-duration centrifugal force. J Neurophysiol 39:970-984

Fernandez C, Goldberg JM (1976b) Physiology of peripheral neurons innervating otolith organs of the squirrel monkey. II. Directional selectivity and force-response relations. J Neurophysiol 39:985-995

Fernandez C, Goldberg JM (1976c) Physiology of peripheral neurons innervating otolith organs of the squirrel monkey. III. Response dynamics. J Neurophysiol 39:996-1008

Fernandez C, Goldberg JM, Abend WK (1972) Response to static tilts of peripheral neurons innervating otolith organs of the squirrel monkey. J Neurophysiol 35:978-997

Festen H, Clemens A (1970) Pattern centre. Adv Oto Rhino Laryngol 17:100-106

Fiorentini A, Ercoles AM (1966) Involuntary eye movements during attempted monocular fixation. Atti Fond Ronchi 21:199-217

Flandrin JM, Courjon JH, Jeannerod M, Schmid R (1979) Vestibulo-ocular responses during the states of sleep in the cat. Electroencephalogr Clin Neurophysiol 46:521-530

Fleisch A (1922a) Tonische Labyrinthreflexe auf die Augenstellung. Pflügers Arch Ges Physiol 194:554-573

Fleisch A (1922b) Das Labyrinth als beschleunigungsempfindendes Organ. Pflügers Arch Ges Physiol 195:499-515

Friedman MB (1975) Visual control of head movements during avian locomotion. Nature (London) 255:67-69

Frost BJ (1978) The optokinetic basis of head-bobbing in the pigeon. J Exp Biol 74:187-195

Fuchs AF (1967) Saccadic and smooth pursuit eye movements in the monkey. J Physiol 191:609-631

Fuchs AF, Robinson DA (1966) A method for measuring horizontal and vertical eye movements chronically in the monkey. J Appl Physiol 21:1068-1070

Gauthier GM, Robinson DA (1975) Adaptation of the human vestibulo-ocular reflex to magnifying lenses. Brain Res 92:331-335

Ghelarducci B, Ito M, Yagi N (1975) Impulse discharges from flocculus Purkinje cell of alert rabbits during visual stimulation combined with horizontal head rotation. Brain Res 87:66-72

Giolli RL (1961) An experimental study of the accessory optic tracts (transpeduncular tracts and anterior accessory optic tracts) in the rabbit. J Comp Neurol 117:77-95

Giolli RA, Creel DJ (1973) The primary optic projections in pigmented and albino guinea pigs: an experimental degeneration study. Brain Res 55:25-39

Giolli RA, Creel DJ (1974) Inheritance and variability in the organization of the retinogeniculate projections in pigmented and albino rats. Brain Res 78:335-339

Giolli RA, Guthrie MD (1969) The primary optic projections in the rabbit. An experimental degeneration study. J Comp Neurol 136:99-126

Giolli RA, Guthrie MD (1971) Organization of subcortical projections of visual areas I and II in the rabbit. An experimental degeneration study. J Comp Neurol 142:351-376

Giolli RA, Braithwaite R, Streeter TT (1968) Golgi study of the nucleus of the transpeduncular tract in the rabbit. J Comp Neurol 133:309-328

Gonshor A, Melvill Jones G (1973) Changes of human vestibulo-ocular response induced by vision-reversal during head rotation. J Physiol 234:102P-103P

Gonshor A, Melvill Jones G (1976a) Short-term adaptive changes in the human vestibulo-ocular reflex arc. J Physiol 256:361-379

Gonshor A, Melvill Jones G (1976b) Extreme vestibulo-ocular adaptation induced by prolonged optical reversal of vision. J Physiol 256:381-414

Granit R, Pompeiano O (eds) (1979) Reflex control of posture and movement. Elsevier, Amsterdam New York Oxford (Progress in Brain Research, vol 50)

Graybiel AM (1977a) Organization of oculomotor pathways in the cat and rhesus monkey. In: Baker R, Berthoz A (eds) Control of gaze by brain stem neurons. Elsevier, Amsterdam New York (Developments in Neuroscience, vol 1, pp 79-88)

Graybiel AM (1977b) Direct and indirect preoculomotor pathways of the brainstem; an autoradiographic study of the pontine reticular formation in the cat. J Comp Neurol 175:37-78
Graybiel AM, Hartwieg EA (1974) Some afferent connections of the oculomotor complex in the cat: an experimental study with tracer techniques. Brain Res 81:543-551
Gresty MA (1975) Eye, head and body movements of the guinea pig in response to optokinetic stimulation and sinusoidal oscillation in yaw. Pflügers Arch Ges Physiol 353: 201-214
Gresty MA (1976) A reexamination of 'neck reflex' eye movements in the rabbit. Acta Otolaryngol 81:386-394
Griffith CR (1920) The organic effects of repeated bodily motion. J Exp Psychol 3:15-46
Groen JJ (1957) Adaptation. Pract Oto Rhino Laryngol 19:524-530
Grüsser OJ, Grüsser-Cornehls U (1969) Neurophysiologie des Bewegungssehens. Bewegungsempfindliche und richtungsspezifische Neurone im visuellen System. Ergeb Physiol Biol Chem Exp Pharmakol 61:178-265
Grüsser OJ, Grüsser-Cornehls U (1973) Neuronal mechanism of visual movement perception and some psychophysical and behavioral correlations. In: Jung R (ed) Handbook of sensory physiology. Springer, Berlin Heidelberg New York vol VII/3, pp 333-429
Grüttner R (1939) Experimentelle Untersuchungen über den optokinetischen Nystagmus. Z Sinnesphysiol 68:1-48
Guedry FE (1965) Psychophysiological studies of vestibular function. In: Neff WD (ed) Contributions to sensory physiology, vol I, pp 63-135. Academic Press, London New York
Guillery RW (1971) An abnormal retinogeniculate projection in the albino ferret (Mustela furo). Brain Res 33:482-485
Guillery RW, Kaas JH (1971) A study of normal and congenitally abnormal retinogeniculate projections in cats. J Comp Neurol 143:73-100
Guillery RW, Kaas JH (1973) Genetic abnormality of the visual pathways in a 'White' tiger. Science 180:1287-1289
Guillery RW, Scott GL, Cattanack BM, Deol MS (1973) Genetic mechanisms determining the central visual pathways of mice. Science 179:1014-1016
Guillery RW, Okoro AN, Witkop CJ (1975) Abnormal visual pathways in the brain of a human albino. Brain Res 96:373-377
Gutman J, Bergmann F, Chaimovitz M, Costin A (1963) Nystagmus evoked by stimulation of the optic pathways in the rabbit. Exp Neurol 8:132-142
Gutman J, Zelig S, Bergmann F (1964) Optokinetic nystagmus in the labyrinthectomized rabbit. Confin Neurol 24:158-162
Haddad GM, Robinson DA (1977) Cancellation of the vestibulo-ocular reflex during active and passive head movements in the normal cat. Neurosci Abstr 3
Haddad GM, Friendlich AR, Robinson DA (1977) Compensation of nystagmus after VIIIth nerve lesions in vestibulo-cerebellectomized cats. Brain Res 135:192-196
Hahnenberger RW (1977) Differences in optokinetic nystagmus between albino and pigmented rabbits. Exp Eye Res 25:9-17
Hartmann R, Klinke R (1976) A method for measuring the angle of rotation (movements of body, head, eye in human subjects and experimental animals). Pflügers Arch Ges Physiol Suppl 362:R52
Henn V, Young LR, Finley C (1974) Vestibular nucleus units in alert monkeys are also influenced by moving visual fields. Brain Res 71:144-149
Highstein SM (1973a) The organization of the vestibulo-ocular and trochlear reflex pathways in the rabbit. Exp Brain Res 17:285-300
Highstein SM (1973b) Synaptic linkage in the vestibulo-ocular and cerebello-vestibular pathways to the VIth nucleus in the rabbit. Exp Brain Res 17:301-314
Highstein SM, Ito M, Tsuchiya T (1971) Synaptic linkage in the vestibulo-ocular reflex pathway of the rabbit. Exp Brain Res 13:306-326

Hikosaka O, Kawakami T (1977) Inhibitory reticular neurons related to the quick phase of vestibular nystagmus — their location and projection. Exp Brain Res 27:377-396

Hill RM (1966) Receptive field properties of the superior colliculus of the rabbit. Nature (London) 211:1407-1409

Hitzig E (1874) Physiologische und klinische Untersuchungen über das Gehirn, 1st edn. Hirschwald, Berlin

Hobbelen JF (1971) Optokinetische oogbewegingen bij het konijn: een onderzoek naar de rol van cortex en colliculus superior. Thesis, Erasmus University Rotterdam

Hobbelen JF, Collewijn H (1971) Effect of cerebro-cortical and collicular ablations upon the optokinetic reactions in the rabbit. Doc Ophthalmol 30:227-236

Hoddevik GH (1977) The pontine projection to the flocculonodular lobe and the paraflocculus studied by means of retrograde axonal transport of horseradish peroxidase in the rabbit. Exp Brain Res 30:511-526

Hoddevik GH, Brodal A (1977) The olivocerebellar projection studied with the method of retrograde axonal transport of horseradish peroxidase. V. The projections to the flocculonodular lobe and the paraflocculus in the rabbit. J Comp Neurol 176:269-280

Hoddevik GH, Brodal A, Kawamura K, Hashikawa T (1977) The pontine projection of the cerebellar vermal visual area studied by means of the retrograde axonal transport of horseradish peroxidase. Brain Res 123:209-227

Hoffmann KP (1973) Conduction velocity in pathways from retina to superior colliculus in the cat: a correlation with receptive field properties. J Neurophysiol 36:409-424

Hoffmann KP, Schoppmann A (1975) Retinal input to direction-selective cells in the nucleus tractus opticus of the cat. Brain Res 99:359-366

Holstege G, Collewijn H (in press) The efferent projections of the nucleus of the optic tract in the rabbit, investigated by the antegrade transport of ^{3}H leucine.

Hood JD, Leech J (1974) The significance of peripheral vision in the perception of movement. Acta Otolaryngol 77:72-79

Hood JD, Pfaltz CR (1954) Observations upon the effects of repeated stimulation upon rotational and caloric nystagmus. J Physiol 124:130-144

Horridge GA (1966a) Optokinetic memory in the crab, carcinus. J Exp Biol 44:233-245

Horridge GA (1966b) Optokinetic memory in the locust. J Exp Biol 44:255-261

Horridge GA, Sandeman DC (1964) Nervous control of optokinetic responses in the crab, Carcinus. Proc R Soc London Ser B 161:216-246

Hubel DH, Wiesel TN (1971) Aberrant visual projections in the Siamese cat. J Physiol 218:33-62

Hughes A (1971) Topographical relationships between the anatomy and physiology of the rabbit visual system. Doc Ophthalmol 30:33-159

Hughes A (1972) Vergence in the cat. Vision Res 12:1961-1994

Hughes A (1975a) A comparison of retinal ganglion cell topography in the plains and tree kangaroo. J Physiol 244:61-63P

Hughes A (1975b) A quantitative analysis of the cat retinal ganglion cell topography. J Comp Neurol 163:107-128

Hughes A, Vaney DI (1978) The refractive state of the rabbit eye: variation with eccentricity and correction for oblique astigmatism. Vision Res 18:1351-1355

Igarashi M, Takahashi M, Homick JL (1977) Optokinetic nystagmus and vestibular stimulation in squirrel monkey model. Arch Oto Rhino Laryngol 218:115-121

Igarashi M, Takahashi M, Homick JL (1978) Optokinetic afternystagmus and postrotatory nystagmus in squirrel monkey. Acta Otolaryngol 85:387-396

Ito M (1972) Neural design of the cerebellar motor control system. Brain Res 40:81-84

Ito M (1977) Neuronal events in the cerebellar flocculus associated with an adaptive modification of the vestibulo-ocular reflex of the rabbit. In: Baker R, Berthoz A (eds) Control of gaze by brain stem neurons. Elsevier, Amsterdam New York (Developments in Neuroscience, vol 1, pp 391-398)

Ito M, Miyashita Y (1975) The effects of chronic destruction of the inferior olive upon visual modification of the horizontal vestibulo-ocular reflex of rabbits. Proc Jpn Acad 51:716-720

Ito M, Miyashita Y, Ueki A (1978) Functional localization in the rabbit's inferior olive determined in connection with the vestibulo-ocular reflex. Neurosci Lett 8:283-287

Ito M, Nisimaru N, Yamamoto M (1973) Specific neural connections for the cerebellar control of vestibulo-ocular reflexes. Brain Res 60:238-243

Ito M, Shiida T, Yagi N, Yamamoto M (1974a) Visual influence on rabbit horizontal vestibulo-ocular reflex presumably effected via the cerebellar flocculus. Brain Res 65:170-174

Ito M, Shiita T, Yagi N, Yamamoto M (1974b) The cerebellar modification of rabbit's horizontal vestibulo-ocular reflex induced by sustained head rotation combined with visual stimulation. Proc Jpn Acad 50:85-89

Ito M, Nisimaru N, Yamamoto M (1976a) Pathways for the vestibulo-ocular reflex excitation arising from semicircular canals of rabbits. Exp Brain Res 24:257-271

Ito M, Nisimaru N, Yamamoto M (1976b) Postsynaptic inhibition of oculomotor neurons involved in vestibulo-ocular reflexes arising from semicircular canals of rabbits. Exp Brain Res 24:273-283

Ito M, Nisimaru N, Yamamoto M (1976c) Inhibitory interaction between the vestibulo-ocular reflexes arising from semicircular canals of rabbits. Exp Brain Res 26:89-103

Ito M, Nisimaru N, Yamamoto M (1977) Specific patterns of neuronal connexions involved in the control of the rabbit's vestibulo-ocular reflexes by the cerebellar flocculus. J Physiol 265:833-854

Ito M, Orlov I, Shimoyama I (1978) Reduction of the cerebellar stimulus effect on rat Deiters neurons after chemical destruction of the inferior olive. Exp Brain Res 33:143-145

Ito M, Jastreboff PJ, Miyashita Y (1979a) Adaptive modification of the rabbit's horizontal vestibulo-ocular reflex during sustained vestibular and optokinetic stimulation. Exp Brain Res 37:17-30

Ito M, Nisimaru N, Shibuki K (1979b) Destruction of inferior olive induces rapid depression in synaptic action of cerebellar Purkinje cells. Nature (London) 277:568-569

Itoh K (1977) Efferent projections of the pretectum in the cat. Exp Brain Res 30:89-105

Jacobson M, Hirose G (1978) Origin of the retina from both sides of the embryonic brain: a contribution to the problem of crossing at the optic chiasma. Science 202:637-639

Julesz B (1964) Binocular depth perception without familiarity cues. Science 145:356-362

Jung R (1948) Die Registrierung des postrotatorischen und optokinetischen Nystagmus und die optisch-vestibuläre Integration beim Menschen. Acta Otolaryngol 36:199-202

Kalil RE, Jhaveri SR, Richards W (1971) Anomalous retinal pathways in the Siamese cat: an inadequate substrate for normal binocular vision. Science 174:302-305

Karten HJ, Fite KV, Brecha N (1977) Specific projection of displaced retinal ganglion cells upon the accessory optic system in the pigeon (Columba livia). Proc Natl Acad Sci USA 74:1753-1756

Keane JR (1972) Flash-evoked nystagmus: absence in man. Neurology 22:551-553

Keller EL (1976) Behavior of horizontal semicircular canal afferents in alert monkey during vestibular and optokinetic stimulation. Exp Brain Res 24:459-471

Keller E, Precht W (1978) Persistence of visual response in vestibular nucleus neurons in cerebellectomized cat. Exp Brain Res 32:591-594

Kleinschmidt HJ (1974) Effekten van langdurige prikkeling op de vestibulo-oculaire reflexen van het konijn. Thesis, Erasmus University Rotterdam

Kleinschmidt HJ, Collewijn H (1975) A search for habituation of vestibulo-ocular reactions to rotatory and linear sinusoidal accelerations in the rabbit. Exp Neurol 47:257-267

Koenig E, Allum JHJ, Dichgans J (1978) Visual-vestibular interaction upon nystagmus slow phase velocity in man. Acta Otolaryngol 85:397-410

Körner F (1975) Untersuchungen über die nichtvisuelle Kontrolle von Augenbewegungen. Adv Ophthalmol 31:100-158
Körner F, Dichgans J (1967) Bewegungswahrnehmung, optokinetischer Nystagmus und retinale Bildwanderung. Der Einfluß visueller Aufmerksamkeit auf zwei Mechanismen des Bewegungssehens. Albrecht von Graefes Arch Ophthalmol 174:34-48
Koerner F, Schiller PH (1972) The optokinetic response under open and closed loop conditions in the monkey. Exp Brain Res 14:318-330
Komatsuzaki A, Harris HE, Alpert J, Cohen B (1969) Horizontal nystagmus of rhesus monkeys. Acta Otolaryngol 67:535-551
Krieger HP, Bender MB (1956) Optokinetic afternystagmus in the monkey. Electroencephalogr Clin Neurophysiol 8:97-106
Kulikowski JJ (1978) Pattern and movement detection in man and rabbit: separation and comparison of occipital potentials. Vision Res 18:183-188
Landers PH, Taylor A (1975) Transfer function analysis of the vestibulo-ocular reflex in the conscious cat. In: Lennerstrand G, Bach-y-Rita P (eds) Basic mechanisms of ocular motility and their clinical implications, pp 505-508. Pergamon Press, Oxford
Lane RH, Kaas JH, Allman JM (1974) Visuotopic organization of the superior colliculus in normal and Siamese cats. Brain Res 70:413-430
Levick WR, Oyster CW, Takahashi E (1969) Rabbit lateral geniculate nucleus: sharpener of direction selective information. Science 165:712-714
Lindeman HH (1969) Studies on the morphology of the sensory regions of the vestibular apparatus. Ergeb Anat Entwicklungsgesch 42:1-113
Llinas R, Walton K, Hillman DE, Sotelo C (1975) Inferior olive: its role in motor learning. Science 190:1230-1231
Lockley RM (1975) The private life of the rabbit, 2nd edn. Avon Books New York
Loe PR, Tomko DL, Werner G (1973) The neural signal of angular head position in primary afferent vestibular nerve axons. J Physiol 230:29-50
Lopez-Barneo J, Darlot C, Berthoz A (1979) Functional role of the prepositus hypoglossi nucleus in the control of gaze. In: Granit R, Pompeiano O (eds) Reflex control of posture and movement. Elsevier, Amsterdam New York Oxford (Progress in Brain Research, vol 50, pp 667-679)
Lorente de Nó R (1931) Ausgewählte Kapitel aus der vergleichenden Physiologie des Labyrinthes. Die Augenmuskelreflexe beim Kaninchen und ihre Grundlagen. Ergeb Physiol 32:73-242
Lund RD (1965) Uncrossed visual pathways of hooded and albino rats. Science 149: 1506-1507
MacKay WA, Murphy JT (1979) Cerebellar modulation of reflex gain. Prog Neurobiol 13:361-417
Mackensen G, Wiegmann O (1959) Untersuchungen zur Physiologie des optokinetischen Nachnystagmus. I. Mitteilung. Die Abhängigkeit des optokinetischen Nachnystagmus von der Drehrichtung und der Winkelgeschwindigkeit des Reizmusters. Albrecht von Graefs Arch Ophthalmol 160:497-509
Mackensen G, Kommerrell G, Silbereisen D (1961) Untersuchungen zur Physiologie des optokinetischen Nachnystagmus. II. Mitteilung. Individuelle Unterschiede des Nachnystagmus, die Abhängigkeit des optokinetischen Nachnystagmus von der Reizdauer. Albrecht von Graefs Arch Ophthalmol 163:170-187
Maekawa KE, Simpson JI (1972) Climbing fiber activation of Purkinje cells in the flocculus by impulses transferred through the visual pathway. Brain Res 39:245-251
Maekawa K, Simpson JI (1973) Climbing fiber responses evoked in vestibulocerebellum of rabbit from visual system. J Neurophysiol 36:649-666
Maekawa K, Takeda T (1975) Mossy fiber responses evoked in the cerebellar flocculus of rabbits by stimulation of the optic pathway. Brain Res 98:590-595
Maekawa K, Takeda T (1976) Electrophysiological identification of the climbing and mossy fiber pathways from the rabbit's retina to the contralateral cerebellar floculus. Brain Res 109:169-174

References

Magnus R (1924) Körperstellung. Springer, Berlin Heidelberg New York
Manni E, Azzena GB, Desole C (1964) Eye nystagmus elicited by stimulation of the cerebral cortex in the rabbit. Arch Ital Biol 102:645-656
Masland RH, Chow KL, Stewart DL (1971) Receptive field characteristics of superior colliculus neurons in the rabbit. J Neurophysiol 34:148-156
McCrea RA, Baker R, Delgado-Garcia J (1979) Afferent and efferent organization of the prepositus hypoglossi nucleus. In: Granit R, Pompeiano O (eds) Reflex control of posture and movement. Elsevier, Amsterdam New York Oxford (Progress in Brain Research, vol 50, pp 653-665)
Meiry JL (1971) Vestibular and proprioceptive stabilization of eye movements. In: Bach-y-Rita P, Collins CC (eds) The control of eye movements, pp 483-496. Academic Press, London New York
Melvill Jones G, Davies P (1976) Adaptation of cat vestibulo-ocular reflex to 200 days of optically reversed vision. Brain Res 103:551-554
Melvill Jones G, Milsum JH (1969) Neural response of the vestibular system to tranlational acceleration. In: Supplement to Conference on systems analysis approach to neurophysiological problems, pp 8-20. Brainerd, Minnesota
Mesulam MM (1978) Tetramethyl benzidine for horseradish peroxidase neurohistochemistry: a non-carcinogenic blue reaction-product with superior sensitivity for visualizing neural afferents and efferents. J Histochem Cytochem 26:106-117
Meyer DL, Meyer-Hamme S, Schaefer KP (1972) Electrophysiological investigation of refractive state and accomodation in the rabbit's eye. Pflügers Arch Ges Physiol 332: 80-86
Miles FA, Fuller JH (1974) Adaptive plasticity in the vestibulo-ocular responses of the rhesus monkey. Brain Res 80:512-516
Miller M, Pasik T, Pasik P (1979) Flicker-induced nystagmus in a ganzfeld situation in monkeys. Exp Neurol 66:533-546
Miyoshi T, Pfaltz CR, Piffko P (1973) Effect of repetitive optokinetic stimulation upon optokinetic and vestibular responses. Acta Otolaryngol 75:259-265
Mizuno N, Mochizuki K, Akimoto C, Matsushima R (1973) Pretectal projections to the inferior olive in the rabbit. Exp Neurol 39:498-506
Mizuno N, Nakamura Y, Iwahori N (1974) An electron microscope study of the dorsal cap of the inferior olive in the rabbit, with special reference to the pretecto-olivary fibers. Brain Res 77:385-395
Moran WB (1974) The changes in phase lag during sinusoidal angular rotation following labyrinthectomy in the cat. Laryngoscope 84:1707-1728
Morasso P, Bizzi E, Dichgans J (1973) Adjustment of saccade characteristics during head movements. Exp Brain Res 16:492-500
Mowrer OH (1936a) A comparison of the reaction mechanisms mediating optokinetic nystagmus in human beings and in pigeons. Psychol Monogr 47:294-305
Mowrer OH (1936b) Maturation vs. learning in the development of vestibular and optokinetic nystagmus. J Genet Psychol 48:383-404
Mowrer OH (1937) The influence of vision during bodily rotation upon the duration of post-rotational vestibular nystagmus. Acta Otolaryngol 25:351-364
Murphy EH, Berman N (1979) The rabbit and the cat: a comparison of some features of response properties of single cells in the primary visual cortex. J Comp Neurol 188:401-428
Murphy JT, Sabah NH (1970) The inhibitory effect of climbing fiber activation on cerebellar Purkinje cells. Brain Res 19:486-490
Nasiell V (1924) Zur Frage des Dunkelnystagmus und über postrotatorischen Nystagmus und Deviation der Augen bei Lageveränderungen des Kopfes und des Körpers gegen den Kopf beim Dunkelkaninchen. Acta Otolaryngol 6:175-177
Neverov VP, Kissljakov VA (1971) The reversive postoptokinetic nystagmus — an experimental model of the oculomotor centres automatic activity. In: Visual information processing and control of motor activity. Bulg Acad Sci, Sofia pp 229-235

Neverov VP, Ueda M, Bureš J (1976) The effect of cortical and collicular spreading depression on the optokinetic and reversive postoptokinetic nystagmus in rabbits. Brain Res 115:318-323

Ohm J (1921) Ueber optischen Drehnystagmus. Klin Monatsbl Augenheilk 68:234-235

Ohm J (1926) Ist der optische Drehnystagmus von einem unbeweglichen Auge auslösbar? Klin Monatsbl Augenheilk 77:330-336

Oyster CW (1968) The analysis of image motion by the rabbit retina. J Physiol 199:613-635

Oyster CW, Barlow HB (1967) Direction-selective units in rabbit retina: Distribution of preferred directions. Science 155:841-842

Oyster CW, Takahashi E, Collewijn H (1972) Direction-selective retinal ganglion cells and control of optokinetic nystagmus in the rabbit. Vision Res 12:183-193

Pasik P, Pasik T, Krieger HP (1959) Effects of cerebral lesions upon optokinetic nystagmus in monkeys. J Neurophysiol 22:297-304

Pasik T, Pasik P, Valciukas JA (1970) Nystagmus induced by stationary repetitive light flashes in monkeys. Brain Res 19:313-317

Pompeiano O, Mergner T, Corvaja N (1978) Commissural, perihypoglossal and reticular afferent projections to the vestibular nuclei in the cat: an experimental anatomical study with the method of the retrograde transport of horseradish peroxidase. Arch Ital Biol 116:130-172

Precht W (1974) Characteristics of vestibular neurons after acute and chronic labyrinthine destruction. In: Autrum H et al. (eds) Handbook of sensory physiology, vol VI/2, pp 451-462. Springer, Berlin Heidelberg New York

Precht W (1975) Cerebellar influences on eye movements. In: Lennerstrand G, Bach-y-Rita P (eds) Basic mechanisms of ocular motility and their clinical implications, pp 261-280. Pergamon Press, Oxford New York Toronto

Precht W (1978) Neuronal operations in the vestibular system. Studies of brain function, vol 2. Springer, Berlin Heidelberg New York

Precht W, Cazin L (1979) Functional deficits in the optokinetic system of albino rats. Exp Brain Res 37:183-186

Precht W, Strata P (1979) Pathways mediating optokinetic responses of cat's vestibular neurons. Neurosci Lett Suppl 3:351

Precht W, Shimazu H, Markham CH (1966) A mechanism of central compensation of vestibular function following hemilabyrinthectomy. J Neurophysiol 29:996-1010

Prince JH (1964) The rabbit in eye research. Thomas, Springfield

Provis JM (1979) The distribution and size of ganglion cells in the retina of the pigmented rabbit: a quantitative analysis. J Comp Neurol 185:121-138

Raphan T, Cohen B (1978) Brain stem mechanisms for rapid and slow eye movements. Annu Rev Physiol 40:527-552

Raphan T, Cohen B, Matsuo V (1977) A velocity storage mechanism responsible for optokinetic nystagmus (OKAN) and vestibular nystagmus. In: Baker R, Berthoz A (eds) Control of gaze by brainstem neurons. Elsevier, Amsterdam (Developments in Neuroscience, vol 1, pp 37-47)

Raphan T, Matsuo V, Cohen B (1979) Velocity storage in the vestibulo-ocular reflex arc (VOR). Exp Brain Res 35:229-248

Rashbass C, Westheimer G (1961a) Disjunctive eye movements. J Physiol 159:339-360

Rashbass C, Westheimer G (1961b) Independence of conjugate and disjunctive eye movements. J Physiol 159:361-364

Roberts TDM (1978) Neurophysiology of postural mechanisms, 2nd edn. Butterworths, London

Robinson DA (1963) A method of measuring eye movement using a scleral search coil in a magnetic field. IEEE Trans Bio-med Electron BME 10:137-145

Robinson DA (1968) Eye movement control in primates. Science 161:1219-1224

References

Robinson DA (1971) Models of oculomotor neural organization. In: Bach-y-Rita P, Collins CC (eds) The control of eye movements, pp 519-538. Academic Press, London New York

Robinson DA (1972) Eye movements evoked by collicular stimulation in the alert monkey. Vision Res 12:1795-1808

Robinson DA (1974) The effect of cerebellectomy on the cat's vestibulo-ocular integrator. Brain Res 71:195-207

Robinson DA (1975) Oculomotor control signals. In: Lennerstrand G, Bach-y-Rita P (eds) Basic mechanisms of ocular motility and their clinical implications, pp 337-374. Pergamon Press, Oxford

Robinson DA (1976) Adaptive gain control of vestibulo-ocular reflex by the cerebellum. J Neurophysiol 39:954-969

Robinson DA (1977a) Vestibular and optokinetic symbiosis: an example of explaining by modelling. In: Baker R, Berthoz A (eds) Control of gaze by brain stem neurons. Elsevier, Amsterdam New York (Developments in Neuroscience, vol 1, pp 49-58)

Robinson DA (1977b) Linear addition of optokinetic and vestibular signals in the vestibular nucleus. Exp Brain Res 30:447-450

Rönne H (1923) Mouvements apparents, produits à la vision par verres de lunettes, et la correction de ces mouvements par les canaux semicirculaires. Acta Otolaryngol 5: 108-110

Roucoux A, Crommelinck M (1976) Eye movements evoked by superior colliculus stimulation in the alert cat. Brain Res 106:349-363

Rubens SR (1945) Cube-surface coil for producing a uniform magnetic field. Rev Sci Instrum 16:243-245

Ryu JH, McCabe BF (1976) Central vestibular compensation: effect of the bilateral labyrinthectomy on neural activity in the medial vestibular nucleus. Arch Otolaryngol 102:71-76

Sanderson KJ (1975) Retinogeniculate projections in the rabbits of the albino allelomorphic series. J Comp Neurol 159:15-27

Sanderson KJ, Guillery RW, Shackelford RM (1974) Congenitally abnormal visual pathways in mink (Mustela vison) with reduced retinal pigment. J Comp Neurol 154:225-248

Scala NP, Spiegel EA (1941) Subcortical (passive) optokinetic nystagmus in lesions of the midbrain and of the vestibular nuclei. Conf Neurol 3:53-73

Scalia F (1972) The termination of retinal axons in the pretectal region of mammals. J Comp Neurol 145:223-258

Schaefer KP (1966) Mikroableitungen im Tectum opticum des frei beweglichen Kaninchens. Arch Psychiatr Nervenkr 208:120-146

Schaefer KP, Meyer DL (1974) Compensation of vestibular lesions. In: Autrum H et al (eds) Handbook of sensory physiology, vol VI/2, pp 463-490. Springer, Berlin Heidelberg New York

Schiller PH, Stryker M (1972) Single-unit recording and stimulation in superior colliculus of the alert rhesus monkey. J Neurophysiol 35:915-924

Schiller PH, True SD, Conway JL (1979) Effects of frontal eye field and superior colliculus ablations on eye movements. Science 206:590-592

Schöne H (1964) On the role of gravity in human spatial orientation. Aerospace Med 35:764-772

Schor CM, Levi DM (1980) Disturbances of small-field horizontal and vertical optokinetic nystagmus in amblyopia. Invest Ophthalmol 19:668-683

Schor RH (1974) Responses of cat vestibular neurons to sinusoidal roll tilt. Exp Brain Res 20:347-362

Semm P (1978) Antidromically activated direction selectiva ganglion cells of the rabbit. Neurosci Lett 9:207-211

Shinoda Y, Yoshida K (1974) Dynamic characteristics of responses to horizontal head angular acceleration in vestibuloocular pathway in the cat. J Neurophysiol 37:653-673

Simpson JI, Alley KE (1974) Visual climbing fiber input to rabbit vestibulocerebellum: a source of direction-specific information. Brain Res 82:302-308

Simpson JI, Hess R (1977) Complex and simple visual messages in the flocculus. In: Baker R, Berthoz A (eds) Control of gaze by brain stem neurons. Elsevier, Amsterdam New York (Developments in Neuroscience, vol 1, pp 351-360)

Simpson JI, Soodak RE, Hess R (1979) The accessory optic system and its relation to the vestibulocerebellum. In: Granit R, Pompeiano O (eds) Reflex control of posture and movement. Elsevier, Amsterdam New York (Progress in Brain Research, vol 50, pp 715-724)

Sjöstrand FS, Nilsson SE (1964) The structure of the rabbit retina as revealed by electron microscopy. In: Prince JH (ed) The rabbit in eye research, pp 455-467. Thomas, Springfield, Ill

Skavenski AA, Robinson DA (1973) Role of abducens neurons in vestibulo-ocular reflex. J Neurophysiol 36:724-738

Skavenski AA, Steinman RM (1970) Control of eye position in the dark. Vision Res 10: 193-203

Skavenski AA, Hansen RM, Steinman RM, Winterson BJ (1979) Quality of retinal image stabilization during small natural and artificial body rotations in man. Vision Res 19: 675-683

Smith KU, Bridgeman M (1943) The neural mechanisms of movement vision and optic nystagmus. J Exp Psychol 33:165-187

Steinhausen W (1933) Über die Beobachtung der Cupula in den Bogengangsampullen des Labyrinths der lebenden Hecht. Pflügers Arch Ges Physiol 232:500-512

Steinman RM, Collewijn H (1980) Binocular retinal image motion during active head rotation. Vision Res 20:415-429

Steinman RM, Cunitz RJ, Timberlake GT, Herman M (1967) Voluntary control of microsaccades during maintained monocular fixation. Science 155:1577-1579

Stewart DL, Chow KL, Masland R (1971) Receptive-field characteristics of lateral geniculate neurons in the rabbit. J Neurophysiol 34:139-147

Stone J (1965) A quantitative analysis of the distribution of ganglion cells in the cat's retina. J Comp Neurol 124:337-352

Stone J (1978) The number and distribution of ganglion cells in the cat's retina. J Comp Neurol 180:753-772

Stone J, Fukuda Y (1974) Properties of cat retinal ganglion cells: a comparison of W-cells with X- and Y-cells. J Neurophysiol 37:722-748

Stone J, Hoffmann KP (1972) Very slow-conducting ganglion cells in the cat's retina: a major, new functional type? Brain Res 43:610-616

Straschill M, Rieger P (1973) Eye movements evoked by focal stimulation of the cat's superior colliculus. Brain Res 59:211-227

Stryker M, Blakemore C (1972) Saccadic and disjunctive eye movements in cats. Vision Res 12:2005-2013

Sunay T, John F, Montandon A (1976) L'habituation vestibulaire pendulaire et rotatoire. ORL 38 (Suppl 1):66-70

Takahashi ES, Hickey TL, Oyster CW (1977) Retinogeniculate projections in the rabbit: an autoradiographic study. J Comp Neurol 175:1-12

Takahashi ES, Oyster CW, Simpson JI, Soodak RE (1979) Size and distribution of retinal ganglion cells projecting to the rabbit medial terminal nucleus. Neurosci Abstr 5: 2736

Takeda T, Maekawa K (1976) The origin of the pretecto-olivary tract. A study using the horseradish peroxidase method. Brain Res 117:319-325

Takemori S, Cohen B (1974) Loss of visual suppression of vestibular nystagmus after flocculus lesions. Brain Res 72:213-224

Tauber ES, Atkin A (1968) Optomotor responses to monocular stimulation: relation to visual system organization. Science 160:1365-1367
Terasawa K, Otani K, Yamada J (1979) Descending pathways of the nucleus of the optic tract in the rat. Brain Res 173:405-417
Ter Braak JWG (1936) Untersuchungen über optokinetischen Nystagmus. Arch Néerl Physiol 21:309-376
Ter Braak JWG, Van Vliet AGM (1963) Subcortical optokinetic nystagmus in the monkey. Psychiatr Neurol Neurochir 66:277-283
Ter Braak JWG, Schenk VWD, Van Vliet AGM (1971) Visual reactions in a case of longlasting cortical blindness. J Neurol Neurosurg Psychiatr 34:140-147
Toates FM (1974) Vergence eye movements. Doc Ophthalmol 37:153-214
Van der Hoeve J, De Kleijn A (1917) Tonische Labyrinthreflexe auf die Augen. Pfügers Arch Ges Physiol 169:241-262
Van Egmond AAJ, Groen JJ, Jongkees LBW (1949) The mechanisms of the semicircular canal. J Physiol 110:1-17
Vaney DI (1980) The grating acuity of the wild european rabbit. Vision Res 20:87-89
Vaney DI, Hughes A (1976) The rabbit optic nerve: fiber diameter spectrum, fiber count, and comparison with a retinal ganglion cell count. J Comp Neurol 170:241-252
Van Hof MW (1966) Discrimination between striated patterns of different orientation in the rabbit. Vision Res 6:89-94
Van Hof MW (1967) Visual acuity in the rabbit. Vision Res 7:749-751
Van Hof MW, Kobayashi K (1972) Pattern discrimination in rabbits deprived of light for 7 months after birth. Exp Neurol 35:551-557
Van Hof MW, Lagers-Van Haselen GC (1973) The retinal fixation area in the rabbit. Exp Neurol 41:218-221
Van Hof MW, Steele Russell I (1977) Binocular vision in the rabbit. Physiol Behav 19: 121-128
Van Hof-Van Duin J (1976a) Development of visuomotor behavior in normal and darkreared cats. Brain Res 104:233-241
Van Hof-Van Duin J (1976b) Early and permanent effects of monocular deprivation on pattern discrimination and visuomotor behavior in cats. Brain Res 111:261-276
Van Sluyters RC, Stewart DL (1974) Binocular neurons of the rabbit's visual cortex: receptive field characteristics. Exp Brain Res 19:166-195
Velzeboer CMJ (1952) Bilateral cortical hemianopsia and optokinetic nystagmus. Ophthalmologica 123:187-188
Vital-Durand F, Jeannerod M (1974) Role of visual experience in the development of optokinetic response in kittnes. Exp Brain Res 20:297-302
Vital-Durand F, Putkonen PTS, Jeannerod M (1974) Motion detection and optokinetic responses in dark-reared kittens. Vision Res 14:141-142
Waespe W, Henn V (1977a) Neuronal activity in the vestibular nuclei of the alert monkey during vestibular and optokinetic stimulation. Exp Brain Res 27:523-538
Waespe W, Henn V (1977b) Vestibular nuclei activity during optokinetic afternystagmus (OKAN) in the alert monkey. Exp Brain Res 30:323-330
Waespe W, Henn V (1979) Motion information in the vestibular nuclei of alert monkeys: Visual and vestibular input vs. optomotor output. In: Granit R, Pompeiano O (eds) Reflex control of posture and movement. Elsevier, Amsterdam New York Oxford (Progress in Brain Research, vol 50, pp 682-693)
Waespe W, Huber Th, Henn V (1978) Dynamic changes of optokinetic afternystagmus (OKAN) caused by brief visual fixation periods in monkey and in man. Arch Psychiatr Nervenkr 226:1-10
Wässle H, Levick WR, Cleland BG (1975) The distribution of the alpha type of ganglion cells in the cat's retina. J Comp Neurol 159:419-438
Walley RE (1967) Receptive fields in the accessory optic system of the rabbit. Exp Neurol 17:27-43

Weber JT, Kaas JH, Harting JK (1978) Retinocollicular pathways in Siamese cats: an autoradiographic analysis. Brain Res 148:189-196

Westheimer G, Blair SM (1973) Oculomotor defects in cerebellectomized monkeys. Invest Ophthalmol 12:618-621

Westheimer G, Blair SM (1974) Unit activity in accessory optic system in alert monkeys. Invest Ophthalmol 13:533-534

Whitteridge D (1960) Central control of eye movements. In: Field F, Magoun HW, Hall VE (eds) Handbook of Physiology, section 1: Neurophysiology, vol II, pp 1089-1109. American Physiological Society, Washington

Wiersma CAG, Hirsch R (1974) Memory evoked optomotor responses in crustaceans. J Neurobiol 5:213-230

Wiersma CAG, Hirsch R (1975a) On the organization of memory in the optomotor system of the crab pachygrapsus crassipes. J Neurobiol 6:115-123

Wiersma CAG, Hirsch R (1975b) Contrast induced zones as the basis of optomotor memory in the crab, Pachygrapsus. J Comp Physiol 102:173-188

Wiesel TN, Hubel DH (1963) Single-cell responses in striate cortex of kittens deprived of vision in one eye. J Neurophysiol 26:1003-1017

Wildberger H, Meyer M (1978) Zur augenmotorischen Störung des Albino. Klin Monatsbl Augenheilk 172:487-490

Wilson VJ, Melvill Jones G (1979) Mammalian vestibular physiology. Plenum Press, New York London

Winkler C (1907) The central course of the nervus octavus and its influence on motility. Proc K Ned Akad Wet II 14:1-44

Winterson BJ, Collewijn H (1979) Beyond the looking glass: direction sensitivity to frontal fields is inverted in units in the nucleus of the optic tract in albino rabbits. Invest Ophthal ARVO Abstr Suppl (1979):102

Winterson BJ, Collewijn H (in press) Inversion of direction-selectivity to anterior visual fields in neurons of the nucleus of the optic tract in rabbits with ocular albinism. Brain Res, in press

Winterson BJ, Collewijn H, Steinman R (1979a) Compensatory eye movements to miniature rotations in the rabbit: implications for retinal image stability. Vision Res 19: 1155-1159

Winterson BJ, Collewijn H, Van der Steen J (1979b) Postrotatory nystagmus, optokinetic afternystagmus and the vestibulo-ocular response in Dutch belted rabbits. Neurosci Abstr 5:1317

Witkop CJ, Hill CW, Desnick S, Thies JK, Thorn HL, Jenkins M, White JG (1973) Ophthalmologic, biochemical platelet and ultrastructural defects in the various types of oculocutaneous albinism. J Invest Dermatol 60:443-456

Wood CC, Spear PD, Braun JJ (1973) Direction-specific deficits in horizontal optokinetic nystagmus following removal of visual cortex in the cat. Brain Res 60:231-237

Wurtz RH, Albano JE (1980) Visual-motor function of the primate superior colliculus. Annu Rev Neurosci 3:189-226

Wyatt HJ, Daw NW (1975) Directionally sensitive ganglion cells in the rabbit retina: specificity for stimulus direction, size and speed. J Neurophysiol 28:613-626

Yamamoto M (1979) Topographical representation in rabbit cerebellar flocculus for various afferents inputs from the brainstem investigated by means of retrograde axonal transport of horseradish peroxidase. Neurosci Lett 12:29-34

Yee RD, Baloh RW, Honrubia V, Lan CGY, Jenkins HA (1979) Slow build-up of optokinetic nystagmus associated with downbeat nystagmus. Invest Ophthalmol 18:622-629

Young LR, Henn VS (1974) Selective habituation of vestibular nystagmus by visual stimulation. Acta Otolaryngol 77:159-166

Young LR, Henn VS (1976) Selective habituation of vestibular nystagmus by visual stimulation in the monkey. Acta Otolaryngol 82:165-171

Zee DS, Friendlich AR, Robinson DA (1974) The mechanism of downbeat nystagmus. Arch Neurol 30:227-237

References

Zee DS, Yee RD, Cogan DG, Robinson DA, Engel WK (1976a) Ocular motor abnormalities in hereditary cerebellar ataxia. Brain 99:207-234

Zee DS, Yee RD, Robinson DA (1976b) Optokinetic responses in labyrinthine-defective human beings. Brain Res 113:423-428

Zuidam I, Collewijn H (1979) Vergence eye movements of the rabbit in visuomotor behavior. Vision Res 19:185-194

Appendix

Investigations on Optokinetic Nystagmus[1]
By J.W.G. ter Braak

From the Department of Physiology, University of Leiden
Head: Prof. Dr. G.G.J. Rademaker

Translated by H. Collewijn

---

1 Original title: Untersuchungen über optokinetischen Nystagmus. Published in Archives Néerlandaises de Physiologie de l'homme et des animaux, Vol. 21, pp. 309-376 (1936)

1. Introduction

Many attempts have already been made to classify the complex of eye movements known as optokinetic nystagmus among the various types of eye movements. However, the different investigators interested in this problem have arrived at widely divergent concepts.

Still widely held nowadays, particularly among clinicians, is the original concept of Barany, according to which the slow phase of the nystagmus is generated because an object which attracts the attention is pursued with the eyes. In this concept, the fast phase is considered as a refixation movement aimed at a new object that draws the attention.

In contrast, Ohm emphatically argues that optokinetic nystagmus has nothing to do with pursuit and fixation of specific objects; according to Ohm optokinetic nystagmus is a phenomenon closely related to vestibular rotatory nystagmus. On the other hand he too supposes that attention is necessary for eliciting OKN and, in agreement with Barany and others, he assumes that the cerebral cortex is indispensable for its generation.

The concept of Bartels should be mentioned as a third. According to this investigator OKN is a primitive mechanism, closely related to "tropisms" and served by subcortical centers and pathways, although under certain circumstances it can be influenced to a certain extent by the cerebrum.

The following investigations, performed mainly in several species of animals and partly also in humans, will show that all three concepts mentioned contain correct elements and that two fundamentally different types of optokinetic nystagmus exist.

2. The Optokinetic Nystagmus in the Rabbit

To those supporting the first concept mentioned in the introduction of optokinetic nystagmus as an alternating pursuit and refixation of objects moving in the same direction, the choice of the rabbit as an experimental animal may come as a surprise.

It is generally recognized that under physiological conditions the rabbit will never pursue distinct objects with the eyes, even when they are of great interest (e.g., food, other animals), nor will the animal align its ocular axis with such objects. Therefore the oculomotor behavior of the rabbit in relation to the visual surroundings is best characterized as a continuous *staring*. Bartels' assertion that OKN is absent in this animal is still generally accepted.

The incorrectness of this statement can be easily observed, when a rabbit is rotated on a turntable with the eyes open. At the beginning of such a rotation a nystagmus is generated, which is caused by vestibular stimuli. However, even when the rotation has attained a constant velocity, this nystagmus is sustained for an indefinite time (e.g., a quarter of an hour). That this nystagmus is indeed optokinetically controlled is demonstrated when the animal is surrounded by a paper cylinder rotating together with the animal. In this case the initial vestibular nystagmus decays after some time, but reappears when the cylinder is removed. The presence of "interesting" objects in the surroundings is completely immaterial in this respect, and such objects do not suppress the nystagmus when they rotate with the turntable within the visual field of the animal.

As optokinetic nystagmus cannot be elicited in the rabbit by the motion of a striped drum or belt in front of the eyes, one might suppose that motion of the *entire* visual surroundings (or at least a very large part of it) is required. These conditions can be achieved for the stationary animal by rotating a large cylinder of paper, provided with optical contrasts on the inside, around the animal. Also under these circumstances, when vestibular effects are excluded, genuine nystagmus is generated.

For the study of this OKN the following experimental equipment was used:

A large paper cylinder with a diameter of 140 cm and similar height, painted on the inside with 44 alternating black and white vertical stripes of equal width (about 10 cm) is suspended from the ceiling with freedom of rotation. The cylinder can be rotated by an electromotor coupled to its lower periphery. With an electrical resistance and a gear box, a large variety of rotational velocities can be achieved in the range of 6 s arc up to 450°/s (corresponding to 60 h and 0.8 s, respectively, per full rotation).

The head of the experimental animal is fixed with a clamp in the axis of the cylinder. The observer stands behind the animal to be able to watch the eye movements closely without obstructing a considerable part of the visual field of the animal.

To make a more precise analysis possible, OKN was recorded. Originally this was done by attaching a silk thread to the anterior pole of the cornea and connecting this to a light writing lever that recorded the eye movements on a conventional kymograph. This method is satisfactory for a crude analysis, but an accurate reproduction of eye movements is not achieved due to the inertia of the lever, etc. Therefore optical recording was chosen for the further investigations.[1]

With an egg membrane a small mirror is attached to the center of the cornea. The mirror reflects a narrow lightbeam through a horizontal slit on a vertically moving strip of photosensitive paper.

When the eye is rotated through a certain angle, the light beam is deviated through an angle twice as large.

If the distance between the mirror and the paper is known, the angular rotation of the eye can be easily derived from the recorded deviations. As the mirror is very light and makes only very small movements, inertial effects can be neglected.

During optical registration the eye whose movements were recorded was completely covered by the egg membrane; therefore the optokinetic stimulus was restricted to the second, free eye.

The inside of the cylinder was always illuminated by an electrical bulb positioned in the axis of the cylinder. As the whole apparatus was placed in a dark room, the stimulus could be suddenly interrupted by extinguishing the light.

With this equipment the *conditions* for the eliciting of OKN were first of all further explored.

---

[1] A similar method was used by Fleisch (1922) for the recording of compensatory eye movements

2.1 The Conditions for the Eliciting of OKN

2.1.1 Size of the Moving Field

As mentioned above, OKN in the rabbit cannot be elicited with the striped drum, striped belt or similar stimuli as most often used with humans, but movement of the whole visual surroundings is effective.

From this one might conclude that a stimulus not involving the whole retina is too weak to elicit nystagmus, but this notion is incorrect. The ability for nystagmus to be elicited is not abolished by the covering of substantial parts of the visual field with *contrastless* screens. In this respect it is insignificant which part of the visual field is excluded. For instance, nystagmus could still be elicited when a circular screen of 8 cm diameter was placed in the visual axis of the eye at a distance of 4 cm. In this way a central disc with a diameter of 90° was excluded. As the cylinder was not larger than 90° in the vertical direction, nystagmus was in this case elicited solely through the lateral remains of the visual field. Also large parts of the peripheral visual field can also be abolished with the same result.

It is even possible to elicit nystagmus when only one point is moving in the visual field. Figure 1 shows a nystagmogram from such an experiment.

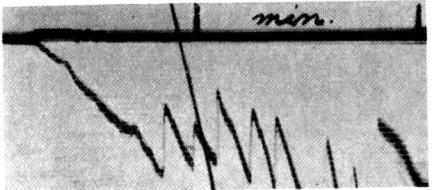

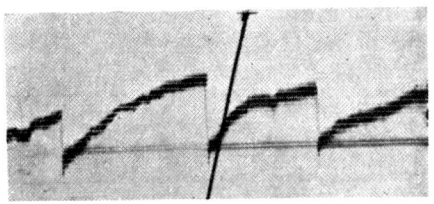

Fig. 1a, b. In the otherwise completely dark visual field of the left eye a lightspot moves with a velocity of 51 min arc/s. Optical recording of the (covered) right eye. Deviation downward represents movement of the eye in anterior direction (translator's remark: this must be a mistake, the context makes it obvious that downward deviation must stand for *posterior* movement of the right eye). Time in min.
a Movement of the light spot in anterior direction: several beats of nystagmus;
b Movement of the light spot in posterior direction: nystagmus in the other direction, the beats are less frequent than in a

In this experiment only a small electrical lightbulb was moved in a totally dark visual field at an angular velocity of 51 min arc/s. *This experiment shows that OKN is generated even when only a tiny part of the retina is stimulated, on the condition that stationary contrasts in the visual field are absent or at least very small compared to the moving contrasts.*

The question is how stationary contrasts can inhibit the generation of nystagmus. This phenomenon can be simply explained. It suffices to realize that the displacement of the retinal image providing the optokinetic stimulus is determined not only by the movements of the contrasts, but also by the movements of the eyes.

Let us assume that an object moves in *anterior* direction in front of the left eye. The retinal image of this point will move in the *posterior* direction, which elicits an anterior movement of the eye. As soon as this eye movement is executed, the retinal images of the stationary contrasts move in anterior direction. This motion constitutes a stimulus for a posterior eye movement, which will cancel the primary anterior eye movement.

The correctness of this explanation can be demonstrated by modifying the experimental conditions so that the movements of the stimulated eye are fully abolished.

Four sharp, elastic steel pins are attached to a brass ring with a diameter about equal to that of the rabbit's cornea with the points aimed at the center. Within this ring a second ring is fitted, which forces the points outward. When these two rings are placed on the (cocainized) cornea, concentrical with its periphery, the points just avoid penetrating it (Fig. 2a). If the inner ring is

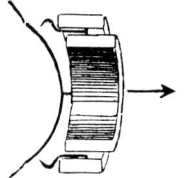

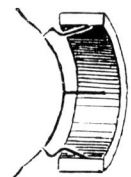

Fig. 2. Diagram of the apparatus for immobilization of the eye (description in text)

then removed, the four points will penetrate the periphery of the cornea superficially, immobilizing the outer ring with respect to the cornea (Fig. 2b). This ring is then rigidly connected to the head-holder of the animal and as a result the eye is fully immobilized with respect to the environment.

The movements of the second, normally moving eye, which is deprived of visual stimulation by an egg membrane, are optically recorded.

The results obtained with this experimental arrangement differ considerably from the ones described so far. It turned out that *the stationary contrasts are totally irrelevant in this situation and that motion of even a very small part of the contrasts in the visual field is capable of eliciting nystagmus.*

This observation allows an important conclusion. If under normal circumstances (i.e., when the stimulated eye can move freely) no *visible* eye movements are evoked by motion of a minority of the contrasts, this does not mean that no eye movements take place at all, as the experiment with the immobilized eye shows that motor commands are actually produced.

However, immediately after its generation the eye movement is inhibited by opposite commands, elicited by the movement of the retinal image of the stationary contrasts. As a result the eye movement remains too small to be observed. Therefore, the rabbit in the normal visual world, in which usually only isolated objects move, is not as inactive as is generally assumed.

2.1.2 Velocity of Moving Contrasts

In the investigation in the rotating cylinder it becomes clear that not every arbitrary rotatory velocity of the drum generates nystagmus. If one starts with a high velocity, e.g., one rotation (360°) per second, and this velocity is gradually lowered, nystagmus is only observed below a certain maximal velocity. The value of this maximal velocity is not equal for every experimental animal and varies considerably. A value higher than 70°/s was rarely found, while in many rabbits nystagmus was generated only at much lower velocities (20°-40°/s; see Fig. 3).

The existence of such a maximal velocity is understandable. For visual perception a certain velocity will induce fusion of the stripes and loss of motion perception, and in optokinetic stimulation a similar thing must happen. According to Roelofs and Van der Bend (1930), the intensity of the optokinetic stimulus is inversely proportional to the velocity of the moving contrasts.

The maximal velocity which elicits OKN in the rabbit is low compared to the maximal velocity which elicits motion perception in man. One might infer from this that a much stronger stimulus is needed to elicit OKN than to elicit a perception of movement. The question is whether the nystagmus stimulus continues to increase indefinitely with the decrease in the velocity of the stripes.

According to Roelofs and Van der Bend (1930), the stimulus intensity will at first increase when the velocity of the stripes decreases, but when

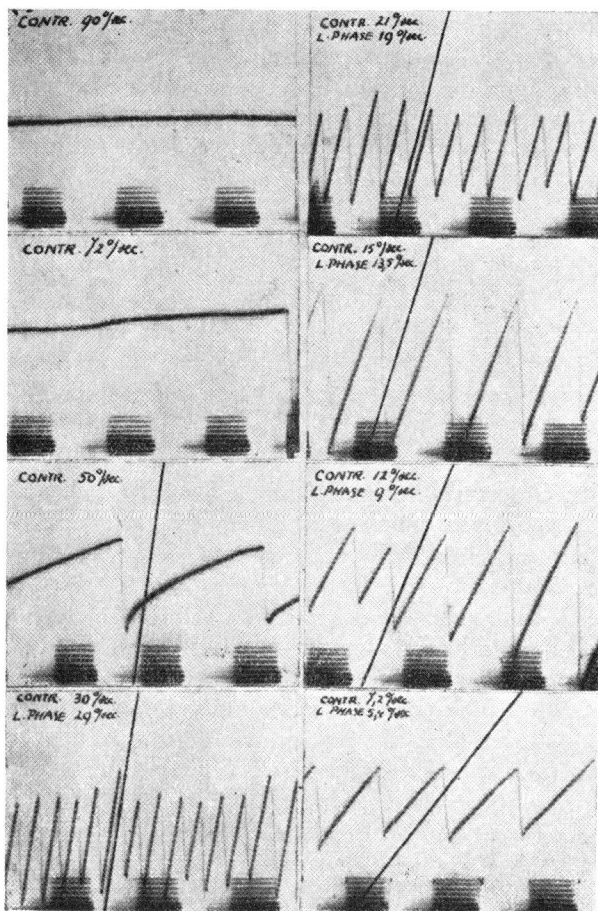

Fig. 3. Optokinetic nystagmus at different angular velocities of the contrasts. The contrasts were moved in anterior direction in the visual field of the right eye. Optical recording of the movements of the (covered) left eye. The *slanting line* drawn in most graphs indicates the theoretical course of the slow phase for the case that the angular velocity of this phase would be equal to the angular velocity of the contrasts. Angular velocity 90°/s: no nystagmus. Angular velocity 72°/s: nystagmus, the velocity of the slow phase is very low. Angular velocity 50°/s: lively nystagmus, the velocity of the slow phase is clearly higher, but still strongly inferior to that of the contrasts. At 30°/s: very marked nystagmus. The velocity of the slow phase is only slightly lower than that of the contrasts. At lower contrast velocity (21°/s, 15°/s, 12°/s and 7.2°/s) the angular velocity of the slow phase is correspondingly lower

this velocity becomes too low to produce a "direct" movement perception they assume that a stimulus for nystagmus no longer exists.

The rabbit is a highly suitable animal for testing OKN at extremely low velocities, as this animal (with the head fixed) makes no spontaneous eye movements and the eyes remain, in the absence of an optokinetic or vestibular stimulus, almost indefinitely in exactly the same position. The optical recording method described allows also the registration of extraordinarily slow eye movements, which cannot be directly observed, on a very slowly moving paper strip.

It turned out that a clear OKN can still be elicited at very low velocities. It was technically not possible to produce velocities smaller than 6.4 s arc/s, i.e., one revolution of the cylinder in 2½ days. As shown in Fig. 4a, at this

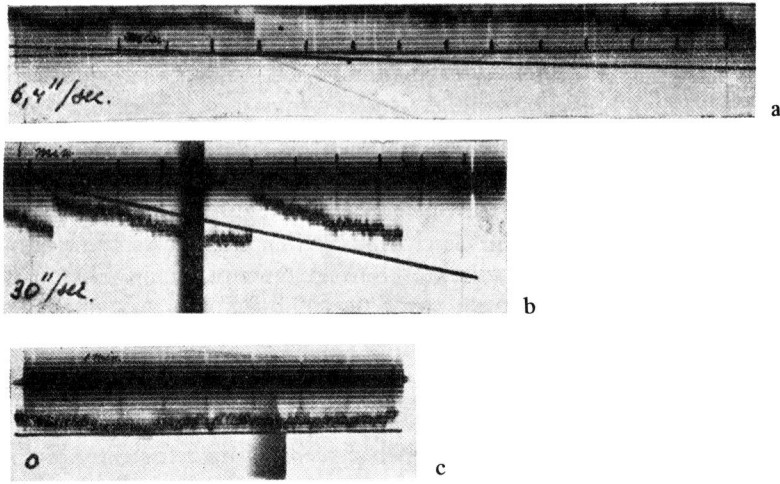

Fig. 4a-c. Optokinetic nystagmus at very low angular velocity of the contrasts. Stimulation of the left eye. Optical recording of the covered right eye. Movement of the contrasts in anterior direction. Time marks in minutes. Significance of the drawn line as in Fig. 3.
a Contrast velocity 6.4 s arc/s. Very slow motion of the eye with about the same angular velocity as the contrasts, interrupted once by a fast phase.
b Contrast velocity 30 s arc/s. The velocities are again almost similar. The slow phase is interrupted three times by a fast phase (duration of the slow phase 3-4 min).
c Control experiment. Contrast velocity zero

velocity an unambiguous nystagmus can still be recorded, although it is admittedly a rather slow type. In this nystagmus the angular velocity of the slow phase is about the same as that of the cylinder and it takes a long time before the slow phase has proceeded so far that it is interrupted by a fast phase. In this case only one fast phase was observed in more than a quarter of an hour! However, since all transitions between this type and the usual nystagmus are found it seems permissible to call this also a nystagmus. Figure 4b shows a nystagmogram at a velocity of 30 s arc/s (velocity of the slow phase and frequency of the nystagmus are higher in this case). Figure 4c shows a control experiment, in which the cylinder is stationary, and in accordance with this, the eye shows no deviation.

At these low velocities humans experience no "direct" motion sensation. The latter is, according to the investigations of Aubert, Bourdon and others experienced *under the most favorable circumstances* only at 1 min arc/s, under unfavorable circumstances (absence of stationary contrasts, such as in the rotating drum) only at 10 min arc/s and higher velocities. Based on data from Roelofs, Zeeman has calculated 1 min arc/s as the theoretical minimal velocity to elicit optokinetic eye movements.

From the description above it follows that either the rabbit perceives much slower motions than the human or that a motor command can be generated before any perception of motion.

The fact that very low velocities can elicit nystagmus does not prove that with decline of rotational velocity the intensity of the optokinetic stimulus is continuously increased. It is also possible, and theoretically even more likely, that the stimulus is optimal at a certain velocity.

In the freely moving eye this distinction is impossible. The stimulus intensity is determined by the velocity of the retinal images, and this changes continuously when the eye responds to the nystagmus stimulus. The distinction can be made also in this case with the technique of stimulating the immobilized eye described in the previous section. Under these conditions the angular velocity of the retinal images is always equal to that of the moving contrasts. It was found *that an optimal velocity of retinal images exists for the generation of OKN*. Other circumstances being equal, the generated nystagmus is optimal (the exact definition of this term will be discussed later) when the angular velocity of the moving contrasts (and thus the retinal images) is between about 10 and 50 min arc/s.

This finding is particularly interesting because the velocities are relatively low, much lower than the velocities commonly used until now (e.g., in the clinic) to elicit OKN. Of course the values found for the rabbit cannot be generalized without caution to other species.

2.1.3 Nature of the Stimulus

In the previous sections it was assumed without discussion that the optokinetic stimulus consists of a movement of *contrasts*. We should now clarify what we mean by "contrasts".

If the optical surroundings or part of them should influence the organism to different degrees depending on whether they are moving or stationary, then the different elements should have a different luminance. If, for example, the optical surroundings consist of a completely homogeneous white field, they can provide an *optical*, but not an *optokinetic* stimulus, since it will make no difference to the optical receptors whether it moves or not. If, on the other hand, half of the surroundings is black and half white, then some of the receptors are stimulated, and some not. If the surroundings are stable, the stimulated receptors remain the same, but when the surroundings move, the number and position of the stimulated receptors change. Thus if the motion of the surroundings provides a stimulus, then the latter can only be related to those receptors whose excitation changes, which are those close to the image of the black-white transition line. Neither the black nor the white field, but in fact only the borderline between black and white is significant for the optokinetic stimulation. Thus, with "contrast" in this article such a borderline is indicated, or more generally a transition between two parts with a different luminosity. It may not be superfluous to point out that contrasts are not only constituted by the sharp black and white transitions usual in schematical experiments, but also by less obvious luminosity differences as generated, for instance, by the granular surface of a sheet of white paper. For example, OKN can be elicited in the rabbit by rotating a cylinder of ordinary rough white drawing paper without any stripes around the animal. To study the effect of certain elementary contrasts (e.g., a black-white border) one should therefore first be satisfied that the black as well as the white field is indeed free of contrasts.

In the experiments to be described now, this was achieved in the following way. A stationary plate of opal glass, covering the major part of the visual field, is illuminated from the back by a stationary electric bulb. *Behind* this plate certain black figures are moving. The animal can thus only see the shadows of these figures on the opal glass plate, and the outlines of these figures are the only moving contrasts.

To exclude a disturbing influence of any stationary contrasts in the glass plate, the stimulated eye is immobilized in the manner previously described. An optimal velocity of the contrasts (30 min arc/s) was always used.

First of all the following question had to be answered. When a contrast, e.g., black-white transition, moves, certain retinal receptors will undergo a change in excitation. This change will consist of an *increase* in excitation if the transition line moves toward the black side, and a *decrease* when it moves in the opposite direction. Do such an increase and decrease have equal value as an optokinetic stimulus?

The investigation has shown that this is not the case. Increase in excitation is a powerful, decrease in excitation on the other hand a very weak or even totally ineffective optokinetic stimulus.

This result was obtained in the investigation of four rabbits. In one of the animals stimulation was done with one single transition line (height 18 cm, at a distance of 12 cm).

With movement toward the black side (increase of excitation) an unambiguous nystagmus was observed (Fig. 5), while movement toward the white side with the same velocity did not induce nystagmus.

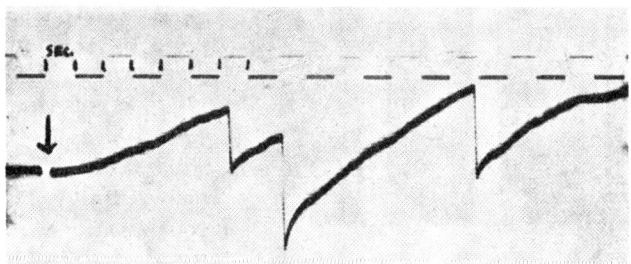

Fig. 5. Stimulation of the immobilized right eye with a single black-white transition. Recording of the movements of the covered left eye. Motion of the contrast line in anterior direction in such a way that the excitation is *increased* (more white enters the visual field). The onset of stimulation is marked by an *arrow*. A clear nystagmus is recorded

As the motion of a single transition is a rather weak stimulus, it seemed desirable to increase the intensity of the stimulus. For this the following experimental arrangement was chosen. Behind the opal glass six vertical black stripes are placed, each 3 cm wide and 18 cm high, separated by spaces of 3 cm. Behind this pattern a second, identical but movable stripe pattern is mounted.

Figure 6 shows that only one of the vertical borders of each moving stripe will be visible as a moving shadow on the opal glass plate, while the second border remains covered by the stationary stripes and that dependent upon the relative positions of the stripe patterns the displacement of the posterior stripes will cause either only an *increase*, or only a *decrease* in the excitation of retinal receptors. Also with this more powerful stimulus could the difference mentioned above be demonstrated unambiguously.

Figure 7 shows the differential effects of increase and decrease in excitation for the same rabbit as illustrated in Fig. 6.

Figure 8 is derived from another rabbit. In this case decrease in excitation has no effect at all, while increase elicits a marked nystagmus.

The conspicuous difference between the two types of stimulation can be explained as follows. When the stimulation of a retinal receptor is suddenly interrupted, the excitation of the receptor does not end abruptly, but decays over a certain time, as shown in the sensory domain by the appearance of an after-image.

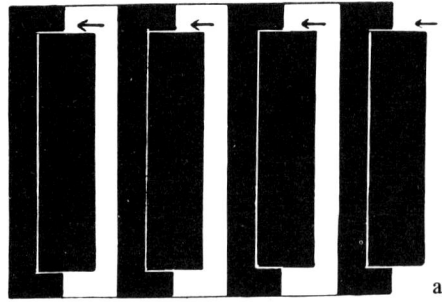

Fig. 6a, b. Diagram of experimental arrangement for stimulation with several contrasts, so that either only increase or only decrease of excitation is achieved. **a** Increase of excitation. **b** Decrease of excitation

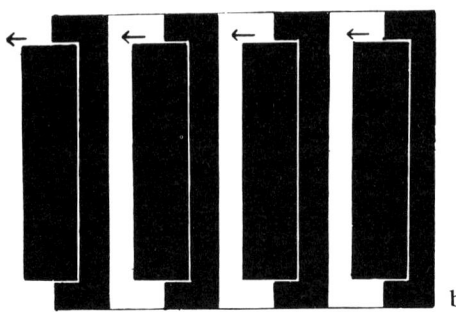

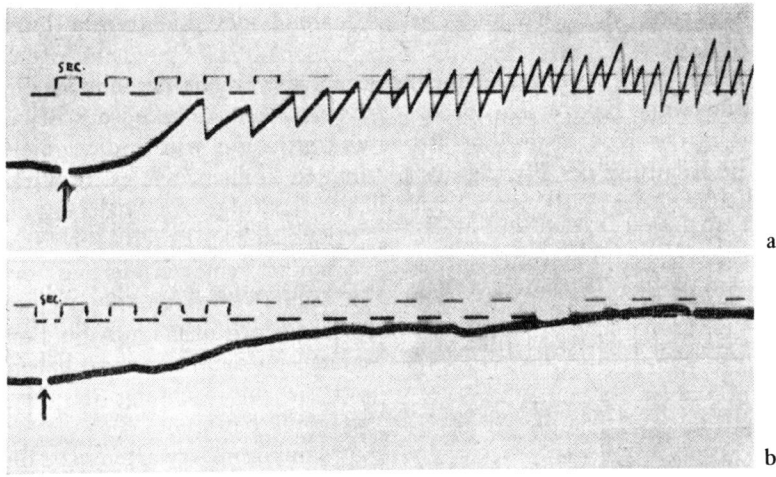

Fig. 7a, b. Stimulation of the immobilized right eye by six elementary contrasts (black-white transitions). Recording of the movements of the covered left eye. Movements of the contrasts in anterior direction with a velocity of 30 min arc/s. The *arrow* indicates the onset of motion.

a Increase in excitation (cf. Fig. 6a). Marked nystagmus.

b Decrease in excitation (cf. Fig. 6b). No nystagmus, only deviation in the direction of the slow phase

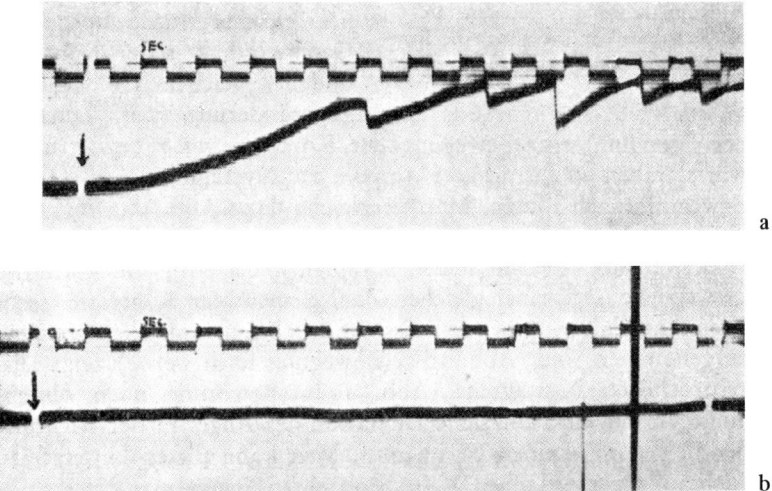

Fig. 8a, b. The same experimental arrangement in another rabbit. During decrease in the excitation (**b**) no reaction of the eye at all can be observed in this case

When, on the other hand, a receptor is suddenly stimulated, excitation reaches its maximum immediately or at least in a much shorter time. A very brief light flash is perceived, a very brief interruption of a light stimulus is not seen.

Thus, if — as postulated — *change* in the excitation is crucial for the generation of OKN, then the much faster change in excitation due to an increased light stimulus will have a larger effect than the slower change in excitation due to decrease of the light stimulus (cf. Fig. 9).

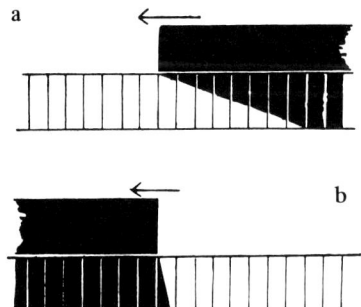

Fig. 9a, b. Diagram of changes in the excitation of retinal receptors. White means: maximal excitation. *Black* no excitation. **a** Decrease in excitation: the excitation subsides only slowly. **b** Increase in excitation: the excitation reaches its maximum quickly

The change of excitation cannot be the only controlling factor, however, otherwise the *direction* of the contrast movement would be irrelevant, and it could not control the direction of the nystagmus in the way it actually does. The sequence in which the different receptors undergo a change in excitation must also have an important effect on central nervous processing, as it determines the direction of the nystagmus.

One might expect the direction of the motion of contrasts to affect only the direction of the nystagmus and not its intensity. However, this is not the case. If one stimulates only one eye optokinetically, it is found that with a similar (e.g., the optimal) contrast velocity and a similar type of change in excitation (e.g., increase of excitation), a motion of the contrasts in the *anterior* direction (nasal) is a much stronger stimulus for nystagmus than a posterior motion. Compare Fig. 10a and 10b, which are recorded in the same

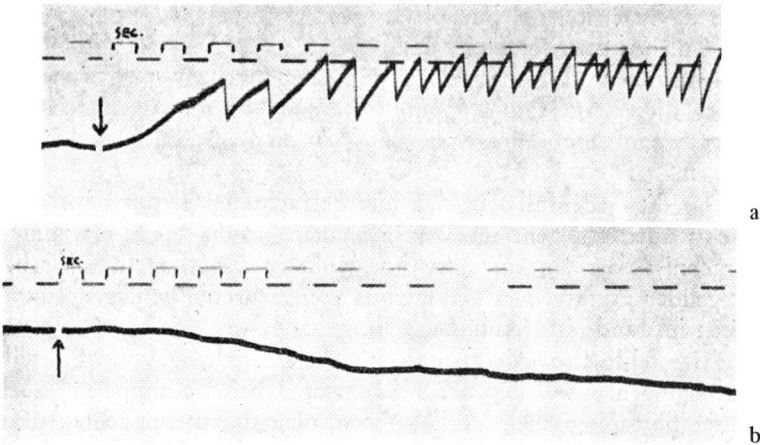

Fig. 10a, b. Stimulation of the immobilized right eye with six elementary contrasts. Recording of the movements of the left eye. The motion of the contrast is arranged in such a way that the excitation is increased. **a** Anterior motion of the contrasts: nystagmus. **b** Posterior motion of the contrasts: only deviation in the direction of the movement

rabbit at a velocity of 30 min arc/s, with similar numbers of elementary contrasts (six black-white transitions) and in both cases with increasing excitation. Figure 10a (*anterior* motion) shows marked nystagmus, Fig. 10b (*posterior* motion) on the other hand shows only a slow deviation of the eye in the direction of the motion, no nystagmus. This difference can also be observed very simply when a rabbit is rotated on a turntable with one eye covered. For example, when the right eye is covered, a (vestibular) nystagmus is observed only during the beginning of rotation to the right, while during rotation to the left nystagmus continues indefinitely. This means that during rotation of the animal with both eyes open, nystagmus is maintained by the left eye during rotation to the left, and by the right eye during rotation to the right.

That the optokinetic stimulus of posterior motion is not wholly without effect is shown by the fact that stationary contrasts impede the generation of nystagmus even when their images move anteriorly on the retina as the eye responds to the nystagmogenic stimulus (cf. Fig. 8).

2.2 Slow and Fast Phase

In the previous section we have only discussed optokinetic nystagmus *as a whole*. Now we have to study the two *components*, the slow and the fast phase, in greater detail.

According to the "classical" concept, which considers OKN as an interplay between fixation (pursuit) movements and refixations, the fast phase is generated because the eye directs itself at a distinct object demanding attention, i.e., the visual axis is aimed at this object. This object is then pursued for some time with the visual axis (slow phase) and when it is "mentally" processed and the next object moving in the same direction draws the attention, the eye rotates with a new fast "refixation movement" toward this second object, and so on. According to this concept an OKN can thus be generated only when a series of objects moves in the visual field.

That this is not true, at any rate for the kind of OKN considered here, follows from the already mentioned observation that a single point moving in darkness is able to elicit several beats of nystagmus (Fig. 1).

In this case there is no occasion whatsoever for refixations which, parenthetically, are never observed in the rabbit even under physiological conditions. (Nystagmus elicited by a single contrastline is shown in Fig. 5).

The fast phase therefore must be elicited either by the same stimulus as the slow phase, or by nonvisual stimuli.

As a source of the latter the signals from the muscular receptors have to be considered in the first place. When the eye is deviated by the slow phase, certain eye muscles are stretched and conditions for the generation of a stretch reflex could be created. The following observations argue against this idea.

If we generate an optokinetic nystagmus and suddenly interrupt the stimulus (e.g., by turning the light off), we observe that the eye (often after a number of beats of afternystagmus, which will be discussed later) deviates in the direction of the slow phase and remains there.

If one waits longer, the eye returns to the midposition with a *slow*, smooth movement (Fig. 11a). If, however, the optical stimulus is switched on again while the eye is still deviated, it can often be observed that the eye returns immediately with a fast movement (Fig. 11b). This observation justifies the

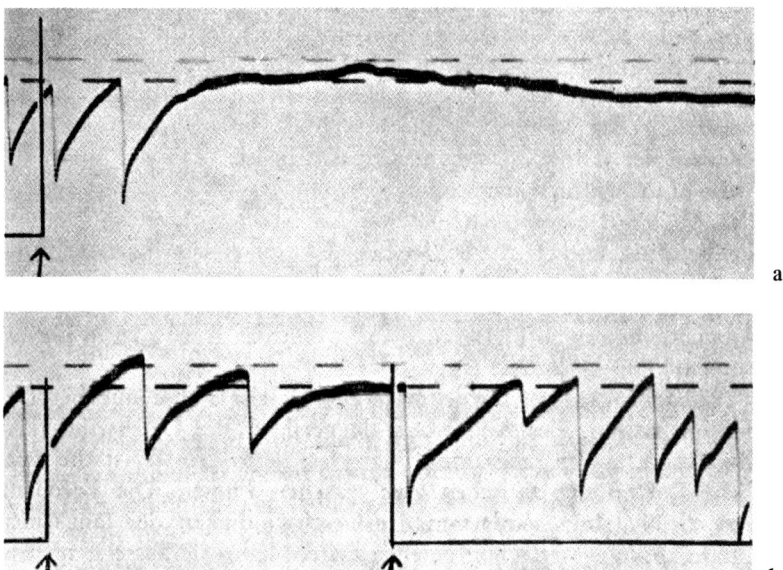

Fig. 11a, b. Optokinetic stimulation of the right eye, recording of the left eye. The *first arrow* indicates that the stimulation is suddenly interrupted.
a After the end of stimulation first two beats of afternystagmus. Then the eye reaches a deviated position in the direction of the original slow phase. Finally the eye returns with a slow movement in the initial position.
b First part as in a. Also in this case beats of afternystagmus followed by a deviation in the direction of the slow phase can be observed after the end of stimulation. When the stimulus is switched on again (*second arrow*) the eye returns with a fast movement to the initial position and the nystagmus starts once again

conclusion that the optical stimulus contributes to the generation of the fast phase. Depending on the position of the eye, the same optical stimulus can sometimes elicit a slow movement in one direction, and at other times a fast movement in the opposite direction.

Which of these possibilities is elected might be determined by a switching mechanism influenced by the stretch receptors in the eye muscles.

On the other hand it seems equally possible that the alternation of phases is determined purely centrally, by an automatic rhythmic activity of the centers. This concept has been especially advocated by Ohm. At the moment no suitable observations are available to distinguish between the possibilities. Finally we have to consider the possibility that a central-automatic as well as a peripheral-sensory control system for eye movements exists, as we know to be the case for the respiratory control system.

The stimuli that trigger the fast reset of the eye from the deviated- to the mid-position are not exclusively optical. Tactile stimuli such as touching the animal or acoustical stimuli such as a sudden noise can elicit a fast phase when the eye is deviated.

As stated above, a fast phase is only generated when the eye is deviated. The lower the velocity of the eye in the slow phase, the longer the time interval between two fast phases. The frequency of the OKN thus depends on the velocity of the slow phase. As we have already seen, the latter can be extremely low; with an angular velocity of the moving contrasts of 6.4 s arc/s the frequency is lower than one every quarter of an hour. At a high velocity of the slow phase it can be more than two per second.

The degree of deviation, and thus the amplitude of the OKN at which the fast phase is generated, is quite variable. First of all there are large individual differences. Some rabbits always produce small average amplitudes (e.g., 1.7°) even when investigated at different times, while others produce a much larger amplitude (e.g., 7°).

Apart from individual differences the amplitude depends on other factors. At a low slow phase velocity the average amplitude is generally lower than at higher velocities. Finally, the amplitude is not even constant in the same animal under the same conditions, and therefore it is only meaningful to specify an average amplitude.

The fast phase always returns the eye in the direction of the initial (middle) position, but often this midposition is not reached, as a new slow phase is started while the eye is still deviated. Certain rabbits show this type of nystagmus very markedly (Fig. 8).

More rarely, the fast phase carries the eye across the mid-position.

The evidence presented demonstrates that the central mechanism for the alternation of phases displays a rather complex behavior.

2.3 Quantitative Relations Between Stimulus and Effect

When a constant optokinetic stimulus is allowed to continue for some time, one observes that the elicited nystagmus reaches a steady state only after a certain period: a kind of "equilibrium" between stimulus and effect is thus achieved. After sudden interruption of the stimulus the nystagmus also does not stop immediately, but decays gradually. In this case also the new "equilibrium" is achieved only after a certain time.

For the examination of the quantitative relations it seems simplest to clarify first of all the relations between stimulus and effect in the steady state and later those at the onset and end of stimulation.

2.3.1 Equilibrium Between Stimulus and Nystagmus, at Different Velocities of the Moving Contrasts

In the discussion of stimulus conditions for OKN it has already been emphasized that not the absolute velocity of the contrasts, but the velocity of the retinal images with respect to the retina is most relevant.

The relations are thus simplest when the immobilized eye is stimulated, since in this case the angular velocities of retinal images and contrasts are always equal.

As a quantitative measure the *angular velocity of the slow phase* is the most significant one, for two reasons.

Firstly, because it is nearly constant in the steady state, while the amplitude and frequency of the nystagmus vary considerably. Secondly, because this velocity is physiologically the most meaningful parameter, if compensation of retinal image displacement is considered as the physiological purpose of OKN. The velocity of the slow phase can be easily measured in the optical recordings by measuring the tangent of the angle of the curve with the horizontal and multiplying it by a certain constant factor.[1]

With this measurement it is found that the velocity of the slow phase is maximal for a specific velocity of the contrasts between 10 and 50 min arc/s.

For this reason this contrast velocity was characterized as "optimal" in the discussion of stimulus conditions. It is important to note in this respect that under these conditions *the velocity of the eye is many times higher than that of the contrasts*.

Figure 12 shows the nystagmus of a rabbit with a contrast velocity of 10 min arc/s. The slanted line drawn in the figure shows the slope of the curve for the case that angular velocities of the eye and the contrasts are equal. The measurement shows that the velocity of the eye is actually 3.7°/s, thus 16 times larger. (Translator's note: this is apparently an error, the ratio between 3.7° and 10 min arc is 22.2). With larger as well as smaller stimulus velocities the slow phase velocity is lower.

With stimulation of the freely moving eye, an essentially different result is found. Figures 3 and 13 show the OKN of two rabbits at different angular velocities of the contrasts. In each figure the slanted line again shows the

---

[1] The angular velocity of the eye is $tg\alpha \dfrac{90°}{\pi dt}$ /s, if α is the angle of the curve with the horizontal, d is the distance of the paper to the mirror and t is the time in which the paper moves 1 cm. A small error is introduced as the deviation of the paper is considered to be proportional to the angle of deviation of the light beam, while it is actually proportional to the tangent of this angle. This error is negligible for the actually occurring, relatively small deviations in comparison with the other inaccuracies of the method

course of the curve if the angular velocities of the eye and the contrasts are equal. Figure 13 demonstrates that *at very different angular velocities of the contrasts (6.4 s arc/s up to about 2°/s) the velocity of the slow phase is almost equal to the velocity of the contrast.*

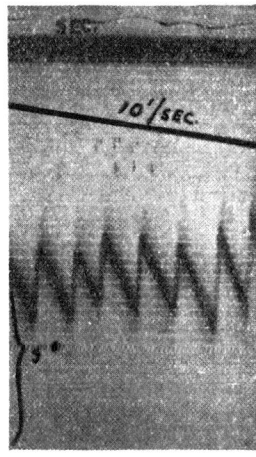

Fig. 12. Optokinetic stimulation of the fixed left eye. Recording of the covered right eye. Contrast velocity 10 min arc/s. The *slanted line* indicates the course of the slow phase if its angular velocity were equal to that of the contrasts. In reality the velocity of the slow phase is 3.7°/s, thus 16 times larger! (Translator's note: the ratio of 3.7° to 10 min arc is actually 22.2, not 16)

With an optimal contrast velocity (Fig. 13: 11 min 36 s arc/s and 51 min arc/s) the velocity of the slow phase is thus much lower than with stimulation of the immobilized eye. This essential difference can be easily accounted for.

When the stimulated eye is free, a movement of this eye with a velocity superior to that of the contrasts will not only cancel, but even invert the initial slip of the retinal images. The movement of the stimulated eye will thus lead to the abolishment and even inversion of the stimulus. Since in this way the stimulus for the eye movement disappears, the velocity of the eye will decrease until it has become somewhat lower than that of the contrasts. Thus the stimulus is reestablished and the velocity of the eye will increase again, and so on.

Thus this *self-regulating mechanism* always keeps the velocity of the eye a little lower than that of the contrasts. As shown in Figs. 13 and 3, this difference is only very small in a certain range, so that it can be contended that optokinetic nystagmus has the tendency *to abolish the shift of the retinal image as much as possible, or in other words, to stabilize the image of the world on the retina.* This amounts to a kind of *optical fixation*, i.e., not fixation in the usual sense, which implies the stabilization of a specific point of the retina, but *fixation of the surroundings as a whole on the retina as a whole.*

While for fixation in the usual sense the *attention*, i.e., the preference for certain points in the visual field above other points is essential, we have in

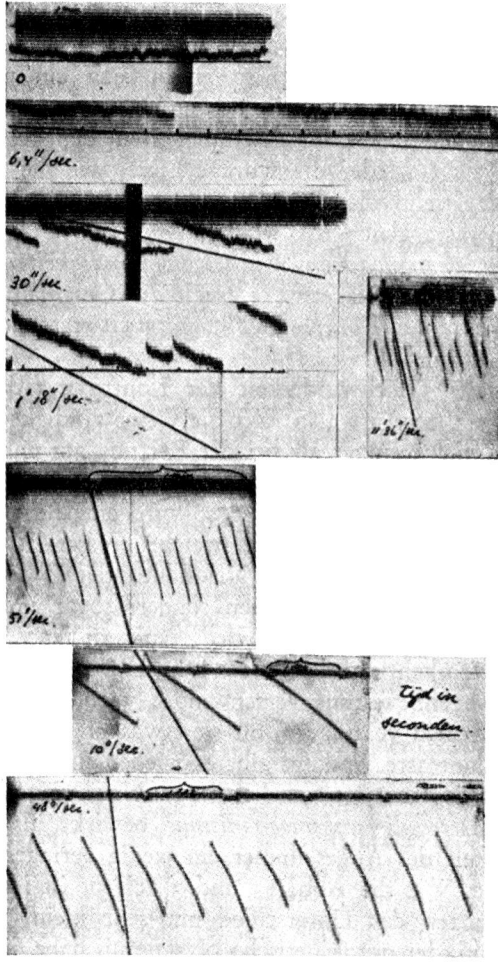

Fig. 13a-e. Optokinetic nystagmus at different angular velocities of the contrasts. The stimulated eye can move freely (cf. the description of Fig. 3).

a-e time in minutes; **f** time also in minutes, but faster moving paper. **g** and **h** time in seconds. **b-f** at low contrast velocities 6.4 s arc/s, 30 s arc/s, 1 min 18 s arc/s, 11 min 36 s arc/s, and 51 min arc/s the velocities of the contrasts and of the slow phase are almost similar. **g** and **h** at higher contrast velocity (10°/s and 48°/s) the eye moves slower than the stimulus. **a** control experiment, velocity is zero

this case a *fixation without attention*, i.e., the significance of the different points in the visual field is only determined by their contrast value.

The relation to the surroundings without control of eye movements by attention is called staring, therefore I would like to characterize the type of fixation described above as stare fixation, in contrast to look-fixation or fixation in the usual sense, which will be discussed further later on. As demonstrated in Fig. 13, at higher contrast velocities the eye can be considerably slower than the contrasts (in this case at 10 and 48°/s), fixation in this case is thus incomplete. Figure 3 on the other hand, derived from another rabbit, shows that fixation can be almost perfect even at higher contrast velocities (in this case up to 40°/s).

It is not surprising that the optokinetic stimulus cannot always generate the required velocity.

It is remarkable that during stimulation of the freely moving eye the velocity of the slow phase is often considerably higher than that achieved by stimulation of the immobilized eye with "optimal" velocity! A satisfactory explanation of this phenomenon cannot be given as yet.

It seems most likely that the immobilization of the eye in itself has some inhibitory effect on the central nystagmus mechanism.

Moreover, the cornea of the immobilized eye is somewhat deformed by the attached equipment, which must affect the refraction and cause defocusing of the retinal image. This could also weaken the stimulus.

As mentioned above, the amplitude of nystagmus shows considerable individual differences under similar stimulus conditions. In general it can be stated that the larger the slow phase velocity, the larger the average amplitude, although exceptions to this rule are far from rare.

2.3.2 Behavior of Nystagmus at the Beginning and End of Stimulation

When a constant optokinetic stimulus is suddenly started (here again this can be done most simply with the immobilized eye) one observes that the nystagmus develops only gradually, i.e., the velocity of the slow phase increases gradually and only reaches a final, maximal value after a certain time (Fig. 14, cf. also Figs. 7a and 10a).

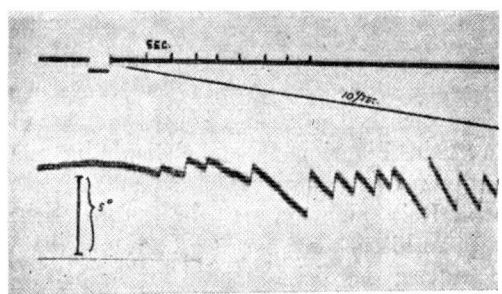

Fig. 14. Optokinetic stimulation of the immobilized left eye. Recording of the covered right eye. Contrast velocity 10 min arc/s. During the continuous stimulation the velocity of the slow phase increases gradually

Similarly, the nystagmus does not disappear immediately when stimulation is ended (by turning off the lights or stopping the rotating drum) but continues for a certain time, with a gradual decrease in slow phase velocity (Fig. 15, cf. also Fig. 11).

This latter phenomenon is the optokinetic *afternystagmus* which was first noticed by Ohm. The duration of this afternystagmus is highly variable and determined primarily by the slow phase velocity immediately before the end of the optokinetic stimulation. The higher this velocity is, the longer the duration of the afternystagmus. Under favorable circumstances the afternystagmus may consist of more than 20 beats. At the end of afternystag-

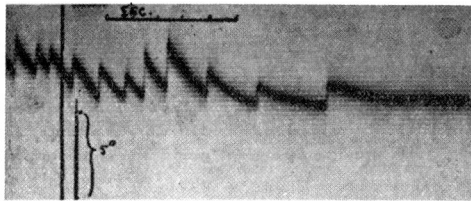

Fig. 15. Optokinetic afternystagmus. The *vertical line* marks the time at which stimulation is ended. After the end of stimulation the nystagmus persists ("afternystagmus"). The velocity of the afternystagmus diminishes gradually

mus the eye usually remains deviated in the direction of the slow phase, to return subsequently with a very slow movement in the opposite direction to the midposition.

The existence of an afternystagmus shows, as also emphasized by Ohm, that the excitation of the oculomotor centers is prolonged for some time after the end of the optical stimulus and decays only gradually. Similarly, the gradual acceleration of nystagmus at the onset of stimulation shows that the excitation in the oculomotor centers only reaches its maximum after some time. The central apparatus of the nystagmus thus shows a certain "inertia".

It is clear that the insertion of a sluggish central apparatus between stimulus and effect makes it more difficult to determine the quantitative relation between these two factors. The velocity of the slow phase at a certain time is determined not only by the stimulus at that moment, but also by preceding stimuli. The velocity of the slow phase can therefore never be a quantitative parameter for the stimulus existing at that moment. That such a parameter is nevertheless feasible can be easily illustrated with a mechanical model. When a body is moved by a constant force, the motion is accelerated up to a certain point where the force is used entirely to overcome the friction. When the force ceases acting, the body will continue to move for some time, until it stops as a result of friction.

It is clear that to derive the magnitude of the force from the motion of the body, the *velocity* of the body can not be used, since it changes as a result of the force and persists when the force is no longer acting.

Therefore we use the *change in velocity* at the onset of the movement, when frictional forces are still small, or in other words the *initial acceleration*, which is at any time proportional to the force acting on the body.

The possibility for a similar approach in optokinetic nystagmus is given by the fact that under favorable conditions the slow phase movement of the eye during a constant optokinetic stimulus is *uniformly accelerated*. Figure 16 is an attempt to illustrate this effect. From the nystagmogram of Fig. 14, recorded after the onset of a constant optokinetic stimulus, the fast phases have been eliminated, i.e., at every fast phase the curve has been shifted vertically so that the next slow phase forms the continuation of the preceding one. In this way one obtains a very regular curve which is highly similar to a parabole. If one constructs a curve of the *velocity* of the slow phase as a

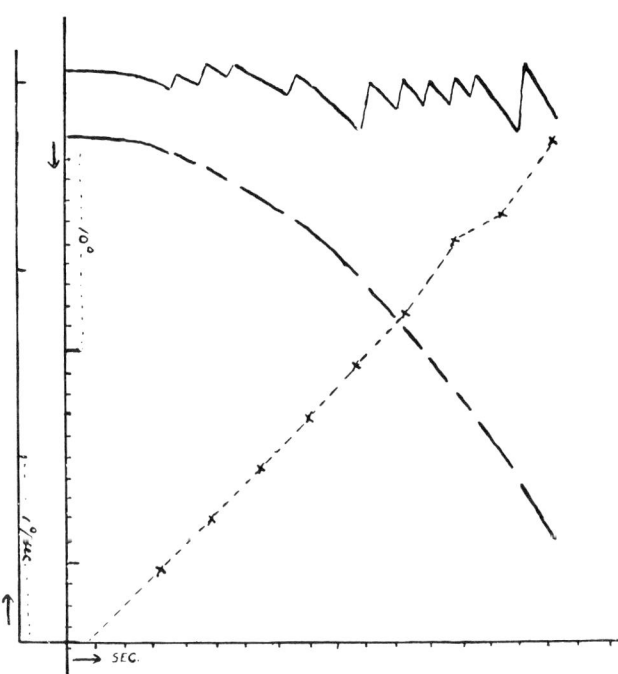

Fig. 16. Graphical reconstruction of the velocity of the slow phase of the nystagmus of Fig. 14, representing the first nystagmic beats in the beginning of the optokinetic stimulation. The *dotted line* represents slow phase velocity as a function of time

function of time, a practically straight line is obtained. Thus, the movement of the eye in the slow phase is *uniformly accelerated*.

Since the *acceleration* is constant, it can be used as a parameter of the likewise constant stimulus. For the nystagmus in Fig. 14 it amounts to 14.9 min arc/s^2. Stimulation was effected in this case at an optimal contrast velocity (10 min arc/s). With contrast velocities above or below the optimum the acceleration of the slow phase is lower.

Obviously the movement of the eye during the slow phase is uniformly accelerated only in the beginning of the stimulation. When the stimulation is continued, the acceleration decreases gradually and in the end the velocity becomes constant (equilibrium between nystagmus and stimulus). We observed something similar in our mechanical model. In that case the velocity of the inertial body became constant, because the force acting on the body was fully used to overcome *friction*. Therefore, something equivalent to mechanical friction must be present in the central nystagmic apparatus, which we shall call "central resistance", to avoid more specific terms for the moment. This "resistance" augments with the increase in slow phase velocity and in the end becomes so large that it is in equilibrium with the optokinetic stimulus and therefore slow phase velocity no longer increases. It is clear that the velocity reached at equilibrium will be larger with a high stimulus intensity than for a low one, and therefore this velocity in the equilibrated stage is also a quantitative parameter for the intensity of the stimulus.

On the other hand, the determination of the stimulus intensity from the initial acceleration is preferable since in this case the "central resistance" may be neglected.

Without a "central resistance" the slow phase velocity would remain unchanged after the end of the stimulus and nystagmus would continue indefinitely. The "resistance" causes a decrease in velocity immediately after the end of the stimulus and eventually the arrest of the eye movement.

It is to be expected that the velocity of the slow phase will not decrease uniformly during the afternystagmus, since, as follows from the previous discussions, the "central resistance" will also gradually decrease when the velocity decreases. The deceleration of the slow phase therefore will not be uniform, but gradually decreasing. In reality the behavior of the afternystagmus is even more complex, as will be discussed in the next section.

2.4 A Theoretical Model of the Central Mechanism of Stare Nystagmus

The purpose of the following discussion is only to present a working hypothesis of the central mechanism of nystagmus, which accounts for the complex phenomena as satisfactorily as possible, *without discussing the reality of the assumed central mechanisms*.

When the eye moves laterally with a smooth movement, more muscle fibers (more motor units) must gradually be activated. This means that the excitation in the center related to these eye muscles (henceforth called center A) will gradually increase. If the eye velocity is *uniform*, the increase in excitation will also be uniform. With the onset of the fast phase, the excitation must cease abruptly, to increase again at the same velocity as before after the end of the fast phase. This process can be most readily understood by assuming that the increase in excitation during the slow phase is governed by a second center (B), which controls center A.

When center B sends a steady stream of impulses to center A, then according to our model a substance a is synthesized, and the quantity (i.e., the concentration) of this substance, which determines the level of excitation, increases with the duration of the impulse stream from center B.

As soon as this concentration reaches a maximum, all of substance a is suddenly destroyed (as a result of a rhythmic activity of center A which is not further discussed), but resynthesized at the same velocity as before if the impulses from center B are continued. Thus, *constant activity* of center B causes *uniformly increasing excitation* of center A, and nystagmus with uniform velocity of the slow phase interrupted by fast phases.

Now we shall consider the activity of center B. This center according to our model receives the nerve fibers which conduct the excitation caused by the optokinetic stimulation.

We may suppose again that the excitation of these fibers liberates a substance b in center B, and that the quantity or concentration increases continually as long as the constant optokinetic stimulus lasts.

With constant optokinetic stimulation we have thus *uniformly increasing* concentration of substance b, uniformly increasing excitation of center B, and a *uniform increase* in the impulse to center A. In center A the concentration of substance a and thus excitation will increase with a *uniform acceleration*, and the *velocity* of the slow phase will also be *accelerated*.

In this way it becomes understandable how a constant optokinetic stimulus can elicit a nystagmus with a uniformly accelerated slow phase.

We still have to account for the "central resistance". For this we have to assume that substance b in center B is in some way destroyed, and specifically that the decay of substance b is accelerated when the concentration of the substance is increased. In the beginning of the optokinetic stimulation the decay rate will still be small, but the decay will gradually increase and eventually become fast enough to reach an equilibrium between synthesis and decay, which means that as much of substance b is produced as is destroyed. The concentration of substance b then remains unchanged (Fig. 17, II), the impulse rate to center A remains constant and the velocity of the slow phase becomes *uniform* (Fig. 17, III). If the optokinetic stimulus is now *switched off*, substance b is no longer synthesized, the decay is no longer replaced and the concentration diminishes gradually to zero (see Fig. 17 I, II).

The impulses to center A will then also decrease, and the concentration of substance a will increase no longer uniformly but at a decelerating rate. The slow phase will slow down accordingly, and its velocity will decrease to zero (Fig. 17, III).

If we examine an optokinetic nystagmus of a relatively small amplitude with optimal stimulation, we find that its main features are in agreement with the phenomena to be expected from the model.

A nystagmus with a larger amplitude usually shows distinct deviations, which may be satisfactorily explained by the (logical) assumption that substance a is destroyed in way similar to substance b, and that similarly the quantity of substance a destroyed per unit of time is proportional to the concentration of substance a.

We can then expect the following complications (Fig. 17, IV).
a) When center B is in equilibrium, and sends a constant stream of impulses to center A, the excitation in center A will not increase uniformly, but more and more slowly. The slow phase in the nystagmogram will thus not be a

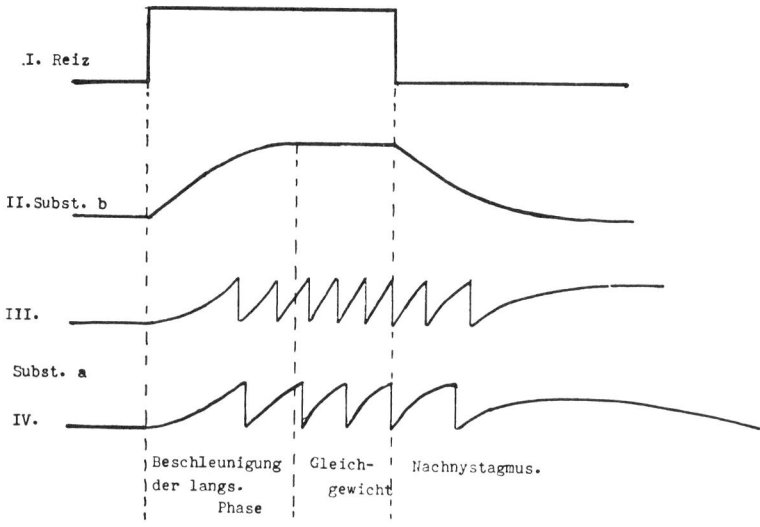

Fig. 17. Schematical diagrams of the hypothetical central processes during and after optokinetic stimulation. *I* Stimulus. *II* Concentration (or total quantity) of substance *b*. *III* Concentration (or total quantity) of substance *a*, with due account for the fast phase, but neglecting the gradual decay. *IV* Concentration (or total quantity) of substance *a*, incorporating the gradual decay

straight line, but a curved line with the convexity upward, as is apparent in certain graphs (Fig. 1b and 8a).

b) If in the synthesis of substance *a* a concentration is reached before the onset of a fast phase at which synthesis and destruction are equally large (equilibrium in center A), the eye will come to rest in a deviated position and stay there. Also this behavior occurs in reality, particularly (as expected) with weak excitation (Fig. 7b).

c) During afternystagmus the activity of center B and therefore the synthesis of substance *a* decreases gradually, which must lead to an equilibrium in center A. The eye will thus come to rest after some time in a deviated position. As the activity in center B continues to decrease, this equilibrium will last only briefly; after this the destruction of substance *a* will exceed its production. The total quantity of substance *a* will thus decrease and therefore the eye will return to the midposition with a smooth movement (see Fig. 11a). This behavior can be consistently observed in afternystagmus.

2.5 Optokinetic and Vestibular Nystagmus

A condition for the generation of optokinetic nystagmus is that the majority of optical contrasts moves relative to the eye.

It is immaterial whether the motion of the contrasts is an absolute one or only a relative one, in which the animal itself moves and the optical surroundings are stationary. However, absolute movement of the majority of contrasts will hardly ever occur under physiological circumstances, relative motion on the other hand very often. If the relative motion of the visual surroundings is caused by a linear motion of the animal in an anterior or posterior direction, this motion will constitute an optokinetic stimulus, but it will not cause nystagmus in the rabbit, as the stimuli for both eyes will work in opposite directions. Only when the motion of the animal is a *rotation*, and thus the world moves forward for one eye and backwards for the other, will optokinetic nystagmus be elicited. Rotations of the animal lead to stimulation of the semicircular canals and thus to vestibular nystagmus.

In physiological conditions we should thus expect combinations of optokinetic and vestibular nystagmus and therefore it is necessary to compare both types of nystagmus. It can be stated rightaway that the recordings of optokinetic and vestibular nystagmus agree fully in their main features, and that it is impossible to distinguish whether a certain nystagmogram was obtained by optokinetic or vestibular stimulation. Admittedly this assertion is only correct for nystagmus of an intermediate slow phase velocity and frequency. If the slow phase velocity and frequency are very low, it can only be an optokinetic nystagmus, if they are on the other hand very large, it must be a vestibular nystagmus. When optokinetic and vestibular stimulation are simultaneously activated, one might expect a kind of superposition of both types of nystagmus. In this case the resulting nystagmogram might show a mixture of two frequencies. This is, however, not the case.

If in a rabbit on a stationary turntable a nystagmus is elicited by a continuous optokinetic stimulus, and subsequently the turntable is rotated in such a direction that the vestibular stimulus will elicit a nystagmus in the same direction as the optokinetic nystagmus, one observes a sudden increase in the slow phase velocity, together with an increase in frequency (Fig. 18a). No superposition of any kind is manifest. If the turntable is rotated in the opposite direction and the vestibular stimulus is relatively weak, one observes a decrease in slow phase velocity and frequency. If the stimulus is stronger, the nystagmus is inverted (Fig. 18b). It is also possible to adjust the stimulus intensity so that the nystagmus is exactly cancelled (Fig. 18c).

These facts make it very probable that the shaping of nystagmus as a rhythmic process is accomplished in a common central apparatus which is activated similarly by optokinetic as well as vestibular stimuli.

To test the correctness of this assertion, we have first to examine certain peculiarities of vestibular rotatory nystagmus.

It is well known that flow of endolymph in the semicircular canal and stimulation of the relevant sensory cells occurs only when the head is sub-

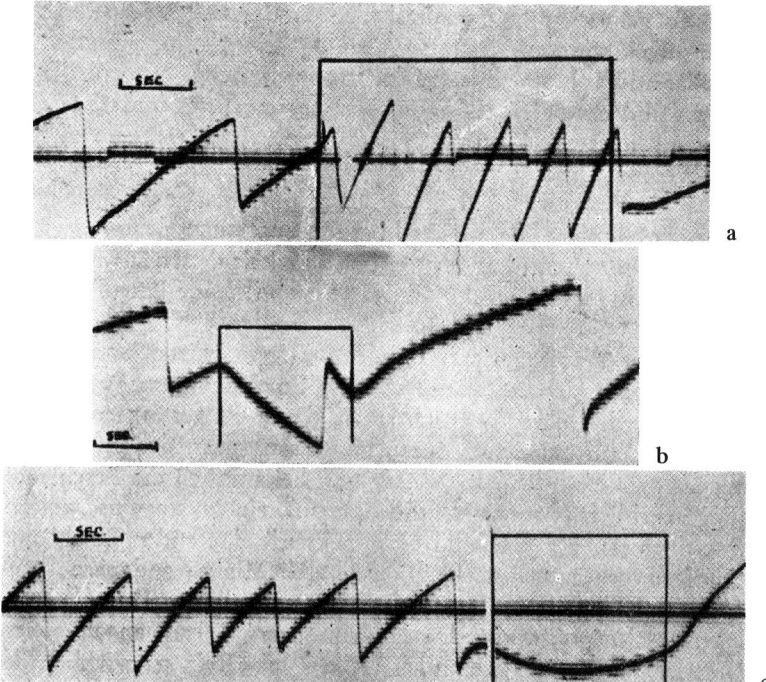

Fig. 18a-c. Combined optokinetic and vestibular stimulation. The rabbit is mounted on a turntable. Optokinetic stimulation is exerted on the immobilized right eye by moving a striped belt in front of this eye anteriorly at a velocity of 50 min arc/s. The optokinetic stimulus remains constant during the entire recording period. The vestibular stimulus consists of a brief rotation of the table (the duration of this rotation is indicated by the *two vertical lines*).

a Rotation of the table to the right: increase of the velocity of the slow phase as well as the frequency. The amplitude remains almost unchanged. After arrest of the rotation the original optokinetic nystagmus is present again.

b Rotation to the left: reversal of nystagmus. After arrest of rotation once again the original type.

c Rotation to the left: the rotatory velocity attained by the table is lower than in **b**. During the rotation cancelling of the nystagmus. After arrest of the rotation once again the original type of nystagmus

jected to a *rotatory acceleration*. On the basis of certain observations and physical arguments one may assume that the flow of endolymph lasts practically as long as the acceleration and that the velocity of this flow increases together with the acceleration acting on the animal. One could conclude from this that the *excitation* of the canal is approximately proportional to the *acceleration*, and that it has about the same duration as the acceleration.[1]

---

[1] This concept is supported by Mowrer's (1935a) observations. According to this investigator the action potentials in the vestibular nerve of *Chrysemys picta* do not last longer than the acceleration of the animal

We shall discuss the correctness of this conclusion only later, and first point out that the effect of the stimulation of the canal, the vestibular nystagmus, lasts — as is well known — *much longer* than the acceleration and that for instance a nystagmus elicited by an acceleration with a duration of a fraction of a second may continue for more than half a minute. To account for this phenomenon a *central aftereffect* of the vestibular stimulus is rather generally assumed. Assuming for the moment that vestibular excitation is indeed proportional to the acceleration, we can give a surprisingly good account of the facts by postulating exactly the same central mechanism for vestibular as for optokinetic nystagmus. A *constant* vestibular stimulus would then also generate a *uniform acceleration* of the slow phase. The *velocity* of the slow phase will thus gradually *increase*, and after *cessation* of the stimulus the nystagmus will *continue* for some time, to then disappear slowly by the action of the "central resistance".

Optical recordings of vestibular nystagmus (Fig. 19) show that during constant acceleration of the animal the acceleration of the slow phase (un-

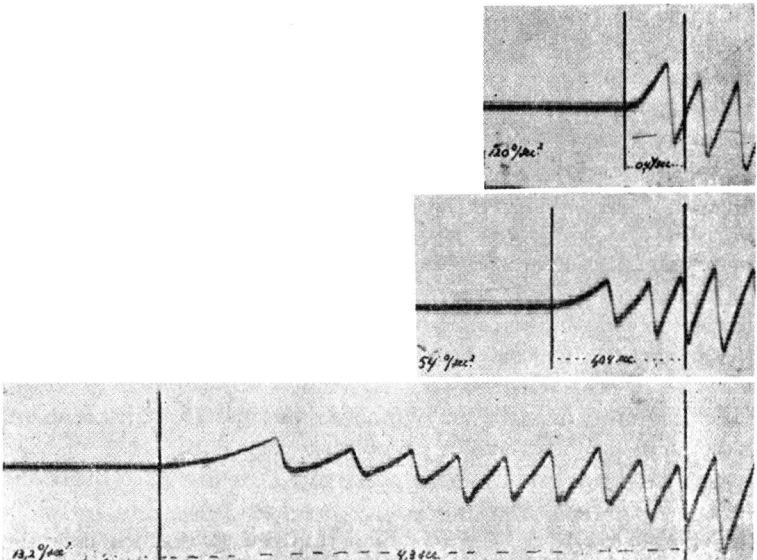

Fig. 19. Vestibular rotatory nystagmus of a rabbit with both eyes covered at different angular accelerations of the animal. The rotational velocity eventually reached by the table is similar in all three cases. In **a** this velocity is attained with a uniform acceleration of $120°/s^2$ within a time of 0.47 s, in **b** with an acceleration of $54°/s^2$ in 1.04 s, in **c** with an acceleration of $13.2°/s^2$ in 4.3 s. The *vertical lines* indicate the beginning and end of acceleration. After the second line the velocity is constant. At the end of the acceleration the slow phase velocity is about equal in all three curves, whereas the acceleration with which this velocity is attained is approximately proportional with the acceleration of the turntable

der certain conditions!) is indeed almost uniform, and that the velocity of the slow phase is proportional to the velocity of the animal. If one compares an optokinetic nystagmus with a vestibular one with a similar slow phase velocity, and the decay of this nystagmus after the termination of the acceleration of the animal, practically no difference between both curves can be observed.

We even have the possibility of *quantitatively comparing* the optokinetic and vestibular *stimulus* by taking the acceleration of the slow phase as a parameter. One finds then that the vestibular stimulus is in general much stronger than the optokinetic one. Whereas for optokinetic nystagmus no acceleration higher than 10 min arc/s^2 is found (with the immobilized eye!), an acceleration of 120°/s^2 (a factor 700 larger) is not unusual for a vestibular nystagmus. However, as the acceleration in a vestibular nystagmus usually only lasts a short time, the eventual *velocity* of the slow phase is of the same order of magnitude. The assumption that the vestibular excitation is proportional to the acceleration of the animal, and that the vestibular and optokinetic stimulus use a common central apparatus thus proves to be very fruitful. The vestibular impulses will in this case be an input to the hypothetical "center B", similar to the optokinetic ones.

There are, however, other possibilities. The investigations of Steinhausen on the labyrinth of the pike have shown that although the flow of endolymph lasts approximately as long as the acceleration, the *deflection of the cupula* lasts much longer, due to the specific physical conditions.

According to his observations and calculations, the deflection of the cupula (and thus the excitation) would not represent the *acceleration*, but the *velocity* of the animal.

If the canal system of the rabbit had similar properties, one would not need the "central resistance" to account for the characteristics of vestibular nystagmus. However, this does not exclude the possibility that the vestibular and optokinetic nystagmus may in part use the same central apparatus. By assuming that in that case the vestibular impulses are relayed not to center B, but to center A, so that the vestibular impulses are treated equally as impulses from center B, the rest of the model remains intact.

Finally, some remarks have to be made about the combination of optokinetic and vestibular stimulation under more physiological conditions.

When a rabbit is rotated with the eyes open on a turntable one observes, as stated before, a continuous nystagmus, which will go on indefinitely without change (Fig. 20b). If the experiment is repeated with the eyes covered, a totally identical nystagmus is recorded at the onset of rotation, but with continued rotation the velocity of the slow phase decreases gradually and finally the nystagmus disappears (Fig. 20a). This means that the nystagmus during rotation with open eyes is *initially* mainly controlled by the

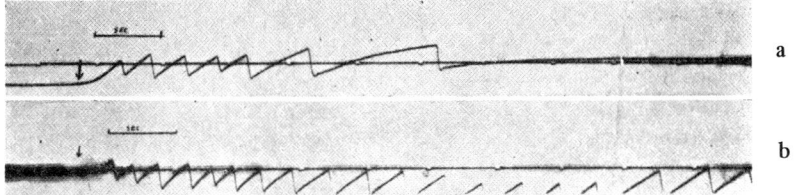

Fig. 20. a Vestibular rotatory nystagmus in a rabbit. The turntable is briefly accelerated to a constant velocity. *The eyes of the animal are covered.* The velocity of the slow phase reaches a maximum in a short time, and then decreases gradually to zero.
b Vestibular-optokinetic nystagmus. Experimental arrangement similar as in a, *but the right eye is opened.* The nystagmus is maintained during the uniform rotation, the velocity of the slow phase remains approximately constant

vestibular stimulus, but that parallel to the *decrease* in vestibular excitation the effect of the optical stimulus *increases* gradually. In this way the velocity of the slow phase can remain constant.

The optokinetic stimulus acting alone would require a longer time to accelerate the slow phase to its final velocity.

Vestibular and optokinetic stimuli together can achieve a nystagmus which continues unchanged during the whole rotation.

The vestibular stimulus, which is strong but short, is particularly suited to *start* the nystagmus; the optokinetic stimulus, which is weak but can continue unlimitedly, is able sustain the nystagmus.

For the reactions shown after the termination of the rotation the presence of optokinetic stimuli during the rotation is also of significance.

When a rabbit is rotated with the eyes covered and stopped when the initial vestibular nystagmus has decayed, the so-called afternystagmus[1] is elicited, which is opposite to the initial nystagmus but otherwise very similar to it (Fig. 21a).

After rotation with the eyes open on the other hand such an afternystagmus is not observed, the eye is at rest immediately after stopping (Fig. 21b). This can be observed at very different rotation velocities. Only when the rotation velocity is high, can a post-rotatory nystagmus be seen.

As an explanation for the absence of afternystagmus after rotation with the eyes open one could think of visual fixation of the surroundings, which suppresses nystagmus. However, this explanation is not correct, because when the eyes are covered during the rotation and opened only at the mo-

---

[1] Here we mean by afternystagmus the nystagmus elicited by the arrest of rotation. Afternystagmus in this case this does not mean, as with optokinetic afternystagmus, nystagmus after the arrest of the stimulus, because the postrotatory nystagmus is caused — at least initially — by the opposite stimulus generated by the stopping. The usual terminology is thus rather confusing

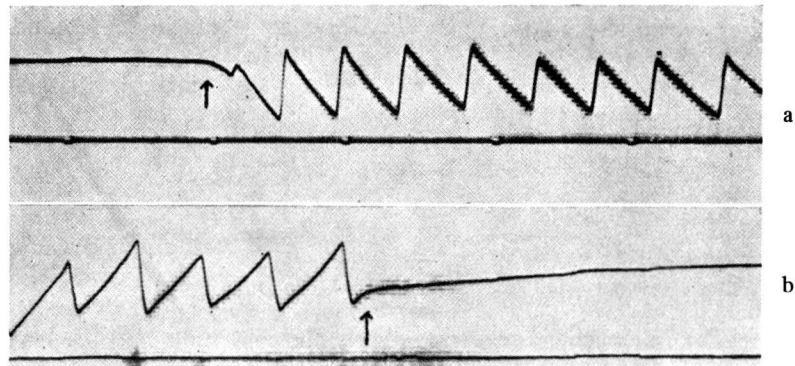

Fig. 21. a Rotation of a rabbit with covered eyes at a velocity kept constant over a long period. At the *arrow* the turntable is suddenly stopped: vestibular postrotatory nystagmus.
b Rotation of the rabbit with the right eye opened, otherwise as in a. During the steady rotation the nystagmus is maintained. At the *arrow* the turntable is suddenly stopped: no afternystagmus

ment of arrest, afternystagmus is not suppressed. If one eye is open during the rotation, while the second (covered) eye is used for the recording, and the first eye is covered immediately after the stopping, no postrotatory nystagmus is recorded, although visual fixation is not possible. Not the optical stimuli *after the stopping*, but rather those *during the rotation* cause the absence of postrotatory nystagmus. As a result of the optokinetic stimulus nystagmus is still present immediately before the end of the rotation. The vestibular stimulus caused by the stopping generates a negative acceleration (deceleration) of the slow phase, which reduces its velocity to exactly zero. In other words, the vestibular stimulus is just sufficient to neutralize the persisting excitation in the center.[1]

When the eyes are covered during the rotation and thus at the end of rotation no nystagmus and no central excitation are present, the velocity of the slow phase is essentially zero and the vestibular excitation caused by the deceleration will generate a nystagmus in the opposite direction.

Thus under physiological conditions, where we always have a combination of optical and vestibular stimuli, neither an optokinetic afternystagmus nor a postrotatory nystagmus occur, but only nystagmus during the whole rotation.

---

1 During *head nystagmus* analogous phenomena have been observed in several animals (Loeb (1907), Visser (1932), Mowrer (1935b)). The explanation given above has already been discussed by Visser (1932) and Mowrer (1935b). However, several other explanations for head nystagmus have to be considered as well (Visser, Mowrer)

If compensation of the shift of retinal images is considered as the physiological purpose of nystagmus, it is clear that this optokinetic-vestibular co-operation is highly effective.

3. Stare Nystagmus in Other Species of Animals

One characteristic of optokinetic nystagmus as analyzed above was the peculiarity that only the contrast relations in the visual field are relevant for its generation, while the selection of specific objects — a process which we call attention — plays no role. Even though the slow phase of this nystagmus can be considered as a kind of fixation, i.e., a stabilization of retinal images, this is not fixation in the usual sense, which always refers to the fixation of distinct objects, selected by attention.

The "fixation without attention" was defined as "stare"fixation and it seems appropriate to me to use also the term stare nystagmus for the future.

With good reason the rabbit was chosen as the first experimental animal, as this animal "stares" continuously, i.e., eye movements guided by attention are never observed.

The question now is whether in those animals that do show eye movements under the influence of attention (dog, cat, monkey) a stare nystagmus is also present. To answer this it would be necessary to eliminate attention, something that obviously cannot be achieved with absolute reliability. When monotonous black and white stripes are used for the optokinetic stimulation a constant effect of attention seems, however, less probable.

Moreover, it is impossible to elicit nystagmus in the species mentioned with the striped cylinder specified by Barany (1921) (which in man can elicit OKN with the aid of attention).

If, however, the animals are investigated inside the striped drum described above, where all contrasts in the visual field move, a regular and sustained nystagmus can be elicited and it is not clear why the enlargement of the moving field would affect the attention. The nystagmus in the rotating drum will therefore in the following be indicated as stare nystagmus, although it is not excluded that attention may influence the nystagmus occasionally.

The stare nystagmus in dogs, cats, and monkeys agrees in many points with the nystagmus of the rabbit as analyzed above. Accordingly, these points are mentioned here briefly:

1. The significance of the size of the moving field has already been discussed. Not the absolute number of moving contrasts, but the ratio between moving and stationary contrasts is decisive.

2. For the generation of nystagmus it is indifferent which part of the retina is stimulated by the optokinetic stimulus.
3. The "central inertia" is manifest also in this case at the onset (gradual acceleration of the slow phase) as well as the arrest (afternystagmus) of the stimulus.

The afternystagmus can be very well observed particularly in the monkey. Under favorable conditions it may consist of about 40 beats.
4. The combination of optokinetic and vestibular stimuli (rotation of the animals with the eyes open) reveals similar close relations between vestibular and optokinetic nystagmus as in the rabbit. In one important respect the performance of stare nystagmus differs from that observed in the rabbit, particularly in the dog and the monkey, and to a smaller extent in the cat.

The determination of the highest contrast velocity able to elicit a nystagmus yields much higher values in these animals. While in the rabbit this highest velocity is only exceptionally as high as 70°/s and usually lower, a velocity of over 360°/s (more than one revolution per second) is capable of eliciting nystagmus in dogs and monkeys; cats are intermediate in this respect. No satisfactory explanation for these differences can yet be given.

The investigation at very low velocities is not possible in dogs etc., as here, in contrast to the rabbit, "spontaneous" fast eye movements occur which impair the observation of very slow smooth eye movements. Investigations on immobilized eyes were not performed in these animals.

Only in dogs and cats has the significance of the direction of the contrast motion been studied. In agreement with the findings in the rabbit it was found that (when only *one* eye was stimulated) a movement of the contrasts in *nasal* direction elicits a nystagmus more easily, i.e., at a higher maximal velocity, than a motion in temporal direction. However, the distinction is not as marked as in the rabbit. Possibly this is related to the different position of the eyes (lateral in the rabbit, frontal in the dog).

Without any doubt a stare nystagmus also occurs in the *human*. Also in this case it is not easy to abolish the influence of attention. Although one can instruct the subject in the rotating drum *not* to look at the moving stripes, but to stare straight ahead, self-observation shows that it is difficult to follow this instruction strictly, as moving contrasts in the center of the visual field draw the attention with a certain compulsion. Diversion of the attention can be most reliably achieved by introducing a stationary *fixation point* in the center of the visual field and instructing the subject to look at this point.

As was first shown by Fisher and Kornmüller (1930), also in these conditions a nystagmus can be observed, which doubtless should be considered as an inhibited stare nystagmus in our terms. This nystagmus, called fixation nystagmus[1] by the authors mentioned, has a very small amplitude and can only be demonstrated by special methods (afterimage technique).

Roelofs and Van der Bend, who also tried to investigate optokinetic nystagmus without facilitation by attention, instruct the subject to look at the center of a stationary *diaphragm*, behind which the stripes are moving.

But it is not so easy to fixate without interruption a nonexisting point when contrasts are moving at the same place and therefore we would not be surprised if the nystagmus observed by the authors was due to a shift of the attention toward the stripes.

Most other investigators concerned with the study of OKN did not attempt to rule out the influence of attention, but on the contrary instructed the subjects to look at the stripes passing by. Some of them (Stenvers (1926), Cords (1926a), Ohm (1929)) even facilitate this task by replacing the monotonous black stripes with "interesting" images. The rotating drums etc. used by these authors are not very suitable for eliciting a stare nystagmus, as the number of moving contrasts is usually very small compared to the stationary contrasts in the visual field.

Without the aid of attention no nystagmus whatsoever could be elicited by such means, as is confirmed also by the negative result in experiments with animals.

The optokinetic nystagmus generated under influence of attention will be discussed in a later section. The conditions under which a nystagmus may be generated in man which is fully equivalent to the stare nystagmus of the rabbit are thus not yet fully known.

Perhaps this may explain why the "central inertia" is so much less manifest in the human than in the rabbit (and also dog and monkey). Admittedly an optokinetic afternystagmus was described first by Ohm in man, but if one compares Ohm's afternystagmus curves with the records obtained from the rabbit (Fig. 15), the difference in favor of the latter is very marked. The existence of afternystagmus in man is even disputed by many authors (Cords (1926b), Nordmann and Lieou (1928)). It is of course possible that the processes in the central apparatus of nystagmus differ essentially in this respect from those in the rabbit, however, the fact that in the sequence rabbit-dog-monkey the importance of afternystagmus increases rather than decreases argues against this possibility. First of all it seems desirable to improve the stimulus conditions for eliciting a pure stare nystagmus in man.

---

[1] The choice of this name seems unfortunate, as this nystagmus is generated not as a result of, but rather despite the fixation

4. The Localization of Stare Nystagmus in the Central Nervous System

As pointed out in the introduction, the majority of investigators (Barany (1921), Stenvers (1926), Ohm (1929), Cords (1926a, b), Strauss and others) consider optokinetic nystagmus as a *cortical* reflex. Although there is no full consensus among these authors on the exact pathway of the reflex arc, they all agree that no optokinetic nystagmus can be generated without mediation of the *visual cortex*.

This conviction is founded on neuroanatomical considerations as well as observations in neurological patients. The latter have been made almost without exception with equipment that is unsuitable for eliciting stare nystagmus (see previous section).

Bartels (1931), on the other hand, is of the opinion that OKN can also be elicited without participation by the cortical visual centers, and that the reflex pathway passes through the midbrain. This concept is based on the fact that optokinetic nystagmus is found even in relatively primitive species, in which a cerebrum has not developed, or only moderately. Van der Spek and Visser (Visser, 1932) have shown that in pigeons, in which the cerebrum is only moderately developed compared to mammals, *an optokinetic head-nystagmus can be elicited also after extirpation of the cerebrum*.

With this experiment the existence of a subcortical optokinetic reflex pathway in birds has been proven.

However, it could be that in mammals, in which the anatomical relations differ considerably from those in birds in the sense that the significance of the visual midbrain is reduced relative to that of the visual cortex, the OKN reflex pathway passes through the visual cortex all the same.

Therefore it was absolutely necessary to investigate the localization of optokinetic stare nystagmus also in the rabbit, cat, dog, and monkey.

a. *Rabbit.* First of all it could be established that also in this animal stare nystagmus can still be elicited after bilateral extirpation of the cerebrum. Essential differences with intact rabbits were not observed, but as the nystagmus of the decerebrated animal was not recorded, some minor difference cannot be excluded. After unilateral extirpation of the cerebrum the nystagmus was asymmetrical in some rabbits. After extirpation of the right hemisphere the nystagmus of the left eye in the posterior direction and of the right eye in the anterior direction could not be elicited or at least not very well. After about a week symmetry had been recovered.

b. *Dog.* Goltz has already pointed out that optical reactions are not totally absent in decerebrated dogs. In addition to pupillary contraction on illumination he found blinking upon strong illumination to be intact. So far it has been assumed that with these two reflexes all possibilities for optical reactions in the cerebrated dog are exhausted. The investigation of a dog in which both hemispheres were removed in two sessions with an interval of 4 weeks (Fig. 22) has shown that also the stare nystagmus belongs among the subcortical optical reactions.

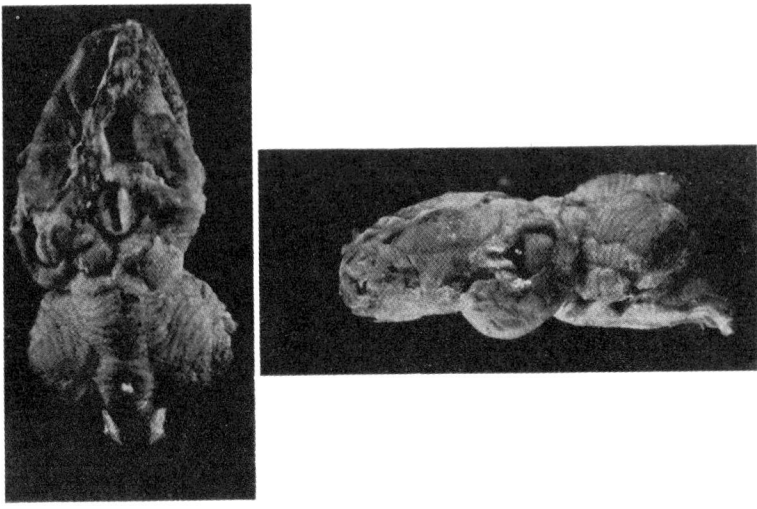

Fig. 22. Brain of a decerebrated dog, which showed starenystagmus. At the *left side* small remains of the temporal lobe (lobus piriformis) are retained

Figure 23 shows a nystagmogram of this optokinetic nystagmus.

The recording technique was in this case different and essentially more crude than the one used for the other nystagmograms.

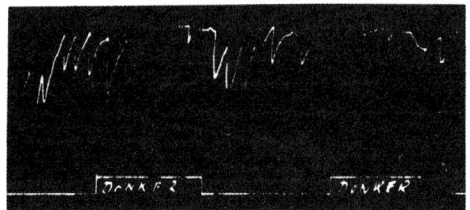

Fig. 23. Stare-nystagmus of the decerebrated dog of Fig. 22. Pneumatic recording of the left eye. Rotation of the striped drum to the left. Nystagmus to the right. Between the marks (*DONKER*): extinction of the light, afternystagmus and deviation of the eye in the direction of the slow phase

Neither the optical recording nor the simple lever technique is suitable for the decerebrated dog, as with these methods the head has to be rigidly fixed and the decerebrated dog vigorously resists such a fixation. Therefore a plaster cap was prepared which exactly fitted on the head and a drum, covered by a thin rubber membrane, was attached to this cap. A silk thread was extended between the anterior corneal pole and the center of the rubber membrane, so that the eye movements were conveyed to the drum. The fluctuations in air pressure thus caused in the drum were transmitted pneumatically by a rubber tube to a conventional Russ-kymograph. During the brief period of the registration the head was loosely held in place with the hand, which was usually allowed by the decerebrated animal.

As demonstrated by the nystagmogram, an afternystagmus is found after the arrest of the stimulus (turning off the lights), which is followed by a deviation in the direction of the slow phase. If the stimulus is switched on at this stage, the first effect is a fast phase in the opposite direction (Fig. 23).

The nystagmogram shows a nystagmus to the right, which is evoked by rotation of the drum to the left. Also with rotation of the drum to the right an OKN (to the left) could be observed, but it was not as distinct and only occurred at a low angular velocity (about 5°/s).

This asymmetry, which persisted for a long period (2 months) after the second operation is probably due to an unintentional lesion of the brain stem.

The nystagmus during rotation of the drum to the left was also not completely normal, i.e., it could only be elicited at relatively low velocities (40°/s), while in intact dogs the maximal velocity is usually 400°/s or more. With respect to the fundamental question of whether a subcortical optokinetic nystagmus exists in the dog these findings are of course of no consequence.

Dogs in which only the *visual cortex* has been removed bilaterally also show the stare nystagmus.

Also in this case the maximal velocity that will elicit OKN is considerably lower than in intact dogs.

Thus it seems that the abnormalities found in decerebrated dogs are not due to some subcortical damage, but indeed to the lack of cortical visual centers. After unilateral decerebration in the dog the stare nystagmus remains permanently asymmetrical. Specifically, during movements of the contrasts toward the operated side nystagmus only occurs with low velocities, while with movement toward the healthy side values similar to those in intact animals are found. This also argues for an influence of the cerebral cortex on subcortical stare nystagmus.

c. *Monkey.* As is well known, the monkey is neuroanatomically and particularly with respect to the central visual system nearly related to man, and therefore it did not seem not superfluous to verify the facts already established for rabbits and dogs also in the monkey. *Macacus rhesus* was chosen as the experimental animal. As mentioned before, this animal shows a beautiful stare nystagmus in a rotating drum. To answer the question of whether this can still be elicited after removal of the cerebral cortex, it is actually sufficient to ablate the visual cortex bilaterally, i.e., the *area striata*. It is generally assumed that the visual cortical projection in the monkey is restricted to the area striata, and therefore an animal in which this area is lacking is visually equivalent to a decorticated one.

Bilateral extirpation of the area striata was performed in three monkeys. This operation is not difficult, as the area striata in the monkey is a relatively well-demarcated zone.

The relations are particularly simple on the convex surface of the hemisphere, where the deep parieto-occipital fissure (monkey sulcus) forms the anterior border (Fig. 24a).

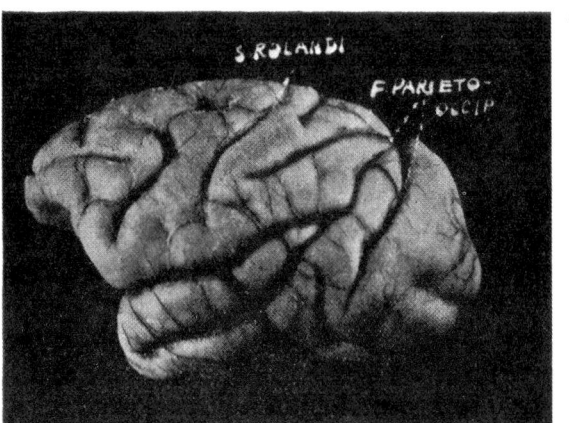

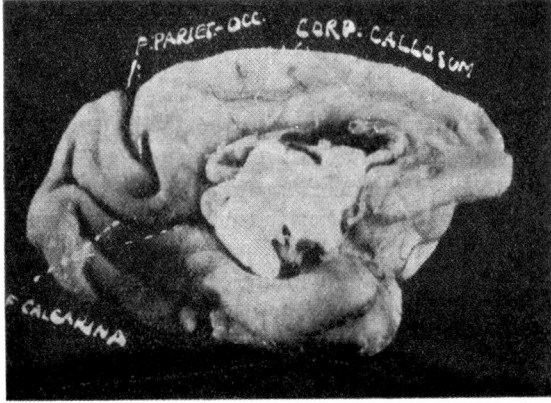

Fig. 24a, b. Intact left hemisphere of *Macacus rhesus*. a Convexity. b Medial aspect

At the medial side the removal is a little more difficult, as the calcarine fissure continues as far as the caudal end of the corpus callosum (Fig. 24b), which hampers the lateral displacement of the occipital lobe.

Figure 25 shows both hemispheres of an operated animal. As this figure demonstrates, the area striata was completely absent on both sides.

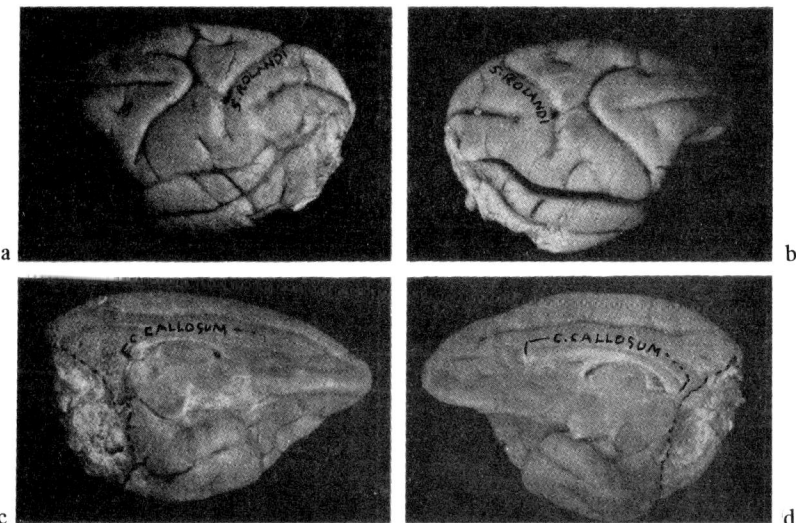

Fig. 25a-d. Hemispheres of a monkey after bilateral extirpation of the area striata. a Left hemisphere: convexity. b Left hemisphere: medial view. c Right hemisphere: conveyity. d Right hemisphere: medial view

This operation was performed in two stages; first the left and then $1\frac{1}{2}$ months later the right area striata was removed. After the second operation the animal was kept alive for more than 2 months. During this period it showed the following behavior: *it gave the impression of being completely blind*. It did not avoid an approaching hand before being touched by it. Food was sought by "touch". Blink reflexes due to threatening movements as well as optical placing reflexes of the front and hindlegs were lacking. Fixation eye movements toward objects displayed in the visual field or pursuit eye movements could not be observed.

In contrast to this, the stare nystagmus in the rotating drum could be elicited with great clarity, by rotation of the drum to the right (nystagmus to the left) as well as by rotation to the left (nystagmus to the right). Moreover, the nystagmus could already be elicited at relatively high drum rotation velocities and a clear difference in this respect with the normal animal could not be established.

As the values found at different times varied appreciably, as in the intact animal, it is meaningless to mention them. In any case the monkey without area striata is obviously different from the dog without visual cortex, in which nystagmus could only be elicited at low velocities. Also the observations on two other monkeys, in which the area striata was also removed bilaterally (in one of them in a single session) led to similar results. Although these observations make it highly likely that the stare nystagmus is a subcortical reflex also in the monkey, this point can only strictly be proven of course by extirpation of the entire cortex.

Observations on completely decerebrated monkeys kept alive for a considerable time are found only occasionally in the literature. Karplus and Kreidl (1914) have reported on a series of such animals, the majority of which died already within the first or second week, while one animal that survived for 26 days was in poor general condition in the last weeks (infection). From the optical reactions only the pupillary light reflex was found positive by these authors; optokinetic reactions were not investigated.

We have been able to keep a decerebrated monkey alive in good general condition for 37 days after the removal of the second hemisphere[1], during which period the animal was investigated repeatedly in the rotating drum.

Figure 26 shows that from the cerebrum only small remains of the temporal lobes were preserved (lobulus piriformis), which was spared in view of their immediate vicinity to the optic tract.

Similarly to the monkeys without area striata, the animal gave the impression of being completely blind. The blink reflexes on threatening movements as well as the visual placing reflexes were absent. The pupillary reflex to illumination was retained. *The stare nystagmus to the right as well as to the left could be elicited.*

An asymmetry was persistently found in this animal; the nystagmus to the *right* (rotation of the drum to the left) was always better elicited and at higher velocities (up to 300°/s) than the nystagmus to the *left* (drum rotation to the right), which could only be elicited by a velocity of 80°/s at the most.

Also the afternystagmus to the right was more marked and of longer duration than the afternystagmus to the left. This asymmetry is most likely due to unintentional subcortical lesions.

Finally some remarks can be made about stare nystagmus in the monkey after *unilateral* extirpation of the cerebrum. The relevant observations were made in the monkey just described, after the first operation (extirpation of the left hemisphere) over period of about 6 weeks, and in a second monkey, in which only the right hemisphere was removed and which died one week

---

1 The cause of death was an acute intestinal obstruction

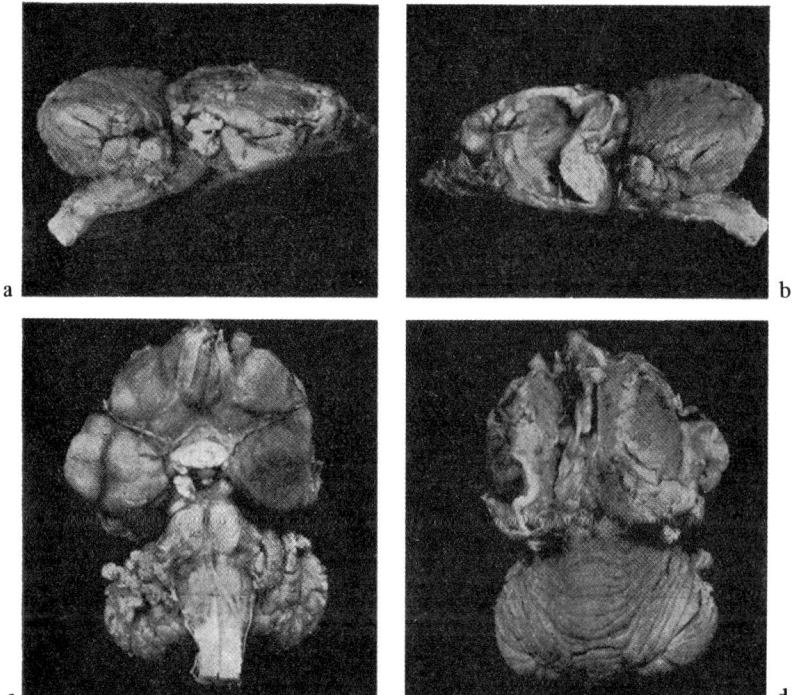

Fig. 26a-d. Brain of an almost completely decerebrated monkey with "stare-nystagmus". **a** Right lateral view. **b** Left lateral view. **c** Basal view: rests of the temporal lobe are retained. **d** Superior view

after the operation. In both cases no asymmetry of stare nystagmus was present at all; the nystagmus could be elicited in both directions at high velocities, and no clear difference with respect to the normal animal could be determined. This finding is of interest namely because on the one hand in the dog a permanent asymmetry of OKN after unilateral extirpation of the cerebrum was found, and on the other hand also in humans with unilateral cerebral lesions an asymmetry has been repeatedly found. After the negative finding in this respect in the monkey it does not seem permissible to consider the asymmetry in man and dog simply as an analogous phenomenon.

The investigations in rabbit, dog, and monkey have thus led to the general result that the reflex pathway for stare nystagmus is subcortical. The precise location of the relevant centers, which are probably situated in the midbrain and pons, cannot be indicated as yet.

Certainly the lateral geniculate nucleus can be excluded, as this is known to degenerate completely after extirpation of the cerebrum or the visual cortex.

Whether the stare nystagmus in man is also a subcortical reflex is a question that can be answered with certainty only in the clinic. So far as it is allowable to extend conclusions from experiments on animals to human physiology, the experiments mentioned certainly support an affirmative answer to this question. The objection that this reflex in man, with his strong development of the cerebrum, may have been "cerebrated", loses much of its strength due to the observations in the monkey.

The demonstration of a subcortical optokinetic nystagmus in man might be possible, if cases of total cortical blindness were investigated appropriately, e.g., within a rotating drum. However, such cases are rare.

Even if one succeeded in eliciting nystagmus in cases of cerebral hemianopsia by optokinetic stimulation of only the "blind" parts on the retina, the case would be proven.

However, in order to do this many a technical difficulty will have to be overcome.

5. Look Nystagmus

For the type of optokinetic nystagmus discussed until now the significance of the stimulus is determined solely by the physical conditions in visual space (number of moving contrasts, velocity and direction of their motion etc.). We now want to discuss a second type of nystagmus, for which the cooperation of the attention is an essential factor. In this case the significance of a certain object as a visual stimulus is not determined primarily by its optical properties, but by its special relation to the human or animal subject, which we shall call from now on *preference*. How such a preference is physiologically established will not be discussed here; one can imagine processes analogous to those in the formation of a conditional reflex.

The eye movements controlled by attention have the tendency to aim and maintain the visual axis at the "preferred" object, so that this object is always projected on the central part of the retina. Two types of these eye movements should be distinguished.

First there is the fast, jerky movement which directs the visual axis toward a "preferred" object in the periphery of the visual field (refixation, search movement).

In the second place there is the relatively slow, smooth movement with which the eye pursues a moving "preferred" object, so that the visual axis remains aimed at the object (pursuit- or tracking movement).

This pursuit movement causes the image of the preferred object to remain *locked* on the central part of the retina (the fovea). Therefore one can consider this as a fixation movement, and in actual fact this is fixation in the conventional sense, for which I propose the name look nystagmus. It seems important at this point to reiterate the distinction between stare and look nystagmus.

Starenystagmus is concerned with the fixation of the entire visual surroundings on the whole retina, look nystagmus is concerned with the fixation of a preferred object on a specific part of the retina. Even when the stare fixation is elicited by the movement of a single object, which is possible only when stationary contrasts in the visual field are absent or when their influence is abolished by the immobilized eye technique, there is a difference with look fixation, because in this case the projection of the object is fixated on an arbitrary part of the retina. For stare fixation the stimulus consists of the movement of images of contrasts over an arbitrary part of the retina whereas for look fixation *movement* of the image is not absolutely necessary.

The preferred object probably evokes a special stimulus as soon as it forms an image extrafoveally, by which a refixation is elicited.

According to this concept the pursuit movement, i.e., the following of a preferred object, is identical with a series of similarly directed small refixations. One could easily conclude from this that only the immediate surroundings of the fovea are of importance for the pursuit, because as soon as the image of the object is removed from the fovea, it will be followed and overtaken by the fovea. A simple experiment can demonstrate that this conclusion is not correct.

Behind a white screen, placed in the center of the visual field of a subject, a vertically oriented pencil is moved in horizontal direction. The middle of the pencil is thus invisible, but the upper and lower ends are not covered by the screen. The subject is instructed to look at the center of the pencil (which he can only imagine). When the pencil is moved behind the screen one observes a smooth pursuit movement of the eyes, which remain directed at the center of the pencil. This observation proves that pursuit movements in the sense of look fixation can also be elicited by stimulation of peripheral parts of the retina. Admittedly the motion of the visible parts of the pencil will also provide impulses for stare fixation, but these cannot possibly be the cause of the pursuit movement, because firstly the latter occurs also when predominantly stationary contrasts are present in the visual field, and secondly it is only observed when the subject is instructed to look at the center of the pencil.

Eye movements guided by attention can be observed not only in man, but also in monkeys, dogs, and cats. They are, however, completely lacking in the rabbit. For the testing of these eye movements a first requirement is of course to choose an appropriate preferred object. For humans this task is obviously very simple, because in this case the preference for any object is established by the simple instruction to look at this object.

With dogs and cats one needs an interesting object, e.g., a piece of meat, another animal, etc.

In general, refixations are more easily elicited in these animals than pursuit movements, as the latter demand a longer period of concentrated attention. Monkeys are known to be always very interested in humans; pursuit can thus be easily elicited when one fixates the head of the animal manually and one moves (not too fast) through its visual field. One can also show the animal its own image in a small mirror; movements of this image induced by rotations of the mirror usually elicit pursuit movements. This discussion of pursuit and refixation movements which are probably familiar to everybody was only necessary because of their close relations to look nystagmus, which will be discussed now.

Look nystagmus can be best studied in man, in whom it is most simply elicited.

If one moves a continuous series of small objects which comprise only a small part of the total contrast of the visual field (e.g., a chain of beads) through the visual field of the subject, who is instructed to look at these objects, one immediately observes a smooth pursuit, which is soon interrupted by a fast movement in the opposite direction, after which a new pursuit movement starts, and so on. As is well known, the "classical" concept (Barany, 1921 and others) identifies the slow phase of this nystagmus with a fixation movement (fixation here in the sense of look fixation!) and the fast phase with a refixation. That the slow phase is a pursuit movement seems very probable; only one serious objection can be raised. If one gives the instruction to follow a single object with the eyes, it will indeed be followed to the extreme borders of the visual field. The slow phase of look nystagmus on the contrary follows a distinct object only over a certain distance. This distinction is, however, a quantitative one.

The single object is only followed up to the border of the visual field when the instruction is explicitly formulated in terms of *following*. If the instruction is only to look at the object, the pursuit movement is in many cases interrupted before the object disappears from the visual field.

This becomes very clear when one *asks not* to follow, but just to look. In this case one observes actually a pursuit movement, which is, however, soon terminated and followed by an opposite fast movement. On the other hand eye movements up to the borders of the visual field can also be elicited with a continuous series of moving objects by the explicit instruction to *follow* the objects.

The concept that the slow phase of look nystagmus is interrupted because a subsequent object draws the attention, and thus that the fast phase is identical with a refixation movement, cannot be correct, because when pursuit is elicited by a single preferred object the eye also returns with a fast phase to the initial position when fixation is interrupted.

Clinical observations (tractus hemianopsia: Stenvers (1924), Ohm (1929)) have also shown that the fast phase cannot be a refixation. Just as with stare nystagmus it must be assumed that the fast and slow phase of look nystagmus are controlled by the same visual stimulus.

If one wants to investigate a "pure" look nystagmus, the conditions should be chosen so that the "preferred" objects form a very small part of the total contrast in the visual field. Only in this case can the stimulus for stare-nystagmus, provided by the movement of the retinal images of these objects, be disregarded relative to the stimulus caused by the opposite movement of the retinal images of the stationary, nonpreferred contrasts. If the number of moving contrasts is increased, a combination of look- and stare nystagmus will be investigated. The nystagmus elicited by the striped drum as specified by Barany, which is mostly used in the clinic, is neither a pure look nystagmus nor a pure starenystagmus.

It is more difficult to elicit look nystagmus in animals than in man.

In dogs an optokinetic nystagmus which can be certainly considered as a look nystagmus was elicited by Rademaker and De Kleyn, and later also by Nordmann and Lieou (1928) as well as Broers and De Kleyn (1934). As the optokinetic stimulus these authors chose a row of living rabbits, which were moved on a turntable in the visual field of the dog. Only in dogs that had a lively interest in rabbits could nystagmus be observed.

In monkeys a look nystagmus can also be evoked with a similar procedure as used to produce pursuit. When a human subject, which always interests the monkey, moves at a distance of several meters through the visual field of the animal while the head of the animal is manually restrained, a pursuit movement can be immediately observed. However, this movement usually is soon interrupted by a fast phase in the opposite direction, so that the gaze of the animal is directed at another part of the body. The latter is then followed by a second pursuit movement, after which another fast phase follows. In this way a nystagmus is generated, which usually consists of 2-3 beats and is terminated when the animal's gaze has passed over the whole person.

The drawback of this method is of course that no nystagmus of extended duration can be studied. On the other hand nystagmus can be induced very consistently in this way in the intact monkey when care is taken that the animal is not distracted, and therefore conclusions can be drawn when this look nystagmus is absent. Attempts to elicit a nystagmus also in the monkey by means of the chain of beads have not led to satisfactory results. Although some occasional beats of nystagmus were observed, a sustained nystagmus could not be produced, presumably because the animal soon withdrew its attention from the chain.

Recordings of look nystagmus in animals are not yet available, therefore the analysis is not as precise as that of stare nystagmus and data on the velocity of the slow phase etc. are still lacking.

One important distinction from stare nystagmus can already be made from observation alone. There is no sign of a central "inertia" either at the onset or the arrest of the stimulation, moreover the complete lack of afternystagmus is very conspicuous. This observation seems to indicate that the central mechanism of look nystagmus is considerably different from that of stare nystagmus. A further elucidation of this point is highly desirable.

6. The Localization of Look Nystagmus in the Central Nervous System

The fact that the great majority of investigators consider optokinetic nystagmus to be a cortical reflex is explained in part by their conviction that the participation of attention is essential for the generation of optokinetic reactions. We have shown that this assumption is not correct; the localization of stare nystagmus in subcortical centers should thus come as no surprise. For the look nystagmus, which fully depends on attention, a cerebral localization is on the other hand much more likely.

Experiments in animals have shown that this supposition is correct. Rademaker and De Kleyn had already established that the optokinetic nystagmus elicited by living rabbits rotated on a turntable is lacking in decerebrated dogs. Likewise the decerebrated dog described before showed no look nystagmus and refixation and pursuit movements were also absent in this animal.

It is not necessary to remove the whole cerebral cortex to abolish look nystagmus as well as refixations and pursuit. It is sufficient to remove the visual cortex. The extent of this cortical area, which is known from Campbell's anatomical investigations in the dog, is shown in Fig. 27. According

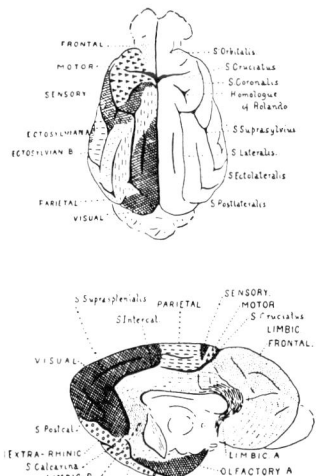

Fig. 27. Cytoarchitectonics of the cerebral cortex of the dog, after Campbell (1905) (visual cortex: *hatched*)

to Minkowski (1911) the data of Campbell (1905) are in good agreement with physiological findings.

In Munk's diagram of the visual area the considerable extension in the frontal direction is not taken into account. But in a number of dogs in which I removed only Munk's visual area, look nystagmus, as well as refixation and pursuit movements, were also absent during the entire observation period (several months after the operation) (Fig. 28). Obviously such negative re-

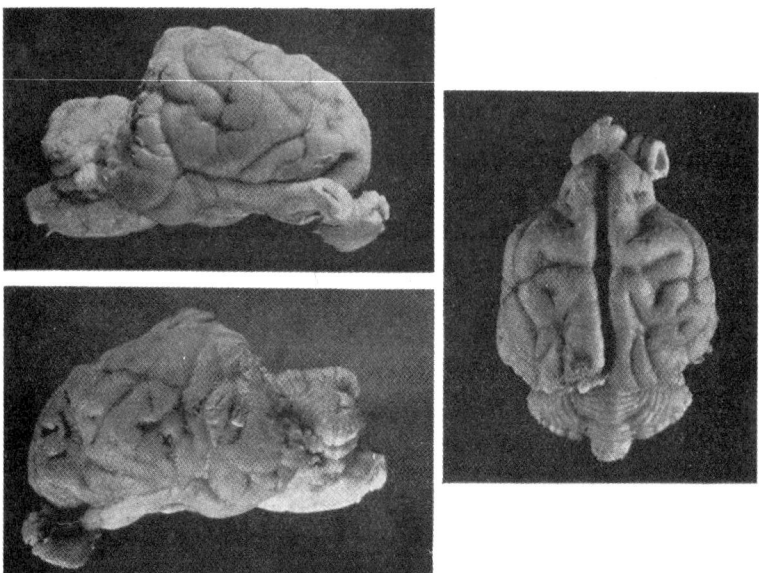

Fig. 28. Brain of a dog after extirpation of both visual areas as defined by Munk

sults should be evaluated with great caution, particularly when one thinks of the difficulty with which look nystagmus is normally elicited, and they do not definitely prove an exclusive localization of look nystagmus in the posterior parts of the visual cortex.

Large parts of the anterior part of the hemisphere, specifically the whole sensorimotor cortex (gyrus sigmoideus and adjacent parts of the gyrus coronalis) could be removed without a noticeable disturbance of look nystagmus, refixations and pursuit movements. Figure 29 shows an example. After unilateral extirpation of the cerebrum or the visual cortex, asymmetrical behavior of the look nystagmus was found, in agreement with the data of Rademaker and De Kleyn. After extirpation of the left half of the cerebrum, no unambiguous look nystagmus was present when the rabbits moved to the left in the visual field of the dog, while during movement to the right a clear nystagmus to the left was elicited.

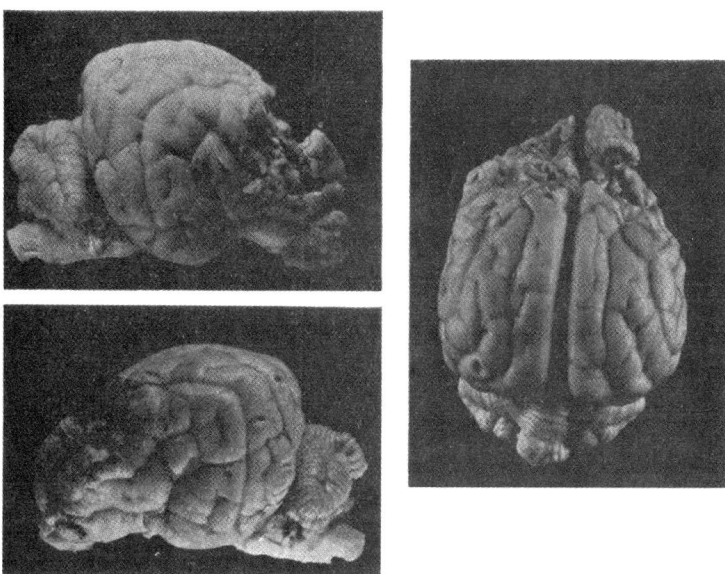

Fig. 29. Brain of a dog after bilateral ablation of the sensorimotor cortex

Broers and De Kleyn (1934) also reported such an asymmetry. On the other hand this asymmetry cannot be observed after unilateral extirpation of the sensorimotor cortex. Experiments in monkeys have led to the following results. In the decerebrated monkey described previously, look nystagmus, refixation and pursuit movements were absent. Bilateral extirpation of the area striata (Fig. 25) also led to permanent loss of these reactions. So far there is full agreement with the results in the dog. A difference is shown after unilateral extirpations. A monkey in which the area striata was removed unilaterally (on the left side) showed a look nystagmus in both directions, on condition of course that the preferred object (a person) was moving in the left half of the visual field. Immediately after unilateral extirpation of the cerebrum (at the left side) the looknystagmus could be elicited only by movement to the right. However, one month after the operation look nystagmus could once more be elicited by motion in both directions, although the nystagmus to the left (movement to the right) was more marked than the nystagmus to the right. Thus, after unilateral extirpations an asymmetry of look nystagmus was not demonstrable in the monkey or was at least less marked than in the dog, which is a phenomenon analogous to that found for stare nystagmus.

The optokinetic nystagmus which is usually investigated in the clinic cannot be regarded as a look nystagmus without qualification. However, as the attention is usually essential for its generation, it seems at first sight very probable that the cerebral cortex is instrumental in this kind of nystagmus and therefore it is important to compare the clinical findings with the experimental results in animals. The clinical neurological literature is mainly concerned with asymmetries of OKN. Several authors have found that in unilateral cerebral lesions OKN cannot be elicited to the side contralateral to the lesion and this phenomenon has even found a regular application in practice. Our findings in the dog seem to agree with this conclusion. Thus it is even more remarkable that in the monkey, which is more closely related to man, this asymmetry is only marginally present even after complete removal of the cerebrum and that in any case the look nystagmus (as well as the stare nystagmus) can still be elicited in both directions. According to Stenvers, not only lesions of the occipital lobe and the area of the gyrus angularis, but also circumscript lesions of the frontal lobe lead to unilateral defects of OKN. Also in this respect there is no agreement with animal experiments, as look nystagmus in dogs can normally also be elicited after bilateral removal of the anterior part of the cerebrum. In the monkey this experiment has not yet been performed. An explanation for this difference cannot yet be given.

Summary

Two types of optokinetic nystagmus have to be distinguished: *stare nystagmus and look nystagmus*.

A. *Stare nystagmus* is characterized by the fact that its generation is fully determined by the physical-optical conditions in the visual field.

The effective stimulus is the motion of retinal images. Stare nystagmus is controlled exclusively by this movement. Other factors such as attention are not required for its generation.

Stare nystagmus was observed by us in man and in addition in the monkey, dog, cat, and rabbit. In the rabbit the mechanism of stare-nystagmus can be studied most easily. The observations in this animal have shown the following.

I. Stare nystagmus is only elicited, when all or at least the majority of the contrasts in the visual field move in the same direction.
II. Stationary objects (contrasts) in the visual field inhibit its generation. This is because their images move in the opposite direction as soon as the eyes follow the moving objects and thus constitute an opposing stimulus.
III. In the absence of stationary contrasts (e.g., in darkness) motion of a single light spot in the visual field is sufficient to elicit nystagmus (the slow as well as the fast phase).

IV. It is indifferent which part of the retina is stimulated by the moving retinal images.
V. A movement of the retinal images which causes an *increase* in excitation of retinal receptors (e.g., when a white stripe on a black background is enlarged on one side) constitutes a *strong* stimulus, a movement which causes a *decrease* in excitation (e.g., when a white stripe on a black background is narrowed on one side) is a weak stimulus.
VI. Motion of retinal images in temporal (i.e., in the rabbit posterior) direction constitutes a strong stimulus, motion in nasal direction is a weak stimulus.
VII. When one eye is immobilized with clamps and contrasts are moved in the visual field of this eye alone, nystagmus is generated in the other eye, on condition that no stationary contrasts are present in the visual field of the latter eye, e.g., when it is covered.
VIII. Stationary contrasts in the visual field of the fixed eye have no inhibitory effect in this case, as their images cannot move over the retina.
IX. The maximal angular velocity of the contrasts at which stare nystagmus is still elicited in the rabbit is about $70°/s$.
X. A minimal angular velocity for eliciting stare nystagmus could not be established. At a contrast velocity of 6 s arc/s (i.e., one revolution of the striped drum in 60 h) a clear nystagmus was still observed; at this velocity movement of the contrasts was no longer perceived by the human eye.
XI. The investigation on the immobilized eye showed that contrast motion at a velocity of 10-50 min arc/s constitutes the strongest optokinetic stimulus.
XII. The slow and fast phases of nystagmus are elicited by the same optical stimulus. Whether the nystagmus starts with a slow or a fast phase depends in the first place upon the initial eye position. Whether this phenomenon is caused by "switching" as a result of proprioceptive signals from the eye muscles or by a purely central automatic mechanism could not be determined. When the eye is deviated, a fast phase can also be induced by acoustic and tactile stimuli.
XIII. As a quantitative parameter of stare-nystagmus the angular velocity of the slow phase can be used.
XIV. The study of the quantitative relations between the optokinetic stimulus and the nystagmus that it generates has shown that the central apparatus contains an "inertia" and that only after some time is an "equilibrium" between stimulus and nystagmus achieved. Although in the beginnung the velocity of the slow phase increases gradually, it does finally reach a constant value. This steady angular

velocity can be used as a quantitative measure for the intensity of the optokinetic stimulus.

XV. During stimulation of the immobilized eye the optimal velocity of the contrasts (10-50 min arc/s) induces a maximal velocity of the slow phase which is many times higher than the velocity of the contrasts.

XVI. During stimulation of the freely moving eye the velocity of the slow phase is in general a little lower than that of the contrasts. The movement of the retinal images is then compensated for as much as possible and the projection of the world on the retina is fixed as much as possible. This "fixation" of the surroundings is achieved by a "self-regulating mechanism". The slow phase cannot be faster in the freely moving eye, since the stimulation is abolished immediately when the velocity of the eye movement becomes equal to that of the contrasts.

XVII. At the beginning of a constant optokinetic stimulation the velocity of the slow phase increases approximately *uniformly*. Therefore the *acceleration* of the slow phase at the beginning of the stimulation can also be used as a quantitative parameter of the optokinetic stimulus.

XVIII. After termination of the optokinetic stimulation the nystagmus persists for some time (optokinetic *after nystagmus*). During this afternystagmus the velocity of the slow phase decreases gradually to zero. The deceleration of the slow phase immediately after the end of the stimulation can be used as a quantitative measure for the central *resistance*.

XIX. "Stare"nystagmus and vestibular rotatory nystagmus are closely related. The conditions for eliciting "stare"nystagmus are under physiological conditions usually not caused by motion of the surroundings, but by motion of the animal, also inducing stimulation of the labyrinth.

Probably the optokinetic and vestibular stimuli are processed in a common center. In general the vestibular stimulus generates a much higher acceleration of the slow phase than the optokinetic stimulus.

At the onset of rotation the nystagmus is predominantly *initiated* by the vestibular excitation, while the optokinetic stimulus *sustains* the nystagmus at a *constant level* during the continued, steady rotation. When the rotation is stopped the vestibular excitation is just sufficient to neutralize the central excitation caused by the preceding stimulation. Under physiological conditions (rotation of the animal with the eyes open) neither an optokinetic afternystagmus nor a vestibular postrotatory nystagmus is present.

B. *In Rabbits, Dogs and Cats the Stare Nystagmus Can Still Be Elicited After Complete Extirpation of the Cerebrum, Thus it is a Subcortical Reflex.* After unilateral removal of the cerebrum the stare nystagmus becomes permanently asymmetrical in the dog, whereas in the rabbit and monkey no lasting differences in relation to the intact animal could be demonstrated.

C. *Look-Nystagmus* is only generated when objects that draw the attention move in the visual field. These objects need to constitute only a very small part of the total amount of contrast in the visual field. This nystagmus is not suppressed by stationary contrasts.

The slow phase of look-nystagmus is identical with a pursuit movement, the fast phase is on the other hand not identical with a refixation. Although the tendency exists in look-nystagmus to project the "preferred" objects on to the fovea, the periphery of the retina is not without significance for its generation.

Look nystagmus is found not only in man, in which it can be studied best, but also in dogs and monkeys. On the other hand it is always absent in the rabbit.

A central "inertia" (afternystagmus etc.) is not evident at all.

D. *After Ablation of the Cerebrum Look Nystagmus is Permanently Absent in the Monkey and the Dog, and the Same is True After Extirpation of Both Visual Areas (area striata).* On the other hand it is retained after ablation of the sensorimotor cortex (in the dog). Look nystagmus is thus a cortical reflex, which is mediated through the visual cortex.

References

Aubert H (1886) Die Bewegungsempfindung. Pflügers Arch Ges Physiol 39:347-370
Barany R (1921) Zur Klinik und Theorie des Eisenbahn Nystagmus. Arch Augenheilk 88:139-142
Bartels M (1920) Aufgaben der Vergleichenden Physiologie der Augenbewegungen. Arch Ophthalmol 101:299-332
Bartels M (1931) Vergleichendes über Augenbewegungen. In: Bethe A, Von Bergmann G, Embden G, Ellinger A (eds) Handbuch der normalen und pathologischen Physiologie, vol XII. Springer, Berlin heidelberg New York, pp 1113-1165
Braak Ter JWG (1935) Optokinetische Nystagmus. Ned Tijdschr Geneeskd 79:1853-1858
Broers H, De Kleyn A (1934) Experimentelle Untersuchungen über den optokinetischen Nystagmus. Acta Brevia Néerl Phys 4:61-62
Campbell AW (1905) Histological studies on the localisation of cerebral functions. Cambridge
Cords R (1926a) Optisch-motorisches Feld und optisch-motorische Bahn. Arch Ophthalmol 117:58-113
Cords R (1926b) Zur Theorie des optomotorischen Nystagmus. Kl Monatsbl Augenheilk 77:781-787
Fischer MH, Kornmüller AE (1930) Optokinetisch ausgelöste Bewegungswahrnehmungen und optokinetischer Nystagmus. J Psychol Neurol 41:273-308
Fleisch A (1922) Das Labyrinth als beschleunigungsempfindendes Organ. Pflügers Arch Ges Physiol 195:499-515
Karplus JP, Kreidl A (1914) Totalextirpationen einer und beider Grosshirnhemispheren an Affen (Macacus Rhesus). Arch Anat Physiol:155-212
Kleyn De A, Rademaker GGJ (1928) Experimenteel onderzoek van den optischen nystagmus. Ned Tijdschr Geneeskd 72:5530-5531
Loeb J (1907) Ueber die Summation heliotropischer und geotropischer Wirkungen bei den auf der Drehscheibe ausgelösten compensatorischen Kopfbewegungen. Pflügers Arch Ges Physiol 116:368-374
Minkowski H (1911) Zur Physiologie der Sehsphäre. Pflügers Arch Ges Physiol 141:171-327
Mowrer OH (1935a) The electrical response of the vestibular nerve during adequate stimulation. Science 81:180-181
Mowrer OH (1935b) Some neglected factors which influence the duration of post-rotational nystagmus. Acta Oto Laryngol 22:1-23
Nordmann J (1928) Bull Soc Ophthalmol 5:
Nordmann J, Lieou YC (1928) Le nystagmus opto-cinétique. Revue d'Oto-Neuro-Ophthalmol 6:81-107
Ohm J (1929) Zur Tätigkeit des Augenmuskelsenders. Selbstverlag
Roelofs CO, Van der Bend JH (1930) Betrachtungen und Untersuchungen über den optokinetischen Nystagmus. Arch Augenheilkd 102:551-625
Steinhausen W (1933) Ueber die Beobachtung der Cupula in den Bogengangsampullen des Labyrinths des lebenden Hecht. Pflügers Arch Ges Physiol 232:500-512

References

Stenvers HW (1924) Ueber die klinische Bedeutung des optischen Nystagmus für die cerebrale Diagnostik. Schweiz Arch Neurol Psychol 14:279-288
Stenvers HW (1926) On the optic (optokinetic, optomotorial) Nystagmus. Acta Oto Laryngol 7:559-567
Visser J (1932) Optische reacties van duiven zonder groote hersenen. Thesis, Leiden
Visser J, Rademaker GGJ (1934) Die optischen Reaktionen grosshirnloser Tauben. Arch Néerl Physiol 19:482-501
Zeeman WPC (1929) Ueber fixieren und optische Augenbewegungen. Arch Augenheilkd 100/101:1-20

Subject Index

Accommodation 5
Adaptation 120–160
 – of maculo-ocular reflexes 127–129
 – of post-rotatory nystagmus 126
Albino rabbits 133, 147–159
Alertness, effects of 31, 33

Binocular vision 3, 26, 27

Cerebellectomy 100–102
Cerebellum 100–106
Cervico-ocular reflexes 31–32
Coordination of eye and head 10, 12, 13, 14, 19, 27

Dark-rearing 115–124
Direction selective units
 – collicular 79
 – geniculo-cortical 78–79
 – in posterior accessory optic system 90–91
 – pretectal 83–90, 154–156
 – retinal 75–77
Directional preference of optokinetic response 65–66, 90, 194–195, 215
Drift 20, 21, 28

Efference copy 109
Efferent connections of nucleus of optic tract 92–98

Flocculus 95, 103–106
Freely moving animals 7–27
Freezing state 3
Frequency response
 – of canal-ocular reflex 29–36
 – of maculo-ocular reflex 41–45
 – of optokinetic reflex 51–54
Frequency specificity of adaptation 140–144

Ganglion cell density 4, 5
Gaze 7, 27

Head nystagmus, linear 7

Immobilized eye 61–63, 185, 198
Inferior olive 92–95
Integration 34, 35, 107–109
Inverted motion vision 136–138
Inverted optokinetic nystagmus in albinism 147–159

Labyrinthectomy 98–100, 111–115
Linear acceleration 41–48
Look nystagmus 50, 225–232

Maculo-ocular reflexes 28, 30, 31, 41–48
Microsaccades 22
Models of the optokinetic system 106–109, 204–206

Nucleus of the optic tract 83–89, 92–98, 154–156

Open-loop optokinetic response 60–65, 107–109, 198–199
Optic projections, primary 77
Optokinetic afternystagmus 69–74, 98, 103, 201–204, 228
Orientation of eyes 2
Oscillation, passive 28–48
Otolith organs 41

Parallel swing 42–44
Pathways of optokinetic reflex 77–98, 153–154
Posterior accessory optic system 90–91
Postrotatory nystagmus 69–74
Prepositus hypoglossi nucleus 92, 96–98
Pursuit 22, 23, 101–103, 226

Recalibration of vestibulo-ocular reflex 125
Recording techniques 7, 8, 9, 21, 29, 183–184
Refractive state 5
Retina 4, 5

Saccades 8, 10–19, 23, 31, 51, 83
Size of optokinetic stimulus 63–65, 184–186
Stability of gaze 7, 8, 11, 20–22, 31
Stare nystagmus 50, 214
Step response
– of canal-ocular reflex 69–74
– of direction selective units
– of maculo-ocular reflex 44–48
– of optokinetic reflex 59
Stimulation, electrical 80–83
Subcortical optokinetic nystagmus 78–79, 217–224
Superior colliculus 79–82
Suppression of vestibulo-ocular reflex 19, 38–41, 103

Thresholds, vestibulo-ocular 37–38
Time constants
– of canal ocular response 70–74
– of cupula 34, 69
Torsional eye movements 31, 43–45, 66

Velocity of optokinetic 54–58, 186–189
Vergence 24–26, 67–68
Vertical eye movements 30, 43–47, 66
Vestibular nuclei 97–99, 114
Visual acuity 4
Visual adaptation of vestibulo-ocular reflex 129–145
Visual field 2, 3
Visual streak 4, 5, 63
Visuo-vestibular interaction 29–31, 33, 38–41, 97, 103–106, 113–114, 117–119, 207–213

Studies of Brain Function

Coordinating Editor: V. Braitenberg
Editors: H. B. Barlow, E. Bizzi, F. Florey,
O.-J. Grüsser, H. van der Loos

Volume 1
W. Heiligenberg

Principles of Electrolocation and Jamming Avoidance in Electric Fish

A Neuroethological Approach
1977. 58 figures, 1 table. XI, 85 pages
ISBN 3-540-08367-7

Contents: General Physiological and Anatomical Background: The Electric Organ. Electroreceptors. Taxonomy of Electrolocating Fish. The Spectral Composition of Electric Organ Discharges. The Neuroanatomy of Electric Fish. – The Mechanism of Electrolocation: Spatial Aspects of Electrolocation. Response Characteristics and Central Projections of Tuberous Electroreceptors. Central Processing of Electric Images. Behavioral Measures of Electrolocation Performance. Electrolocation Performance in the Presence of Electric Noise and Mechanisms of Jamming Avoidance. Neuronal Mechanism Linked to Jamming Avoidance and Electrolocation Under Jamming Conditions. Hypotheses and Results. Speculations on the Evolution of Pulse- and Wave-Type Electric Fish. – References. – Subject Index.

Volume 2
W. Precht

Neuronal Operations in the Vestibular System

1978. 105 figures, 3 tables. VIII, 226 pages
ISBN 3-540-08549-1

Contents: Primary Vestibular Neurons. – Central Vestibular Neurons. – Vestibulocerebellar Relationship. – Vestibuloocular Relationship.

Volume 3
J. T. Enright

The Timing of Sleep and Wakefulness

On the Substructure and Dynamics of the Circadian Pacemakers Underlying the Wake-Sleep Cycle
With a Foreword by E. Flory and an Appendix by J. Thorson
1980. 103 figures, 2 tables. XVIII, 263 pages
ISBN 3-540-09667-1

Contents: Introduction. – A Description of Activity-rhythm Recordings and Their Implications. – The Pacemaker and its Precision. – A Class of Models for Mutual Entrainment of an Ensemble of Neurons. – A "Type Model" and its Behavior: Partial and Loose-Knit Mutual Entrainment. – Precision of Model Pacemakers. – Influences of Constant Light Intensity. A Brief Detour: Further Thoughts About the Discriminator of the Models. – General Features of Entrainment: The Type Model. – Responses to Single Light Pulses. Part I: Nocturnal Rodents. – Responses to Single Pulses. Part II: Diurnal Birds. – Plasticity in Pacemaker Period: A Dynamic Memory. – Predictions from Coupled Stochastic Systems. – Further Predictions: A Modest Success and Two Problem Cases. – Morphology of the Models: Where is the Pacemaker? – A. Reprise and Synopsis: On the Avantages of Apparent Redundancy. – References. – Author Index. – Subject Index.

Volume 4
H. Braak

Architectonics of the Human Telencephalic Cortex

1980. 43 figures, 1 table. X, 147 pages
ISBN 3-540-10312-0

Contents: Introduction. – Types of Nerve Cells Forming the Telencephalic Cortex. – The Three Standard Techniques Used in Architectonics. – The Main Subdivisions of the Telencephalic Cortex. – The Allocortex. – The Proisocortex. – The Mature Isocortex. – Brain Maps. – Notes on Techniques. – References. – Subject Index.

Springer-Verlag
Berlin
Heidelberg
New York

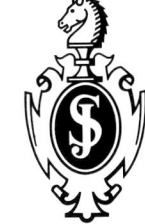

Handbook of Sensory Physiology

Editorial Board: H. Autrum, R. Jung, W. R. Loewenstein, D. M. MacKay, H.-L. Teuber

Volume 7, Part 6

Comparative Physiology and Evolution of Vision in Invetebrates

A: Invertebrate Photoreceptors

Editor: H. Autrum
With contributions by numerous experts
1979. 314 figures, 17 tables. XI, 729 pages
ISBN 3-540-08837-7

Contents: Introduction. – Photic Responses and Sensory Transduction in Protists. – Intraocular Filters. – The Physiology of Invertebrate Visual Pigments. – The Physics of Vision in Compound Eyes. – Receptor Protentials in Invertebrate Visual Cells. – Pseudopupils of Compound Eyes. – Apposition and Superposition Eyes. – Spectral Sensitivity and Color Vision in Invertebrates. – Extraocular Photoreception. – Extraocular Light Receptors and Circadian Rhythms. – Genetic Approach to a Visual System. – Author Index. – Subject Index.

B: Invertebrate Visual Centers and Behavior I

Editor: H. Autrum
With contributions by numerous experts
1981, 319 figures, 10 tables. X, 635 pages
ISBN 3-540-08703-6

Contents: Neuroarchitecture of Brain Regions that Subserve the Compound Eyes of Crustacea and Insects. – Neural Principles in the Visual System. – Polarization Sensitivity. – Optics and Vision in Invertebrates. – Author Index. – Subject Index.

C: Invertebrate Visual Centers and Behavior II

Editor: H. Autrum
With contributions by numerous experts
1981. 213 figures. Approx. 660 pages
ISBN 3-540-10422-4

Contents: Light and Dark Adaption in Invertebrates. – Comparative Physiology of Vision in Molluscs. – Organization and Physiology of the Insect Dorsal Ocellar System. – Spatial Vision in Arthropods. – Author Index. – Subject Index.

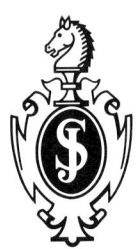

Springer-Verlag
Berlin
Heidelberg
NewYork